Practical Case Studies in Heart Disease

Practical Case Studies in Heart Disease

Editor: Lila Edwards

AMERICAN
MEDICAL PUBLISHERS
www.americanmedicalpublishers.com

AMERICAN
MEDICAL PUBLISHERS
www.americanmedicalpublishers.com

Cataloging-in-Publication Data

Practical case studies in heart disease / edited by Lila Edwards.
p. cm.
Includes bibliographical references and index.
ISBN 979-8-88740-655-8
1. Cardiovascular system--Diseases. 2. Heart--Diseases.
3. Cardiology. I. Edwards, Lila.
RC667 .H43 2023
616.1--dc23

American Medical Publishers,
41 Flatbush Avenue,
1st Floor, New York,
NY 11217, USA

ISBN 979-8-88740-655-8 (Hardback)

Contents

Preface

Heart diseases refer to conditions that affect the heart, its vessels, muscles, valves, or internal electric pathways responsible for muscular contraction. Coronary artery disease is the most common type of heart disease and it may lead to chest pain, stroke, or heart attack. Other major heart diseases include irregular heartbeats (arrhythmias), endocarditis, congestive heart failure, and congenital heart disease. High blood pressure, poor diet, obesity, smoking, high cholesterol, and lack of exercise can all increase the risk of developing various heart diseases. Stress tests, chest X-rays, cardiac CT scans, and electrocardiograms (EKGs/ECGs) can be used to diagnose heart diseases. The treatment of heart diseases is usually based on the type and cause of heart damage. Healthy lifestyle choices such as quitting smoking, exercising regularly, eating a low-fat and low-salt diet, and catching on enough sleep are crucial components of its treatment. This book provides significant information to help develop a good understanding of heart diseases. The extensive content of this book provides the readers with a thorough understanding of the condition. For all readers who are interested in the study of heart diseases, the case studies included in this book will serve as an excellent guide to develop a comprehensive understanding.

This book unites the global concepts and researches in an organized manner for a comprehensive understanding of the subject. It is a ripe text for all researchers, students, scientists or anyone else who is interested in acquiring a better knowledge of this dynamic field.

I extend my sincere thanks to the contributors for such eloquent research chapters. Finally, I thank my family for being a source of support and help.

Editor

1

Double Vessel Coronary Angioplasty in a Patient with Anomalous Single Coronary Artery Arising from the Right Cusp and Premature Atherosclerotic Coronary Artery Disease

Varun Kumar,[1] **Shalini Gupta**,[2] **and Krishna Prasad**[2]

[1]*Department of Cardiology, Orchid Medical Centre, Ranchi, India*
[2]*Department of Anaesthesia, Orchid Medical Centre, Ranchi, India*

Correspondence should be addressed to Varun Kumar; drvarun_gupta@yahoo.co.in
Academic Editor: Takatoshi Kasai

We report a rare case of a 39-year-old male who presented with acute inferior wall myocardial infarction (IWMI). Coronary angiography revealed an anomalous single coronary artery arising from the right coronary cusp. Premature atherosclerotic coronary artery disease (CAD) with critical stenosis in the mid right coronary artery (RCA), proximal posterior left ventricular (PLV) artery, and distal left circumflex (LCX) artery was detected during angiography. The patient managed successfully by percutaneous coronary interventions (PCI) with drug-eluting stents (DESs) by radial approach.

1. Introduction

Single coronary artery anomaly (SCAA), first described in 1903, is a rare inborn anomalous condition in which a single coronary artery originates from a single coronary ostium and gives rise to the entire coronary circulation. It has an estimated incidence of about 0.024%–0.066% among patients undergoing coronary angiography (CAG) [1, 2]. Based on the site of origin and anatomic distribution of the branches, SCAA may be classified into three groups: I, II, and III. Each group is further divided into subgroups: group I into R-I and L-I; group II into R-IIA/B/P and L-IIA/B/P; and group III into R-III category, where R and L refer to the location of the ostium in the right and left coronary sinus, respectively [2].

Most patients (80.6%) with coronary anomalies are asymptomatic and are usually detected accidentally during CAG; however, some (19.4%) may present with life-threatening symptoms, such as angina, syncope, myocardial infarction, congestive heart failure, and even sudden cardiac death [3]. Further, there is an increased susceptibility of anomalous coronaries to atherosclerosis as compared to normal coronaries [4].

The huge variation in the anatomic courses of SCAA can present a challenge. Therefore, the presence and course of an anomalous origin of coronary should be thoroughly examined and recognized during CAG so that the future clinical risk may be estimated and the strategy for the best suitable treatment including coronary angioplasty be planned.

We report a case of SCAA of type R-II P arising from the right cusp, associated with premature atherosclerotic coronary artery disease (CAD) that was successfully treated with percutaneous coronary intervention (PCI) with drug-eluting stents (DESs).

2. Case

A 39-year-old male patient presented with acute onset of chest pain since past 4 hours along with sweating. The patient was a chronic smoker with no significant medical and family history. Physical examination showed a pulse rate of 62 beats/min, blood pressure of 130/80 mmHg, and bilateral clear lungs with no jugular venous distension. Auscultation of the heart revealed normal S1 & S2 with no murmurs. Electrocardiogram (ECG) revealed acute inferior wall myocardial

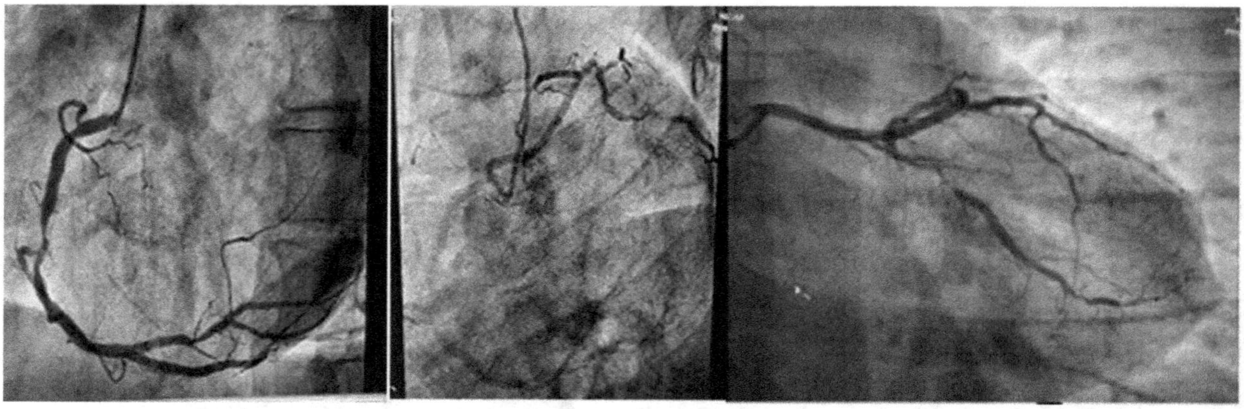

Figure 1: Coronary angiogram images.

infarction (IWMI) with ST segment elevation in the inferior leads, II, III, and aVF, and reciprocal ST segment depression in the lateral leads, I and aVL. Echocardiogram (echo) showed akinesia of the RCA territory with a low left ventricle ejection fraction (LVEF) of 40%. Laboratory testing revealed a positive troponin result and low- and high-density lipoprotein cholesterol level of 134 mg/dL and 40 mg/dL, respectively. However, the serum homocysteine and apolipoprotein B levels were in normal range. As the patient refused primary percutaneous coronary intervention, he initially underwent thrombolysis with tenecteplase. He later consented to CAG that was performed by right radial approach using "Tiger catheter." An injection into the left sinus of Valsalva did not reveal the ostium of left coronary artery (LCA), but when the right coronary ostium was hooked with the same catheter, it revealed a single coronary artery arising from the right cusp (Figure 1). Right coronary artery angiogram showed 90% stenosis in mid-RCA and 80% stenosis in the proximal posterior left ventricular (PLV) artery. A slight anticlockwise rotation of the same catheter in the right coronary sinus resulted in hooking of the LCA, revealing a retroaortic course (R-II P) with LCA dividing into left anterior descending (LAD) and left circumflex (LCX) arteries. Further angiogram showed 90% stenosis in the distal LCX artery.

Based on the angiography results, the patient underwent double-vessel PCI with stenting of RCA, PLV, and LCX arteries with DESs. Cannulation was done, using JR 3.5 guiding catheter by radial approach. A 0.014-inch guidewire (Balance Middleweight (BMW); Guidant Corporation, Indianapolis, IN, USA) was used to cross the lesions. Posterior left ventricular artery was stented with a 2.5×12 mm DES and postdilated with a 2.5×8 mm noncompliant (NC) balloon up to 16 atm. Mid-RCA was stented with another DES (3.5×24 mm) at nominal pressure and postdilated with a 3.5×10 mm NC balloon up to 18 atm. After postdilatation, the patient developed severe coronary spasm just proximal to the stent margin (Figure 2). The coronary spasm was managed with intracoronary nitroglycerin, nicorandil, and diltiazem. The LCA was hooked with the same JR 3.5 catheter with slight anticlockwise rotation, and the BMW wire was used to cross the LCX lesion, while another BMW wire was kept in LAD for support. Stenting of LCX was performed with a 2.5×18 mm DES and postdilatation with a 2.75×10 mm NC balloon up to 18 atm. Post PCI with stenting, thrombolysis in myocardial infarction (TIMI) grade 3 flow was achieved in all three vessels (RCA, PLV, and LCX); the post-PCI angiogram of LCX is shown in Figure 2(b).

The patient was put on intravenous nicorandil for 24 hours. His condition was stable postoperatively, and he was discharged on the third postoperative day with standard medications including aspirin, ticagrelor, statin, angiotensin-converting enzyme inhibitor, and beta blocker. Before discharge, he underwent coronary computed tomography angiography (CCTA) which delineated the single coronary artery, its ostium, and the path of three coronary arteries (Figure 2(c)). The segment that had spasm during the procedure looked normal, and all the three stents were patent. Follow-up echo showed mildly hypokinetic RCA territory with LVEF of 52%. The patient was doing well on further follow-up post discharge.

3. Discussion

In the current case, our patient presented with chest pain and sweating with acute IWMI on ECG, akinetic RCA territory on echo, and lowered LVEF. Further CAG revealed SCAA and double-vessel premature atherosclerotic CAD with severe stenosis (>70%) in RCA, LCX, and PLV.

Cases of premature atherosclerotic CAD (due to an unhealthy lifestyle) and SCAA have been reported in the literature [5]. In our case, the patient had a history of chronic smoking. Smoking has been found to be a significant risk factor associated with premature atherosclerosis in young adults (≤55 years) [6].

According to the SCAA classification, our case corresponded to the rare R-II P subtype. In a large study with 126,595 patients who underwent catheter CAG, CAA incidence was 1.3% (87% origin and distribution anomalies, 13% coronary artery fistulae), and only 19 cases were identified as SCAA R-II subtype (0.015%) [3].

Single coronary artery anomaly can be diagnosed by different diagnostic modalities including conventional CAG, the first diagnostic tool and a gold standard for early detection and evaluation of CAD. Once anomalous coronary arteries are suspected, other excellent noninvasive tools with

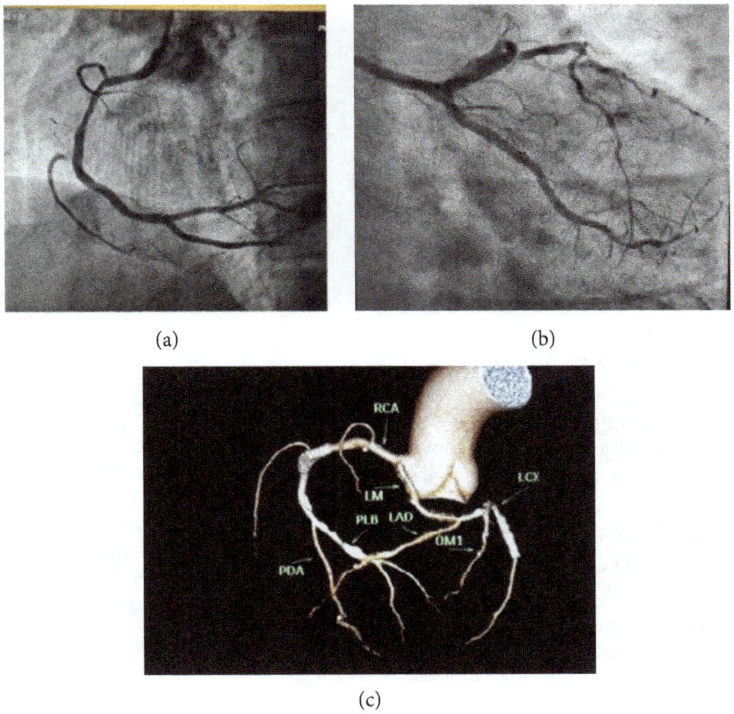

Figure 2: (a) Post-PCI image of RCA showing coronary spasm just proximal to RCA stent after postdilatation. (b) Post-PCI angiogram of LCX. (c) Coronary computed tomography angiography done prior to discharge, delineating the origin and the course of the anomalous artery and patent stents. PCI: percutaneous coronary interventions; RCA: right coronary artery; LCX: left circumflex artery.

better spatial resolution, such as CCTA, may also be used to better determine the complex course of the abnormal arteries and provide three-dimensional information that may have prognostic value [7]. In the present case, our patient was earlier diagnosed with SCAA by CAG and later complemented with CCTA that helped us precisely delineate the origin and the course of the anomalous artery.

Current guidelines favor surgical therapy for anomalous LMCA originating from the right sinus with an interarterial course, but clear guidance is lacking on other subtypes [8]. Although stenoses of anomalous vessels have been described previously, treatment of atherosclerotic lesions by PCI has rarely been reported. Angioplasty in SCAA may pose certain technical challenges in cannulation of the coronary ostium as well as difficulties in providing optimal catheter support during the procedure [9]. Procedural risk also remains very high as dissection of ostia of single coronary artery may result in occlusion of vessel [10]. It is therefore important to have increased awareness about the procedure and complete assessment of the anatomy of the coronary artery in order to prevent complications. Several studies have described different types of guide catheters including JR catheter using radial approach. This approach has been used successfully in accessing anomalous left sinus of Valsalva [11, 12]. Using transradial approach, especially in RCA interventions, negates the distal anatomy effect on the behavior of proximal catheter. Further, radial access also provides superior backup support from the contralateral aortic wall, in contrast to the support provided from femoral approach. A previous case report successfully demonstrated PCI using radial approach and RCA cannulation using JR curve [12]. Although we performed PCI with JR 3.5 guiding catheter by radial approach, we had to keep another BMW wire in LAD for support while performing PCI of LCX. Despite our careful assessment of the course of the anomalous coronary and careful conduction of PCI, the patient experienced severe coronary vasospasm just proximal to the stent margin after postdilatation. Coronary vasospasm may be considered as an important cause of myocardial ischemia and sudden death in patients with anomalies' origin of coronary artery and should be managed immediately with medications [13]. The coronary vasospasm in our patient was managed with intracoronary vasodilators such as nitroglycerin, nicorandil, and diltiazem with good clinical outcome. Adequate TIMI grade 3 flow was achieved in all three coronary vessels in our patient.

4. Learning Points

A single coronary artery anomaly may cause fatal outcome, and if this is associated with atherosclerotic multivessel disease, then the patient should immediately undergo PCI or surgery to prevent life-threatening complications. Our case report demonstrated successful management with PCI of a patient having rare R-II P type anomalous single coronary artery arising from the right cusp, presenting with acute IWMI and severe arterial stenosis in the RCA, PLV, and LCX.

Acknowledgments

We would like to thank BioQuest Solutions for data analysis and editorial services.

References

[1] W. Desmet, J. Vanhaecke, M. Vrolix et al., "Isolated single coronary artery: a review of 50 000 consecutive coronary angiographies," *European Heart Journal*, vol. 13, no. 12, pp. 1637–1640, 1992.

[2] M. J. Lipton, W. H. Barry, I. Obrez, J. F. Silverman, and L. Wexler, "Isolated single coronary artery: diagnosis, angiographic classification, and clinical significance," *Radiology*, vol. 130, no. 1, pp. 39–47, 1979.

[3] O. Yamanaka and R. E. Hobbs, "Coronary artery anomalies in 126,595 patients undergoing coronary arteriography," *Catheterization and Cardiovascular Diagnosis*, vol. 21, no. 1, pp. 28–40, 1990.

[4] G. Somashekhara, "Clinical and angiographic profile of coronary artery anomalies in patients undergoing coronary angiography," *Journal of Cardiovascular Medicine and Surgery*, vol. 3, pp. 167–174, 2017.

[5] A. Gholoobi and H. Poorzand, "Single coronary artery anomaly: report of an extremely rare variation," *Asian Cardiovascular & Thoracic Annals*, vol. 25, no. 6, pp. 459–462, 2017.

[6] V. J. Leijdekkers, A. C. Vahl, J. J. M. Leenders, P. C. Huijgens, R. O. B. Gans, and J. A. Rauwerda, "Risk factors for premature atherosclerosis," *European Journal of Vascular and Endovascular Surgery*, vol. 17, no. 5, pp. 394–397, 1999.

[7] C. Liesting, J. J. Brugts, M. J. Kofflard, and A. Dirkali, "Acute coronary syndrome in a patient with a single coronary artery arising from the right sinus of Valsalva," *World Journal of Cardiology*, vol. 4, no. 8, pp. 264–266, 2012.

[8] M. R. Patel, G. J. Dehmer, J. W. Hirshfeld, P. K. Smith, J. A. Spertus, and Coronary Revascularization Writing Group, "ACCF/SCAI/STS/AATS/AHA/ASNC/HFSA/SCCT 2012 appropriate use criteria for coronary revascularization focused update: a report of the American College of Cardiology Foundation Appropriate Use Criteria Task Force, Society for Cardiovascular Angiography and Interventions, Society of Thoracic Surgeons, American Association for Thoracic Surgery, American Heart Association, American Society of Nuclear Cardiology, and the Society of Cardiovascular Computed Tomography," *The Journal of Thoracic and Cardiovascular Surgery*, vol. 143, no. 4, pp. 780–803, 2012.

[9] M. Çalışkan, O. Çiftçi, H. Güllü, and M. Alpaslan, "Anomalous right coronary artery from the left sinus of Valsalva presenting a challenge for percutaneous coronary intervention," *Türk Kardiyoloji Derneği Arşivi*, vol. 37, no. 1, pp. 44–47, 2009.

[10] M. Sato, T. Okada, A. Ohara, T. Aoki, and I. Kawamoto, "Percutaneous coronary intervention of a single coronary artery arising from the right sinus of Valsalva," *Journal of Cardiology*, vol. 54, no. 2, pp. 322–325, 2009.

[11] L. Charan, S. Shiradkar, P. G. Kerkar, and A. Ashish, "Stenting of anomalous left main coronary artery stenosis in an adult with a retroaortic course," *Cardiology Research and Practice*, vol. 2011, Article ID 296946, 3 pages, 2011.

[12] R. Mahla, H. Mahla, D. Choudhary, and P. Nahata, "Percutaneous coronary intervention in single coronary artery from right sinus: radial route is right," *J Clin Imaging Sci*, vol. 5, p. 65, 2015.

[13] J. Nakazato, K. Hirata, and M. Wake, "Coronary spasm as the cause of myocardial ischaemia in a patient with anomalous origin of the left anterior descending artery from the proximal right coronary artery," *BMJ Case Reports*, vol. 2014, 2014.

2

Ordinary AV Nodal Reentry Tachycardia-Unusual Ablation

Franz Haertel,[1] P. Christian Schulze,[1] Anett Große,[1] Dirk Prochnau,[2] and Ralf Surber[1]

[1]*University Hospital Jena, Department of Internal Medicine I, Cardiology, Am Klinikum 1, 07743 Jena, Germany*
[2]*Department of Internal Medicine, Cardiology, Sophien-und Hufeland-Klinikum, Henry-van-de-Velde-Straße 2, 99425 Weimar, Germany*

Correspondence should be addressed to Franz Haertel; franz.haertel@med.uni-jena.de
Academic Editor: Yigit Canga

A 72-year-old woman was referred to us with typical symptoms of paroxysmal supraventricular tachycardia for electrophysiological diagnostics and catheter ablation. During the first session of catheter ablation, a probing of the right ventricle was not successful. Therefore, an angiography of the central veins was performed. A rare anatomical variation with atresia of the inferior vena cava below the hepatic veins with azygos persistence was detected. The blood of the lower half of the body was drained via the dilated azygos into the superior vena cava; the blood of the liver veins enters into the right atrium directly. By atypical catheter placement over the azygos vein in the right ventricle and coronary sinus, an AV nodal reentry tachycardia (AVNRT) could be confirmed as the mechanism of tachycardia. However, a stable position of the ablation catheter could not be achieved by the femoral approach, so the successful AV node modulation with ablation of the slow pathway was performed via jugular access.

1. Introduction

Vena azygos persistence is considered an extremely rare, asymptomatic venous anomaly. As relevant anatomical access routes may not be available, particularly the transseptal access to the left atrium, it will pose a complex challenge for the interventionalist. With the number of cases of interventions gradually increasing, this anomaly must be given special consideration.

2. Case Report

A 72-year-old woman presented herself for a scheduled consultation in the outpatient clinic. During that meeting, both hypertensive derailment (blood pressure > 180/100 mmHg) and tachycardia with frequencies up to 200/min were noticed. A regular, supraventricular tachycardia (SVT) was diagnosed. The patient was referred to the central emergency department, where conversion to regular sinus rhythm was achieved by administration of adenosine. There was no ventricular preexcitation during sinus rhythm. Therefore, an atrioventricular nodal reentrant tachycardia (AVNRT) was suspected. The cardiac examination was uneventful with regular heart sounds with no pathological murmurs. Clinical examination of the respiratory tract, abdominal, and neurological status was unremarkable. Echocardiography revealed left ventricular hypertrophy with preserved systolic function, most likely due to hypertensive heart disease. No valvular disease was detected, and the dimensions of the atria were within normal range. In the current 12-lead electrocardiogram, we detected a normal sinus rhythm with a first-degree atrioventricular block (PR interval 216 ms) as shown in Figure 1.

Subsequently, the patient was admitted to our cardiac unit for an elective ablation of the SVT. The patient gave informed consent to procedure and was brought to the electrophysiology laboratory. After establishing access to the femoral vein, an atypical anatomy of the large veins was suspected as the right atrium was not accessible conventionally. Next, a venous angiography was performed (Figure 2) which

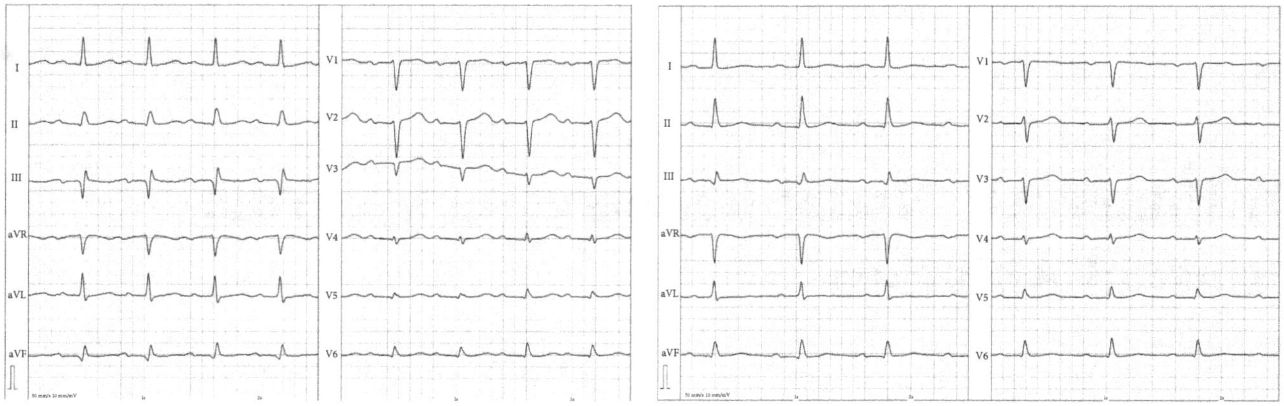

(a) (b)

FIGURE 1: (a) 12-lead surface ECG before the intervention.(b) 12-lead surface ECG after the intervention with no change in the PQ interval.

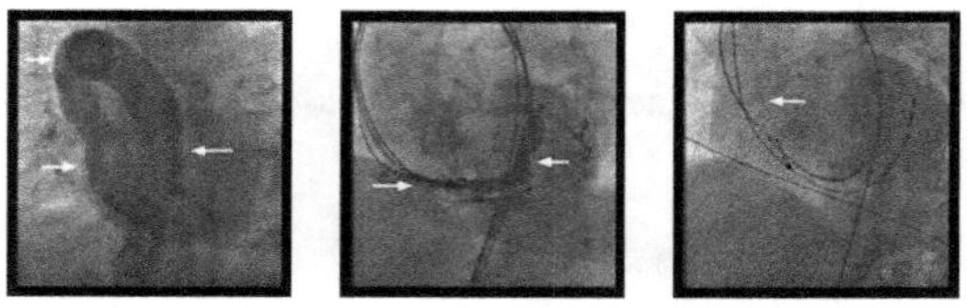

(a) (b) (c)

FIGURE 2: (a) Fluoroscopy of a dilated vena azygos (arrows) with inflow into the superior vena cava and the right atrium (p.a. projection). (b) Fluoroscopy of the coronary sinus (arrows), LAO 30°. (c) Fluoroscopy of the ablation catheter (arrow) via internal jugular vein placed in the area of the coronary sinus ostium (posteroseptal) during ablation, LAO 30°.

revealed that the coronary sinus was accessible through the azygos vein (Figure 2). Typical AVNRT was inducible as per standard protocol. However, a stable position of the ablation catheter could not be achieved by femoral access. As a consequence, the ablation could not be performed. A chest radiograph featured a suspicious configuration of the upper right mediastinum (Figure 3). Further diagnostics using contrast CT angiogram confirmed a rare anomaly: atresia of the inferior vena cava below the hepatic vein with azygos persistence (Figure 4).

In a second session, catheter positioning in the coronary sinus was achieved via the right internal jugular vein and the catheter in the right ventricle via the femoral vein. The ablation catheter was also positioned via the internal jugular vein. Recording of His bundle activity prior to ablation could be achieved 15 mm above the ostium of the coronary sinus only with the ablation catheter and resulted in an atrioventricular (AV) interval of 128 ms and His-ventricular (HV) interval of 48 ms (Figure 5). A stable position of the ablation catheter was established in the same location posteroseptally at the ostium of the coronary sinus (Figure 2). The ablation was performed using a multicurve steerable ablation catheter (RF MARINR; Medtronic®) which enables variable curve size adjustment (range: from small tight curve to larger reach) and out-of-plane incremental lateral deflection including side-to-side tip rotation aiding placement in varied anatomy. This specific model used for the ablation is 7Fr and featured a 4 mm tip electrode with an embedded thermocouple temperature sensor. Tissue contact during

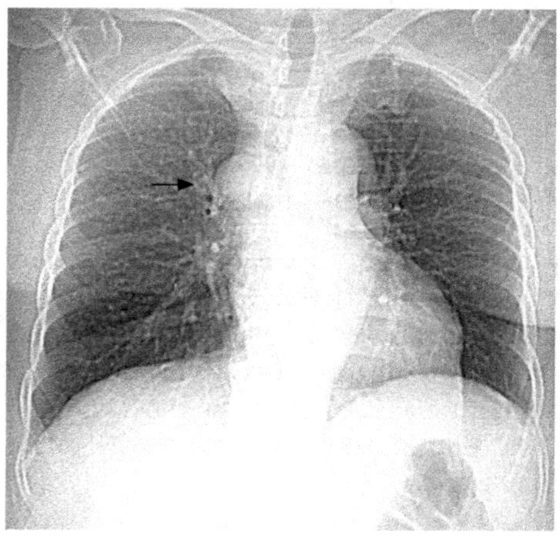

FIGURE 3: Chest radiograph showing a prominent upper right mediastinum (arrow) as the correlation of the azygos continuation entering the vena cava superior in a cross-sectional view.

ablation was adequate, verified by an impedance drop of >10% and occurrence of junctional beats during radiofrequency (RF) delivery in a typical right posteroseptal position at the ostium of the coronary sinus (Figure 6). Thereafter, no tachycardia could be induced, dual AV node physiology was no longer present, and the first-degree AV block remained unchanged (Figure 1). The patient was discharged without any complications; to this day, her clinical status remains stable with no recurrence of AVNRT.

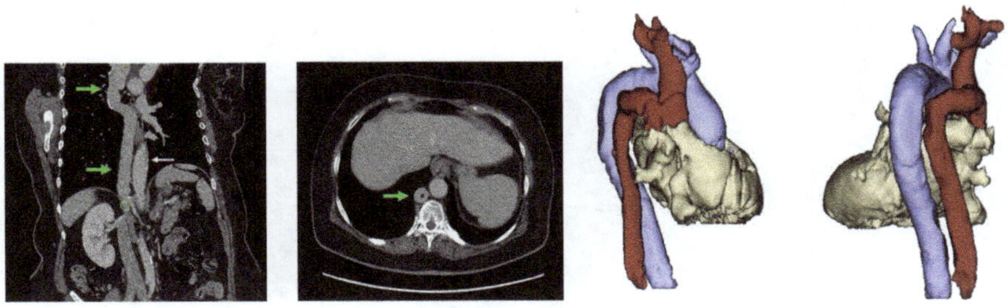

(a) (b) (c)

FIGURE 4: (a) Stretched reconstruction of a venous CT with azygos continuation (green arrows), aorta (white arrow), and diaphragmatic passage of the azygos (green circle). (b) Axial CT view, venous phase, showing a prominent azygos vein (green arrow). (c) 3D reconstruction showing the azygos continuation/superior vena cava (red) and the aortic arch (blue) in a right lateral and posterior view.

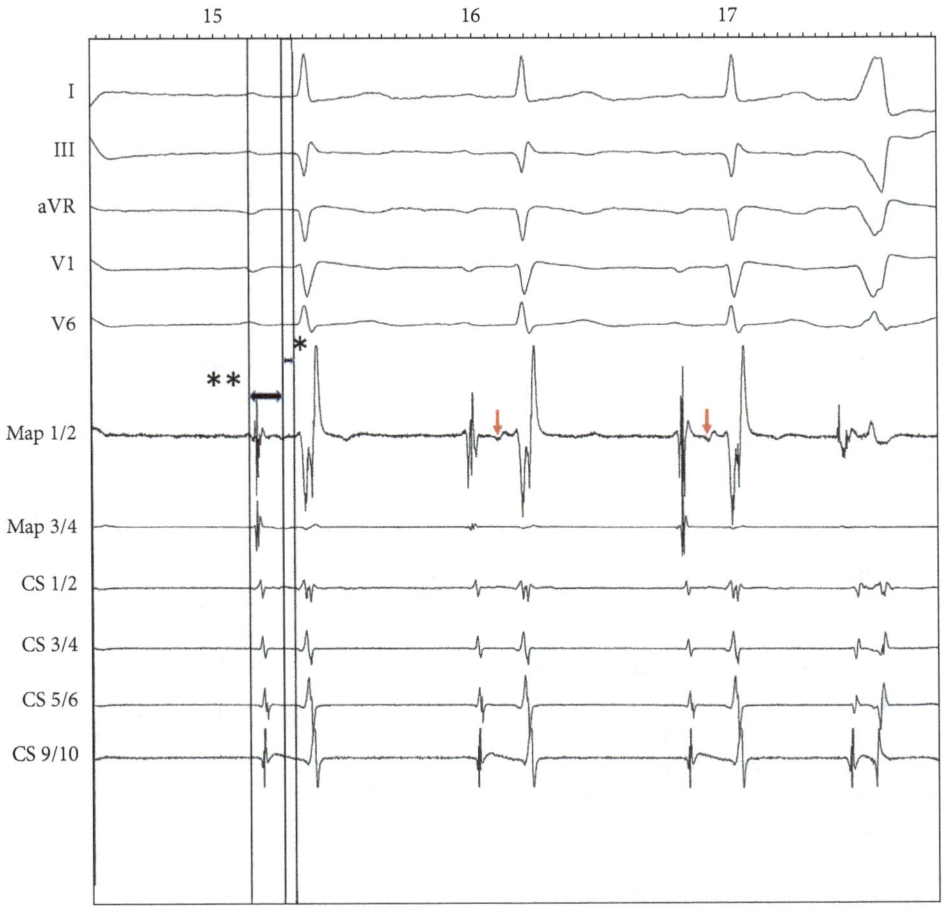

FIGURE 5: His bundle electrogram (red arrows) immediately performed before the second ablation attempt (**atrioventricular (AV) interval of 128 ms; *His-ventricular (HV) interval of 48 ms).

3. Discussion

Vena azygos persistence usually occurs in combination with other congenital anomalies of the heart such as cyanotic or acyanotic congenital cardiac disorders and abnormalities of cardiac position such as dextrocardia and polysplenia or asplenia [1–3]. However, in this case, no other anomalies were found.

In the literature, a frequency ranging from 0.2 to 3.0% was reported as the incidence of systemic venous anomalies in patients undergoing cardiac catheterization [1, 4]. The most frequently seen variants are the persistence of the left superior vena cava, with or without a right superior vena cava, and azygos or hemiazygos continuation of an interrupted inferior vena cava [4]. For patients admitted to the cardiac unit of our hospital, an incidence of <0.2‰ was recorded for azygos continuation.

For symptomatic AVNRT patients, catheter ablation is currently considered as a standard treatment. Common access to the heart is attained from a femoral approach.

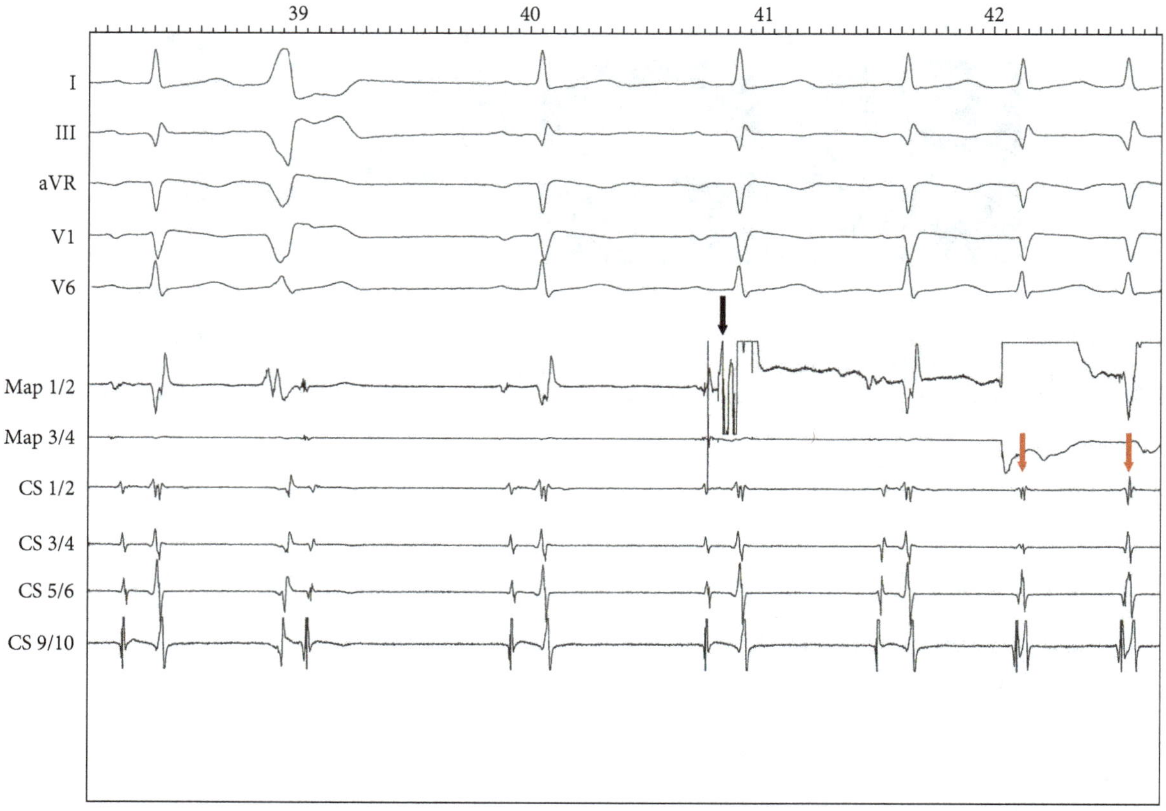

FIGURE 6: Electrogram of the ablation (black arrow: ablation start; red arrows: junctional beats after application of radiofrequency (RF)). A small A and a large V potential were recorded immediately before the ablation.

The technique is proven to be safe and effective. However, individual cases of electrophysiologic examination and ablation of different arrhythmias have been described, demonstrating the feasibility of the ablation procedure under unusual anatomical circumstances, where even a transseptal approach with jugular access was attempted. As a particular challenge, the positioning and manipulation of the recording and mapping catheters are more difficult or even impossible due to their design, with a longer course, and angulation of the azygos vein connecting to the superior vena cava. At times, no electrical activity can be registered, and the catheter cannot be advanced to the His bundle position within the heart [5]. In the presented case, we could only achieve an effective position of the ablation catheter in a second ablation attempt from a combined jugular and femoral venous access that resulted in success.

Further cases of challenging ablation procedures in literature in which vascular access was not attainable using the standard approach by inserting the catheter into the femoral vein and advancing it through the inferior vena cava due to a prominent communication between the inferior vena cava and the superior vena cava via an azygos persistence include Wolff-Parkinson-White syndrome via right subclavian vein [5], atrioventricular junction ablation with an inferior approach for treatment of symptomatic, refractory atrial fibrillation in a VVIR-pacemaker patient [6], cryoablation for atrial fibrillation via right internal jugular vein using a transseptal sheath and BRK needle (Abbott Vascular) [7], ablation of AVNRT in a patient with dextrocardia after inserting the ablating catheter and two quadripolar catheters into the femoral and jugular veins [8], ablation of isthmus-dependent atrial flutter having the ablation catheter advanced from a femoral access [9], and ablation in a patient with coexistence of two different atrioventricular nodes (twin AV nodes) and AVNRT with venous access through the right internal jugular and left subclavian veins [10].

4. Conclusion

In the case of the above described anomaly, it was not possible to establish access to the right atrium via the femoral route. This anomaly should be put into consideration during procedures such as pulmonary vein isolation, left atrial appendage (LAA) occluder implantation, and interventional therapy on the mitral valve. The probing of the right atrium, ventricle, and coronary sinus is clearly more difficult from an inferior approach. In complex anatomical settings of electrophysiological cases, the use of a 3D mapping system should be considered.

Additional Points

Learning Points. With increasing percutaneous interventions, anatomical variations of the great veins should be considered. Probing and interventional procedures in the left atrium are not possible via the inferior vena cava in patients with azygos persistence. While they are possible through alternative routes via the internal jugular vein, they are challenging to perform and do not always result in success.

Acknowledgments

We thank Katarina Braune for the critical review of this case report.

References

[1] R. C. Anderson, P. Adams Jr., and B. Burke, "Anomalous inferior vena cava with azygos continuation (infrahepatic interruption of the inferior vena cava): report of 15 new cases," *The Journal of Pediatrics*, vol. 59, no. 3, pp. 370–383, 1961.

[2] V. P. Chuang, C. E. Mena, and P. A. Hoskins, "Congenital anomalies of the inferior vena cava. Review of embryogenesis and presentation of a simplified classification," *The British Journal of Radiology*, vol. 47, no. 556, pp. 206–213, 1974.

[3] A. L. Suthar, N. C. Nanda, and P. J. Harris, "Two-dimensional and Doppler echocardiographic identification of infrahepatic interruption of inferior vena cava with azygos continuation," *Pacing and Clinical Electrophysiology*, vol. 6, no. 4, pp. 963–971, 1983.

[4] T. C. Demos, H. V. Posniak, K. L. Pierce, M. C. Olson, and M. Muscato, "Venous anomalies of the thorax," *American Journal of Roentgenology*, vol. 182, no. 5, pp. 1139–1150, 2004.

[5] J. M. Guerra Ramos, E. R. Font, and I. M. A. Moya, "Radiofrequency catheter ablation of an accessory pathway through an anomalous inferior vena cava with azygos continuation," *EP Europace*, vol. 6, no. 2, pp. 134–137, 2004.

[6] M. S. Randhawa, H. C. Taylor, and R. D. Mosteller, "Anatomic twist to a straightforward ablation," *Indian Pacing and Electrophysiology Journal*, vol. 13, no. 2, pp. 94–98, 2013.

[7] A. Baszko, P. Kałmucki, R. Dankowski, M. Łanocha, T. Siminiak, and A. Szyszka, "Transseptal puncture from the jugular vein and balloon cryoablation for atrial fibrillation in a patient with azygos continuation of an interrupted inferior vena cava," *Europace*, vol. 17, no. 7, pp. 1153–1156, 2015.

[8] R. Pecoraro, A. Proclemer, A. Pivetta, and P. Gianfagna, "Radiofrequency ablation of atrioventricular nodal tachycardia in a patient with dextrocardia, inferior vena cava interruption, and azygos continuation," *Journal of Cardiovascular Electrophysiology*, vol. 19, no. 4, p. 444, 2008.

[9] J. Guenther, N. Marrouche, and J. Ruef, "Ablation of atrial flutter by the femoral approach in the absence of inferior vena cava," *Europace*, vol. 9, no. 11, pp. 1073-1074, 2007.

[10] H. N. Pak, C. Hwang, and Y. H. Kim, "Twin atrioventricular node associated with interruption of the inferior vena cava and atrioventricular nodal reentrant tachycardia," *Journal of Electrocardiology*, vol. 39, no. 4, pp. 400–403, 2006.

3

Profound Vagal Tone and Bradycardia Mimicking Asystole: A Resuscitation Case Report

J. Mannion, L. Chapman, K. Deasy, and N. S. Colwell

Cardiology Department, Tipperary University Hospital, Clonmel, Tipperary, Ireland

Correspondence should be addressed to J. Mannion; jamesm2016@gmail.com

Academic Editor: Christopher S. Snyder

A 48-year-old man presented with dizziness. When he arrived at the emergency department, he collapsed and became pulseless. Prior to his collapse, he was asymptomatic and now even participated in multiple marathon and ultra-running events per year. However, he previously experienced a vasospastic inferior STEMI eight years prior from cocaine use. As a result, he had an ischaemic cardiomyopathy with LVEF of 45%. He never took any further illicit substances after the STEMI; instead, he changed his lifestyle completely and commenced extreme endurance sports. After one hour of alternations between VF/VT rhythms and asystole, a rhythm check demonstrated a single complex with a corresponding pulse. He had received 12 mg of epinephrine up to that point as per local resuscitation guidelines. Upon diagnosing extreme bradycardia, 2 mg of total atropine administration resulted in ROSC. We theorise that this bradycardia was a result of increased vagal tone as ROSC was quickly achieved following atropine administration.

1. Case

1.1. Introduction. We present a case of a marathon/ultra-runner with profound vagal tone contributing to bradycardia and mimicking asystole during a resuscitation code. Further, this bradycardia was not responsive to epinephrine and required atropine to obtain return of spontaneous circulation (ROSC).

A 48-year-old man presented to the emergency department (ED) because of an episode of severe dizziness while out jogging with his friend. His symptoms briefly improved en route to the ED, but returned abruptly upon arrival. He experienced syncope and was found to be pulseless. Subsequently, a cardiac arrest call was initiated. His initial rhythm was ventricular tachycardia (VT) which evolved into ventricular fibrillation (VF). Defibrillation was performed, but the patient was "asystolic" and cardiopulmonary resuscitation (CPR) was resumed.

1.2. Examination. Examination revealed a fit man in his 40s wearing running clothing which was wet with sweat, but no obvious abnormalities. There was good bilateral air entry with ventilation via bag mask ventilation with head tilt-chin lift, with no evidence of tension pneumothorax.

1.3. Past Medical History. His history included an ST elevation myocardial infarction (STEMI) induced by coronary artery spasm secondary to cocaine use at age 33 treated with thrombolysis.

He had a coronary angiogram 8 years after the initial STEMI with no obstructive coronary disease. His baseline chart ECG was sinus rhythm, rate 46 with an incomplete right bundle branch block (RBBB), with fusion beats (Figure 1).

There was no family history of heart disease. After a normal exercise stress test and cardiology review, he had taken up endurance athletics which became more extreme over time, including marathon and ultrarunning multiple times per year. He quit smoking at the time of his STEMI, having accumulated 18 pack years.

His medications included aspirin 75 mg, ramipril 1.25 mg, and rosuvastatin 20 mg.

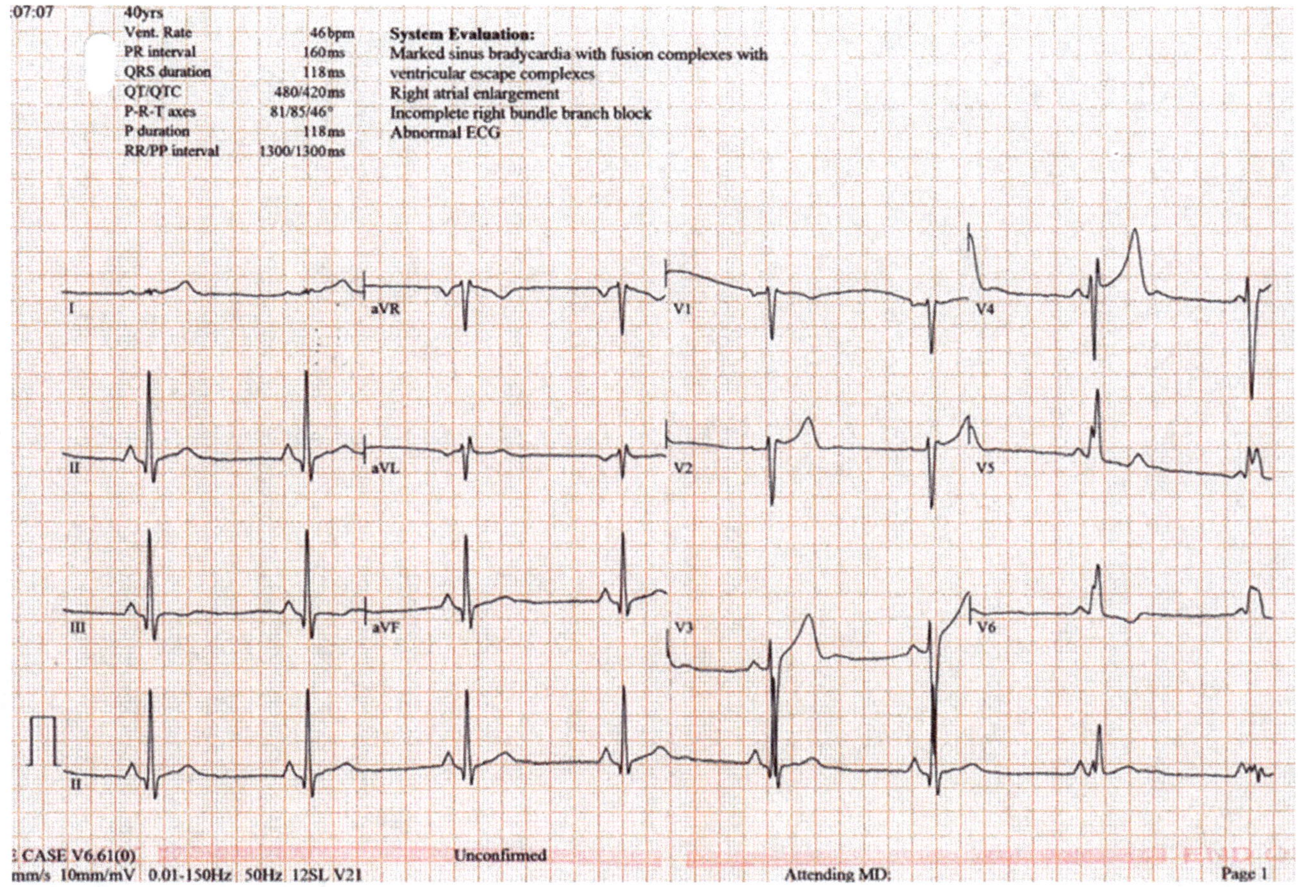

Figure 1: Baseline patient ECG from medical records. Baseline ECG from 2013, with pulse of 46, incomplete RBBB and fusion complexes. We see that our patient had a low resting heart rate in 2013 and has been training for and competing in extreme endurance races such as ultrarunning for the 7 following years.

Upon discovery of his history 10 minutes into the cardiac arrest, a leading diagnosis of VT/VF secondary to ischaemic scar was made.

1.4. Investigations. Initial investigations were conducted during the cardiac arrest. These investigations included rhythm strips, bloods, arterial blood gases, and focused echocardiography.

Rhythm strips: Alternating VF and asystole (rhythm strip A and B, Figure 2)

Focused arrest echocardiography: No myocardial hypertrophy, pericardial effusion, tamponade, or right-sided dilation

Arterial blood gas (20 minutes into CPR): pH 7.15 (7.35-7.45), pC02 10.2 kPa (4.6-6.4), p02 11.1 kPa (11.0-14.4), sodium 137 (136-145), potassium 3.0 mmol/L (3.5-5.1), chloride 96 mmol/L (98-107), ionized calcium 1.10 mmol/L (1.15-1.33), glucose 7.2 mmol/L (3.6-5.3), lactate 10.1 mmol/L (0.0–1.3), anion gap 28 mmol/L (10-20), bicarbonate—standard 8.1 mmol/L (21-28), bicarbonate actual 16.1 mmol/L (21-28)

Full blood count, liver and kidney panel: WCC 6.5×10^9 /L (4-10), neutrophils 2.11×10^9/L (2-7), Hb 13.2 g/dL (13-17), MCV 93.8 fL (83-101), platelets 174×10^9/L (150-400), and CRP < 5; urea, creatinine, electrolytes, coagulation profile, and liver function panel could not be analysed due to haemolysis

Troponin I: 0.09 μg/L (<0.04), with repeat at 2 hours 1.28 μg/L

Urine toxicology: negative for cocaine, opioids, THC, and amphetamines

1.5. Management. Based on his lactic acidosis and possible electrolyte losses, we replaced electrolytes with both 5 g magnesium sulphate and 40 mmol potassium chloride intravenously, in addition to fluid resuscitation during CPR.

At the one-hour mark, after a further defibrillation and 12th dose of 1 mg epinephrine, a spontaneous complex was sighted during the asystole fortuitously just as CPR was going to resume. A post-shock profound bradycardia secondary to extreme baseline vagal tone and myocardial stunning was suspected and high-dose atropine administered (1 mg followed by another 1 mg when a response was noted). Sinus rhythm with a good rate was restored, and the patient underwent investigations such as chest X-ray and ECG (Figure 3). The patient was transferred to the ICU for post-cardiac arrest care, while on IV antiarrhythmics and ionotropic support to maintain adequate heart rate and mean arterial pressure.

He had a coronary angiogram two days later when extubated and stable, which showed no obstructive disease. He

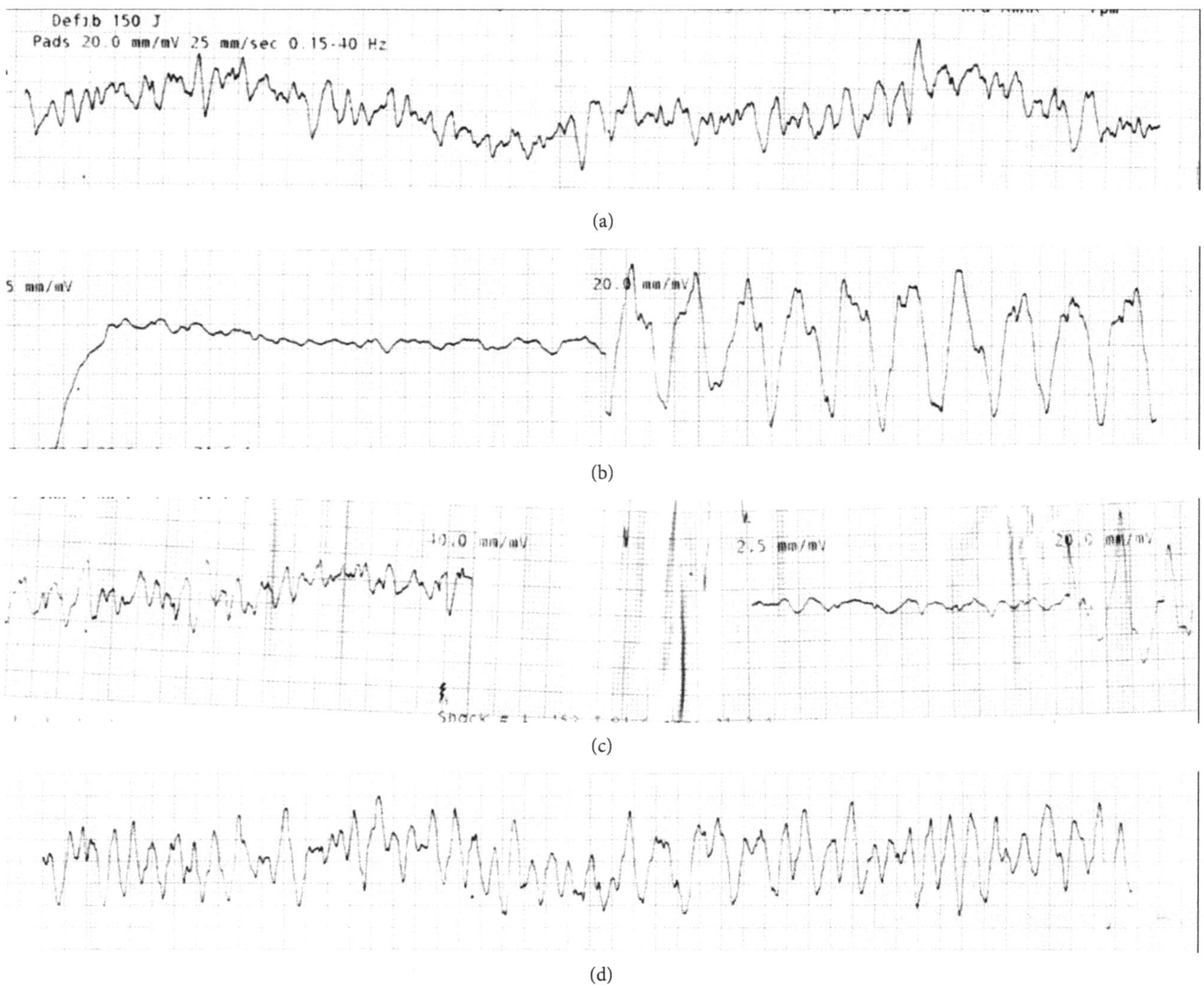

Figure 2: Cardiac arrest rhythm strips. (a) First rhythm strip with ventricular fibrillation identified prior to the first shock. (b) Asystole following defibrillation, this is followed by the arrest team resuming chest compressions. (c) Ventricular fibrillation again during later rhythm check, followed by defibrillation, asystole again, and resumed chest compressions. (d) Further alternation with ventricular fibrillation after prolonged CPR.

also had an implantable cardioverter defibrillator device implanted for secondary prevention.

1.6. Follow-Up. Discharge medications included aspirin 75 mg, bisoprolol 1.25 mg, sacubitril/valsartan 24/26 mg BD, esomeprazole 20 mg, rosuvastatin/ezetimibe 40/10 mg, and paracetamol 1 g QDS/PRN. As an outpatient, he was linked in with our local heart failure service and had a follow-up cardiac MRI which showed an improved LVEF of 38% with no inducible ischaemia on stress perfusion imaging.

2. Discussion

Factors such as witnessed collapse, rapid provision of high-quality CPR, initial shockable rhythm, and short duration of resuscitation are good prognosticators for survival. Despite 60 minutes of CPR, our patient had a good outcome. Each case must have the entire clinical picture assessed when deciding on duration of CPR [1].

Post-defibrillation asystole can occur, and in 25% of cases, it can take >120 seconds to return to an organised rhythm [2]. If this was the only factor in our patient's case, we may expect a detectable rhythm during the rhythm check prior to the next shock; however, this was not detected. Animal models of "accentuated antagonism" suggest that chronotropic response to adrenergic stimulation can inversely depend on underlying vagal activity. This may explain our profound response to atropine in the absence of significant epinephrine response [3]. Paradoxical bradycardia in the setting of epinephrine administration is a rare but recognised phenomenon [4].

Evidence suggests that atropine plays no role in an asystole and is managed with epinephrine and good quality CPR. The newest AHA ACLS guidance for symptomatic bradycardia recommends 1 mgas of atropine initial push [5].

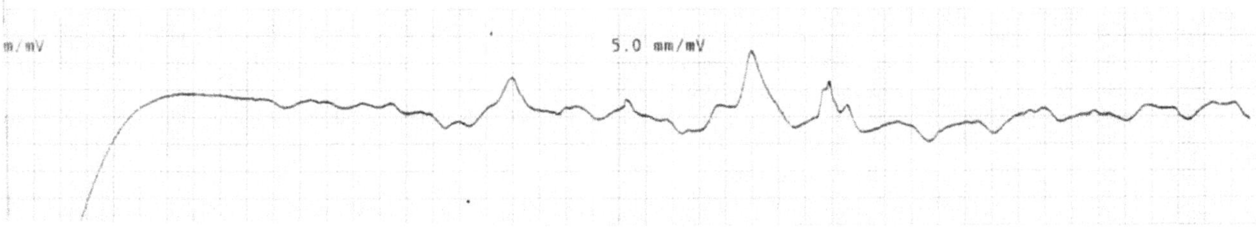

(a)

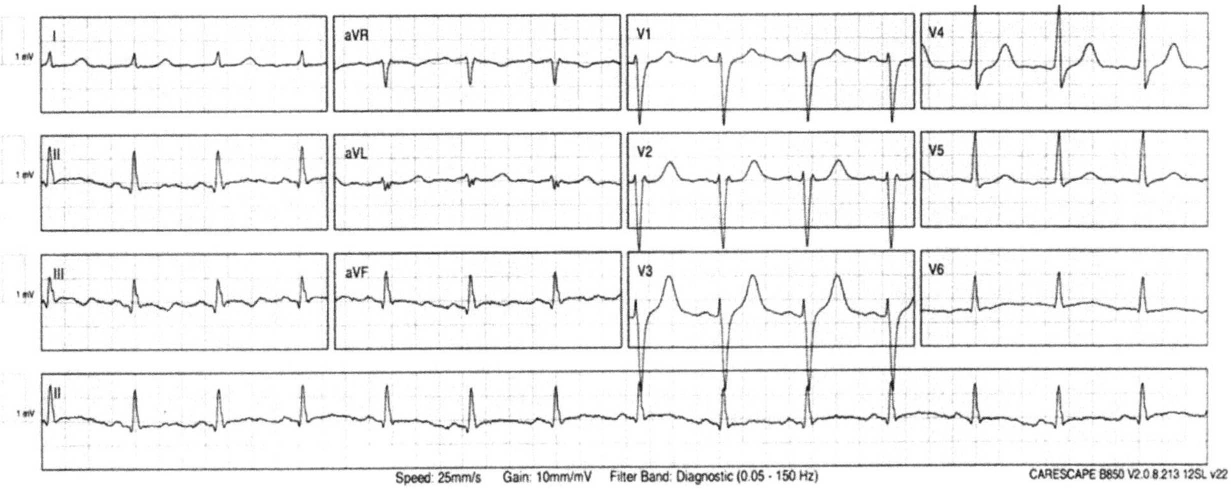

(b)

Figure 3: Extended pulse check followed by post-ROSC 12-lead ECG. (a) Rhythm strip with extended observation, demonstrating an intrinsic rhythm, identified complex with corresponding pulse shown with a red arrow. (b) 12-lead ECG of patient with sinus rhythm restored with a rate of 83.

3. Conclusions

Apparent asystole may not be asystole. Occasionally, profound vagal tone and bradycardia can mimic asystole. This case demonstrates a rare constellation of factors and highlights the phenomenon of profound bradycardia mimicking asystole, as the patient was unresponsive to multiple doses of epinephrine but had rapid clinical improvement following atropine administration.

Abbreviations

ED: Emergency department
VF: Ventricular fibrillation
VT: Ventricular tachycardia
ROSC: Return of spontaneous circulation
ACLS: Advanced cardiovascular life support
ECG: Electrocardiograph
HFrEF: Heart failure with reduced ejection fraction
HFmrEF: Heart failure with midrange ejection fraction.

Consent

Informed consent has been obtained for publication in a medical journal.

Disclosure

Case abstract was presented at the Heart Rhythm Society Conference 2021 as a poster presentation, and abstract has been published in Heart Rhythm Journal, accessible here: doi:10.1016/j.hrthm.2021.06.691.

References

[1] S. Yan, Y. Gan, N. Jiang et al., "The global survival rate among adult out-of-hospital cardiac arrest patients who received cardiopulmonary resuscitation: a systematic review and meta-analysis," *Critical Care*, vol. 24, no. 1, p. 61, 2020.

[2] A. Pierce, L. Roppolo, P. Owens, P. E. Pepe, and A. H. Idris, "The need to resume chest compressions immediately after defibrillation attempts: an analysis of post-shock rhythms and duration of pulselessness following out-of-hospital cardiac arrest," *Resuscitation*, vol. 89, pp. 162–168, 2015.

[3] T. Kawada, T. Sonobe, Y. Hayama et al., "Accentuated antagonism of vagal heart rate control and less potent prejunctional inhibition of vagal acetylcholine release during sympathetic nerve stimulation in the rat," *Autonomic Neuroscience*, vol. 218, pp. 25–30, 2019.

[4] T. Larsen, K. Kaszala, A. Tan, K. A. Ellenbogen, and J. F. Huizar, "Paradoxical reflex bradycardia after epinephrine infusion for arrhythmia induction in the electrophysiology laboratory," *HeartRhythm Case Reports*, vol. 4, no. 10, pp. 455–458, 2018.

[5] R. Merchant, A. Topjian, A. Panchal et al., "Part 1: executive summary: 2020 American Heart Association guidelines for cardiopulmonary resuscitation and emergency cardiovascular care," *Circulation*, vol. 142, 16 supplement 2, pp. S337–S357, 2020.

4

Cardiac Amyloidosis Presenting as Biventricular Systolic Heart Failure

Monique Oye,[1] **Aaron Richardson**,[2] **Edin Sadic**,[2] **Ahmad Alkhasawneh**,[3] **and Gladys Velarde**[2]

[1]*Department of Internal Medicine, UF Health Jacksonville, Jacksonville, FL, USA*
[2]*Division of Cardiology, UF Health Jacksonville, Jacksonville, FL, USA*
[3]*Department of Pathology, University of Florida Health Jacksonville, Jacksonville, FL, USA*

Correspondence should be addressed to Monique Oye; monique.oye@jax.ufl.edu

Academic Editor: Antonio de Padua Mansur

A previously healthy octogenarian presented with new onset heart failure symptoms. Comprehensive multimodality imaging including complete echocardiography with longitudinal strain analysis, cardiac magnetic resonance imaging (cMRI), nuclear medicine pyrophosphate (99-mcTcPYP) scan along with biomarker, monoclonal protein analysis, and fat pad biopsy confirmed diagnosis of transthyretin cardiac amyloidosis.

1. History of Presentation

An 81-year-old female of Jamaican descent with no prior past medical history or hospitalizations presented to the hospital with complaints of four-week history of dizziness, dyspnea on exertion, and lower extremity edema. She denied angina, productive cough, and neurologic symptoms. She was hypertensive with blood pressure of 147/101 mm Hg, regular heart rate of 94 beats/minute, afebrile with 100% oxygen saturation on room air. The electrocardiogram showed sinus rhythm without acute changes. Chest radiograph revealed cardiomegaly and pulmonary congestion. Chemistry panel was unremarkable with normal renal and hepatic function, with no electrolyte abnormalities. NT-Pro-B-type natriuretic peptide was elevated at 6,000 pg/mL. Troponin T was mildly elevated at (0.07 μg/L). Patient was admitted to cardiology service for further evaluation.

2. Investigations

A 12-lead electrocardiogram (ECG) obtained on presentation revealed normal sinus rhythm, low QRS voltage, poor R-wave progression, and Q waves in anteroseptal leads (Figure 1). Transthoracic echocardiography (TTE) revealed a severely decreased ejection fraction (EF) of 10-15%, with biventricular systolic dysfunction, moderate mitral regurgitation, severe tricuspid regurgitation, a trace pericardial effusion, and marked biatrial enlargement. Left ventricular (LV) cavity size was noted to be small, with abnormal left ventricular mass and increased relative wall thickness of 0.78.

Right ventricle was moderately enlarged, and right ventricular systolic function was severely impaired. The PA systolic pressure was estimated to be 40 mmHg based on complete tricuspid regurgitation spectral doppler signal. Diastolic profile was suggestive of restrictive LV filling pattern. There was abnormal global longitudinal (GL) strain with apical longitudinal strain preservation, a pattern suggestive of cardiac amyloidosis (CA) (Figures 2 and 3).

To rule out obstructive coronary artery disease, a left heart cardiac catheterization with coronary angiography was performed. This showed angiographically normal coronaries (Figure 4) and an LVEDP of 12-14 mmHg.

Cardiac MRI was then pursued, which revealed areas of subendocardial delayed gadolinium enhancement within the left ventricle not conforming to a vascular territory. This was also noted throughout the left atrium and along the septal subendocardial surface of the right ventricle (Figure 5). These

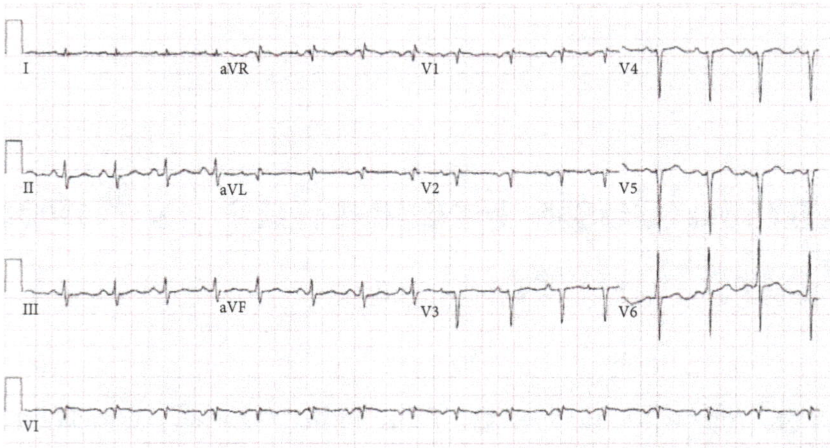

Figure 1: Electrocardiogram obtained on admission. Low voltage is noted in leads I, AVL; however, no left ventricular hypertrophy is noted. Q waves are seen in leads V1 and V2.

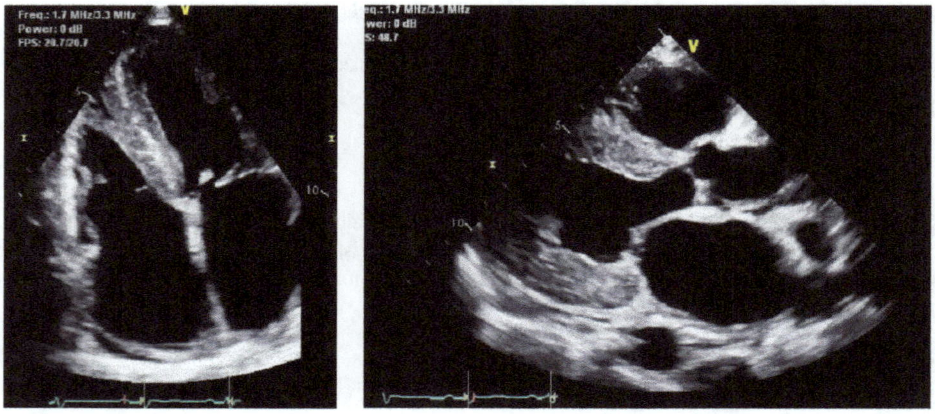

(a) (b)

Figure 2: 4-chamber (a) and a parasternal long axis echocardiogram view. Significant increased left ventricular wall thickness and biatrial enlargement can be seen.

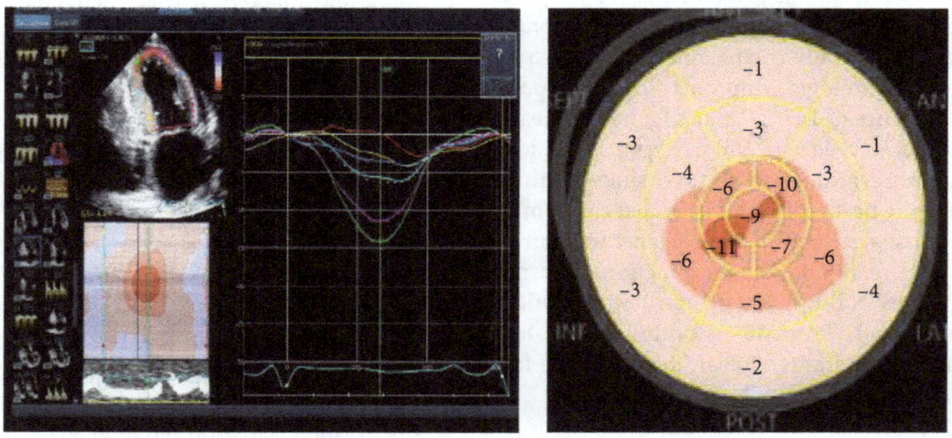

(a) (b)

Figure 3: Decreased global longitudinal strain pattern on echocardiogram. There is apical sparing of longitudinal strain, a finding typically seen in cardiac amyloidosis.

features favored a diagnosis of infiltrative cardiomyopathy. Laboratory markers were ordered to assess for evidence of a monoclonal protein. Serum immunofixation electrophoresis (IFE) revealed a monoclonal spike (0.38 g/dL) in the gamma region corresponding to an IgG ambda paraprotein. Urine IFE had no evidence of monoclonal paraprotein.

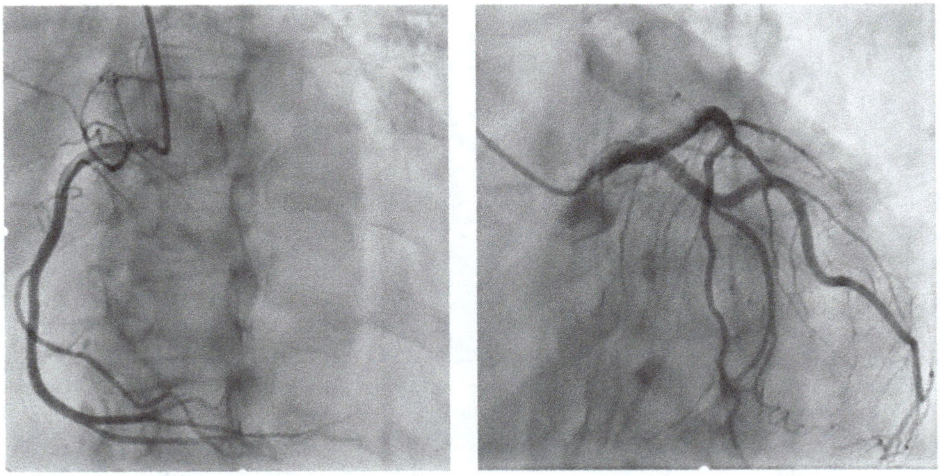

(a) (b)

FIGURE 4: Left anterior oblique caudal images from left heart catheterization. The right coronary system (a) and left coronary system (b) appear angiographically normal.

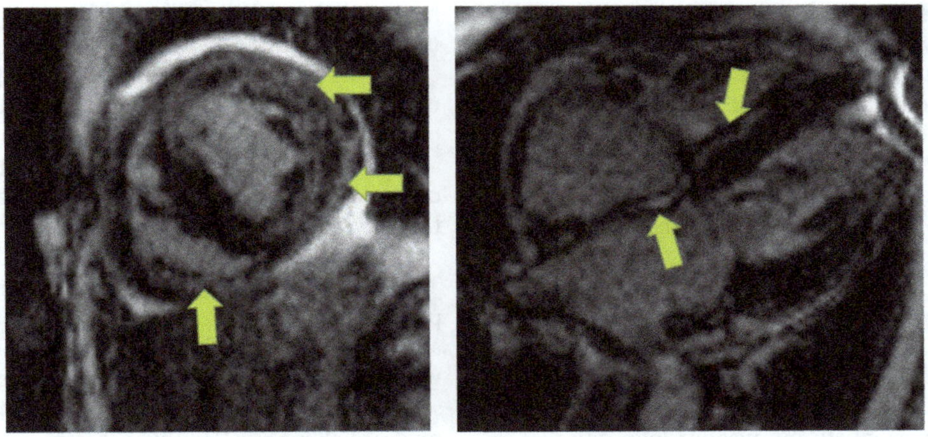

(a) (b)

FIGURE 5: Delayed gadolinium enhancement cardiac MRI images. The image on (a) shows a short axis view, (b) is a 4-chamber view. Extensive midmyocardial and atrial wall enhancement secondary to amyloid deposition is noted (green arrows) which is a signature of cardiac amyloidosis.

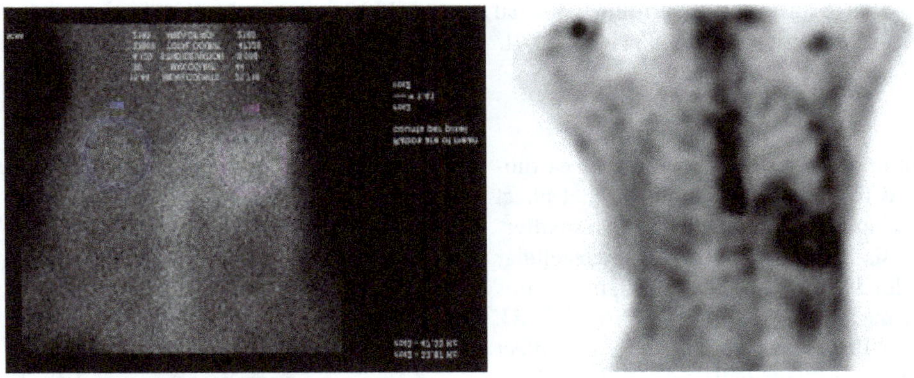

(a) (b)

FIGURE 6: Pyrophosphate scan (99mTc-PYP). Increased cardiac uptake can be seen in the image in (a) denoted by purple circle.

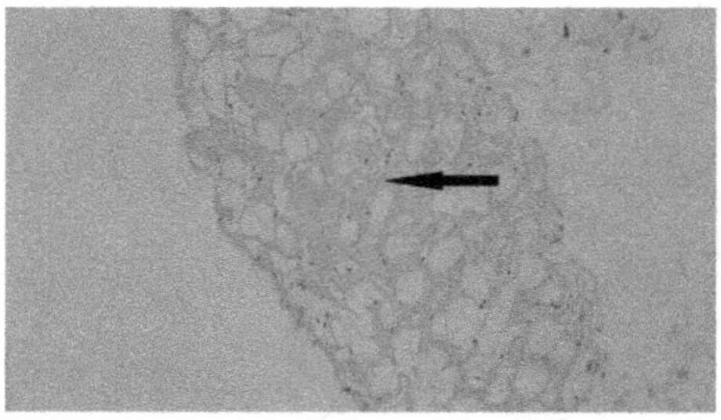

Figure 7: Amyloidosis in abdominal fat. Abdominal fat pad biopsy revealed pretentious infiltrate (arrow) which shows apple-green birefringence on red stain, consistent with amyloidosis (H&E stain, 100x).

Kappa/Lambda free light chain ratio was normal at 1.58 mg/L, which made AL subtype less likely.

In the setting of monoclonal gammopathy of undetermined significance (MGUS) a nuclear medicine pyrophosphate scan (99mTc-PYP) was performed to distinguish between light chain (AL) amyloidosis and transthyretin (TTR) amyloidosis. 99mTc-PYP scan showed grade 2/3 myocardial radiotracer uptake suggestive of TTR amyloidosis (Figure 6). The heart to contralateral (H/CL) ratio was 1.41. Fat pad aspirate biopsy showed positive staining for Congo red (Figure 7). Bone marrow biopsy did not reveal overt evidence of involvement by plasma cell neoplasm. Genetic testing did not reveal any mutations of the TTR gene. Patient was ultimately diagnosed with wild-type transthyretin amyloidosis (wt-ATTR).

3. Management

The patient presented in New York Heart Association (NYHA) functional Class III. Her heart failure symptoms were managed primarily with intravenous loop diuretics to achieve euvolemia. An attempt was made to start standard guideline directed therapy with beta-blockers and angiotensin converting enzyme inhibitors (ACEI), when diagnosis was in question, but she was unable to tolerate them due to hypotension.

With the use of diuretics, her functional status markedly improved, and she was able to return to performing her usual daily activities. Her symptoms improved to NYHA Class II.

4. Discussion

Amyloidosis is a commonly underdiagnosed cause of cardiomyopathy [1]. The two most common subtypes that affect the heart include light chain (AL) amyloidosis and transthyretin (ATTR) amyloidosis [1]. AL is caused by extracellular deposition of misfolded immunoglobulin light chains secreted by clonal plasma cells in the bone marrow [2]. AL cardiac amyloidosis (CA) is a rare condition that can affect nearly every organ in the body, leading to multiorgan failure. The clinical course of AL CA is more virulent and accelerated. Treatment for AL subtype typically includes chemotherapy ± autologous stem cell transplant.

ATTR results from deposition of misfolded TTR, a protein tetramer that is produced in the liver and deposits as insoluble amyloid in extracellular spaces causing damage to the heart and or peripheral nerves. ATTR CA can be wild-type (ATTR-wt, age-related) or variant (ATTRv, hereditary) [1]. ATTR-wt-CA, previously known as senile systemic amyloidosis, is usually diagnosed at an older age, has a male predominance, and is caused by age-related misfolding of genetically unaltered TTR.

ATTRv-CA is an autosomal-dominant disease in which gene mutations lead to changes in the protein TTR [3]. The presentation of hereditary ATTRv-CA depends on the type of mutation present. Some cause familial amyloid polyneuropathy (FAP), others familial amyloid cardiomyopathy (FAC), and some FAP/FAC overlap syndromes. It is usually diagnosed at younger ages, and signs of neuropathy (i.e., carpal tunnel syndrome) typically precede cardiomyopathy by years in advance [1]. In the United States, transthyretin isoleucine 122 (Val122Ile) is a common variant of hereditary ATTRv-CA, and this genetic mutation disproportionally affects African American patients [4]. This variant results in a late-onset, restrictive cardiomyopathy that can mimic other forms of heart failure, such as hypertensive heart disease, leading to underdiagnosis [4].

To avoid misdiagnosis, genetic testing for the Val122Ile mutation can play a role in identification and treatment for patients as well as their family members. Novel treatments are being developed for amyloidosis (ATTR) subtypes that can slow the progression of cardiomyopathy by working as transthyretin silencers and stabilizers [1].

Clinically significant cardiac involvement in both types of TTR typically presents as a syndrome of heart failure with preserved ejection fraction [2], abnormal troponin levels, and markedly elevated pro-bnp levels. However, heart failure with reduced ejection fraction can be seen in the advanced stages of the disease. The gold standard for diagnosis is endomyocardial biopsy. However, recent advances in imaging have provided noninvasive modalities that are helpful in identifying cardiac amyloid. Characteristic patterns on electrocardiogram, echocardiogram, and cardiac MRI can assist in earlier detection. Red flag features for cardiac amyloid typically seen on echocardiogram include increase in left ventricular (LV) wall thickness (relative wall thickness > 0.6), small LV chamber size, speckled myocardium, atrial enlargement, and diastolic dysfunction with a restrictive diastolic pattern [1]. Additionally, relative apical sparing of longitudinal strain (LS) is considered a specific finding [5]. Previous studies have demonstrated that relative sparing of LS in the LV apex using 2-D speckle tracking is highly sensitive (93%) and specific (82%) for the diagnosis of cardiac amyloid [5].

Cardiac MRI is another useful imaging modality showing various patterns of late gadolinium enhancement. However, it is unable to distinguish between the AL and TTR subtype [6].

Nuclear imaging technique with bone-seeking radiotracers have become a diagnostic method for ATTR-CA and is able to distinguish it from AL-CA with high specificity [7]. Different radiotracers can be used including technetium-3,3-diphosphono-1,2-propanodicarboxylic acid (^{99m}Tc-DPD) and ^{99m}Tc-PYP. ^{99m}Tc-DPD scintigraphy is currently the most studied isotope in ATTR-CA and has widespread use among amyloid centers in Europe [8]. It is not approved for clinical use in the United States, where ^{99m}Tc-PYP scanning is more commonly utilized. There has yet to be a direct comparison of the different radiotracers to determine if one has greater specificity in diagnosing ATTR-CA [8]. The exact mechanism by which these bone-seeking radiotracers accumulate in the myocardium of patients with cardiac amyloidosis remains unclear; however, studies suggest an association between radiotracer myocardial uptake and amyloid fibril type in patients with ATTRv [9].

Our patient was an elderly African American female, presenting de novo with significantly increased ventricular wall thickness and heart failure of uncertain etiology. While keeping more prevalent pathologies in the differential; it is important to consider amyloidosis as a potential etiology in this demographic despite her age, sex, and race. While it is true that ATTR-wt CA appears to be more common in older white men, it has also been shown to be present in up to 50% of elderly women admitted with heart failure in at least one prospective study where 99mTc-PYP imaging was used with high accuracy of detection of ATTR-wt cases [10]. Similarly, studies evaluating ATTR-wt have almost exclusively consisted of Caucasian patients. However, population-based data from the United Kingdom have reported an equal prevalence of ATTR-wt among races [9]. Underrecognition of this disease may explain why African Americans are poorly represented in American studies of ATTR wt-CA [11].

Regardless of patient's age, TTR genetic testing should be performed in all patients with ATTR-CA since the results have significant implications for family members at risk as mentioned earlier.

Our case illustrates the occurrence of advanced biventricular systolic heart failure in an elderly woman with ATTR-CA. Her course had been rather indolent, but this condition can be in fact undiagnosed or underdiagnosed for years as many "subtle" signs can be attributed to the aging process.

Her case is unique as this condition typically present with heart failure with preserved ejection fraction (HFpEF). The right ventricle (RV) is usually normal or thickened, especially in the anterior wall, and if the RV is involved, signs of pulmonary hypertension may be observed. In the advanced phases of the disease, biventricular systolic function deteriorates. This has substantial clinical implications, as treatment strategies may become even more limited.

Usual guideline directed medical therapy with angiotensin-converting enzyme inhibitors (ACE-I), and beta-blockers for heart failure with reduced EF (HFreF) have not been shown to offer clinical benefit. In fact, most medications have potential to cause harm as they may exacerbate hypotension when amyloid-associated autonomic dysfunction is present or further limits cardiac output due to relatively fixed stroke volumes secondary to restrictive filling [7]. Accurate diagnosis of ATTR-CA is important to avoid the potentially deleterious effects of using these medications in this group of patients. Furthermore, the benefits of implantable cardioverter defibrillator (ICDs), particularly for primary prevention of sudden cardiac death in patients with HFreF and ATTR-CA, have not been well established. ICDs are recommended only in cases of aborted sudden cardiac death with expected survival >1 year or significant ventricular arrhythmias [7] Our patient did not have ventricular arrhythmias, and ICD placement was deferred. She was referred to the heart failure clinic on discharge for outpatient follow-up and potential treatment with novel ATTR therapies.

5. Conclusions

This case highlights the different imaging modalities that can be used to diagnose cardiac amyloidosis. Echocardiogram and electrocardiogram findings in conjunction with cardiac MRI can assist with the initial diagnosis when amyloidosis is suspected. Nuclear imaging with 99mTc-PYP can further distinguish between different types of amyloidosis (AL vs. ATTR).

Although endomyocardial biopsy is the gold standard diagnostic test, hematology testing, fat pad, genetic testing, and bone marrow biopsies can aid in confirming the diagnosis without putting patients at risk for complications with endomyocardial biopsy. Early detection can lead to an increased number of patients being referred for treatment.

Additional Points

Take Home Messages/Learning Objectives. (i) Recognize the different imaging modalities used in the diagnosis of cardiac amyloidosis. (ii) Recognize how to distinguish the different subtypes of cardiac amyloidosis. (iii) Recognize the common echocardiogram findings seen in cardiac amyloidosis.

References

[1] J. Rubin and M. S. Maurer, "Cardiac amyloidosis: overlooked, underappreciated, and treatable," *Annual Review of Medicine* vol. 71, no. 1, pp. 203–219, 2020.

[2] T. P. Quock, T. Yan, E. Chang, S. Guthrie, and M. S. Broder, "Epidemiology of AL amyloidosis: a real-world study using US claims data," *Blood Advances*, vol. 2, no. 10, pp. 1046 1053, 2018.

[3] H. Yamamoto and T. Yokochi, "Transthyretin cardiac amyloidosis: an update on diagnosis and treatment," *ESC Heart Fail.*, vol. 6, no. 6, pp. 1128–1139, 2019.

[4] K. B. Shah, A. K. Mankad, A. Castano et al., "Transthyretin cardiac amyloidosis in black Americans," *Circulation: Heart Failure*, vol. 9, no. 6, p. e002558, 2016.

[5] D. Phelan, P. Collier, P. Thavendiranathan et al., "Relative apical sparing of longitudinal strain using two-dimensional speckle-tracking echocardiography is both sensitive and specific for the diagnosis of cardiac amyloidosis," *Heart*, vol. 98, no. 19, pp. 1442–1448, 2012, Epub 2012 Aug 3.

[6] S. P. Lee, J. B. Park, H. K. Kim, Y. J. Kim, M. Grogan, and D. W. Sohn, "Contemporary imaging diagnosis of cardiac amyloidosis," *Journal of Cardiovascular Imaging*, vol. 27, no. 1, pp. 1–10, 2019.

[7] M. M. Kittleson, M. S. Maurer, A. V. Ambardekar et al., "Cardiac amyloidosis: evolving diagnosis and management: a scien-

tific statement from the American Heart Association," *Circulation*, vol. 142, no. 1, pp. e7–e22, 2020.

[8] V. Singh, R. Falk, M. F. Di Carli, M. Kijewski, C. Rapezzi, and S. Dorbala, "State-of-the-art radionuclide imaging in cardiac transthyretin amyloidosis," *Journal of Nuclear Cardiology*, vol. 26, no. 1, pp. 158–173, 2019.

[9] B. Pilebro, O. B. Suhr, U. Näslund, P. Westermark, P. Lindqvist, and T. Sundström, "(99m)Tc-DPD uptake reflects amyloid fibril composition in hereditary transthyretin amyloidosis," *Upsala Journal of Medical Sciences*, vol. 121, no. 1, pp. 17–24, 2015.

[10] E. González-López, M. Gallego-Delgado, G. Guzzo-Merello et al., "Wild-type transthyretin amyloidosis as a cause of heart failure with preserved ejection fraction," *European Heart Journal*, vol. 36, no. 38, pp. 2585–2594, 2015.

[11] L. H. Connors, F. Sam, M. Skinner et al., "Heart failure resulting from age-related cardiac amyloid disease associated with wild-type transthyretin: a prospective, observational cohort study," *Circulation*, vol. 133, no. 3, pp. 282–290, 2016.

5

Cardiac Magnetic Resonance for Diagnosis of Neuroendocrine Tumor Metastases to the Right and Left Ventricles with Carcinoid Heart Disease

Daniel Barnebee[1] **Brian Morse**[2] **Jonathan R. Strosberg,**[3] **Marijan Pejic,**[4] **and Daniel Jeong**[2]

[1]*University of South Florida College of Medicine, Tampa, FL, USA*
[2]*Department of Diagnostic Imaging and Interventional Radiology, H. Lee Moffitt Cancer Center and Research Institute, Tampa FL, USA*
[3]*Department of Gastrointestinal Oncology, H. Lee Moffitt Cancer Center and Research Institute, Tampa FL, USA*
[4]*Department of Radiology, University of South Florida College of Medicine, Tampa, FL, USA*

Correspondence should be addressed to Daniel Jeong; daniel.jeong@moffitt.org

Academic Editor: Kuan-Rau Chiou

A 76-year-old male with a small bowel neuroendocrine tumor with hepatic metastases presented with new onset lower extremity swelling, bloating, and weight gain which ultimately lead to cardiac magnetic resonance (CMR) to evaluate for cardiac involvement of disease. CMR showed right and left ventricular myocardial metastases along with findings suggestive of carcinoid heart disease. The patient had severe tricuspid valve regurgitation necessitating surgical valve repair. The patient underwent bioprosthetic tricuspid valve replacement and debulking of the metastases with surgical pathology confirming neuroendocrine tumor metastases. Follow-up clinical evaluations at 3, 6, and 9 months postoperatively showed improvement in cardiac function and stable hepatic tumor burden. This case demonstrates the utility of CMR to diagnose myocardial metastases and carcinoid heart disease complicated by severe tricuspid regurgitation, which guided surgical management.

1. Introduction

Neuroendocrine tumors (NETs) are a diverse group of tumors arising from neuroendocrine cells, and they can cause primary tumors in many different organs including the lungs, small intestine, rectum, pancreas, and other organs [1]. Within this spectrum of disease, neuroendocrine tumors can range from indolent disease to highly aggressive carcinomas. While NETs have an overall incidence of 5.86 per 100,000 people, NETs of the GI tract and lungs (carcinoid tumors) are a type of neuroendocrine tumor with an annual incidence of 4.7 per 100,000 people [2–5]. The most common primary sites of a carcinoid tumor include the small intestine, rectum, and appendix, and hepatic metastases are present in 45% of cases at the time of initial diagnosis [6].

NETs of the midgut (distal small intestine) commonly release vasoactive substances including 5-hydroxytryptamine (serotonin), histamine, tachykinins, and prostaglandins [7]. When these vasoactive substances escape hepatic degradation, the resultant carcinoid syndrome manifests as facial flushing, secretory diarrhea, and bronchoconstriction [2, 7–9]. Secretion of serotonin and other vasoactive substances into the systemic circulation can also result in carcinoid heart disease, a condition characterized by fibrotic damage to the right heart valves (tricuspid and pulmonary). Patients with symptoms of florid carcinoid syndrome have a 50% chance of developing carcinoid heart disease [7].

In rare cases, NETs can metastasize to the heart [10, 11]. Cardiac metastases have been reported as myocardial nodules or pedunculated masses extending into the cardiac

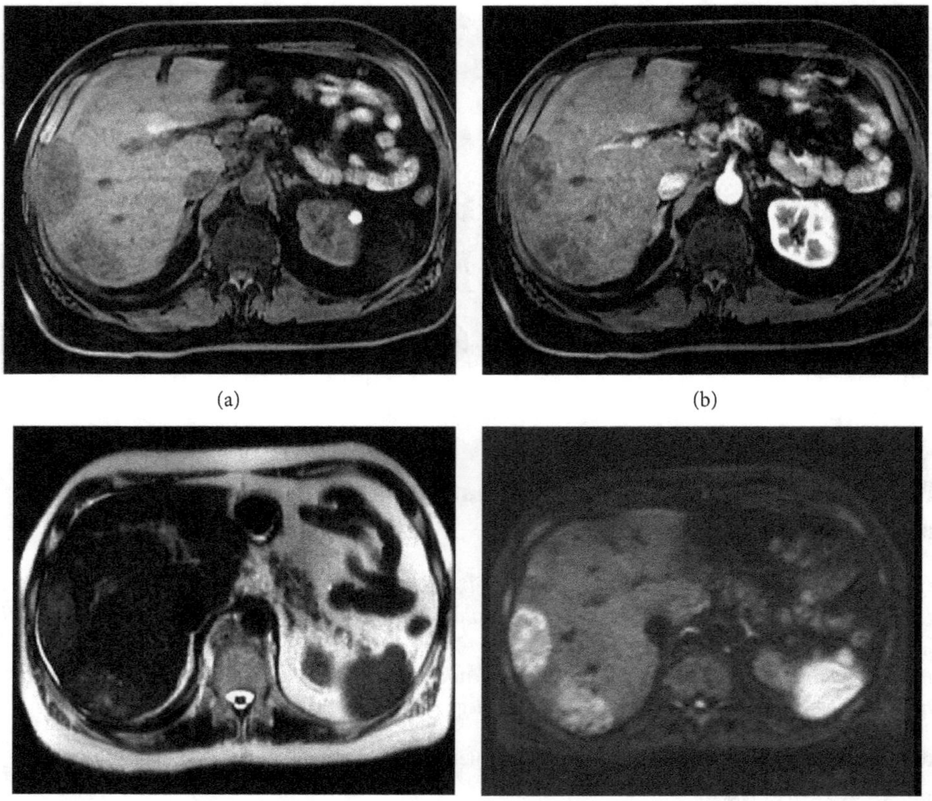

(a) (b) (c) (d)

Figure 1: Hepatic metastases on MRI. (a) Axial T1-weighted fat-suppressed precontrast image and (b) postcontrast arterial phase image demonstrating multiple right hepatic lesions with internal enhancement. (c) Axial T2-weighted image shows mildly high signal within the hepatic lesions. (d) Axial diffusion weighted image ($B = 800$) with high signal within the right hepatic lesions compatible with restricted diffusion.

chamber, and these can mimic myxomas on echocardiography [12]. NET cardiac metastases often occur after hepatic metastases and have been associated with pericardial effusions [10, 13]. Rare cases of NET metastasizing to the heart have been reported, and cardiac MRI findings of carcinoid cardiac metastases are rarely presented [10, 14, 15]. No specific cases of RV myocardial metastasis extending to the tricuspid valve annular region have been reported.

2. Case Presentation

A 76-year-old male with stage IV, small bowel NET metastatic to the liver had been followed by our institution for 4 years with stable hepatic metastatic disease on octreotide long-acting release (LAR) therapy. Originally, the tumor Ki-67 index was 5% and 24-hour urine 5-hydroxyindole acetic acid (5-HIAA) was 105 mg. The patient presented with mild progression of disease on abdominal magnetic resonance imaging (MRI) (Figure 1) after approximately 4 years of stable disease. Six months following this abdominal MRI, the patient developed bilateral lower extremity swelling, weight gain, and bloating lasting over 1 month. The serum brain-natriuretic peptide (BNP) value was 161 pg/ml (normal range < 100 pg/ml). N-terminal proBNP and other cardiac biomarkers were not available. Transthoracic echocardiogram showed tricuspid regurgitation and right ventricular wall thickening with an echogenic mass in the RV free wall extending to the RV outflow tract. There was severe malcoaptation of the thickened tricuspid valve leaflets. Tricuspid regurgitation was described as widely open regurgitation with a peak regurgitant flow velocity of 203 cm/s. Of note, the aortic and mitral valves were structurally normal without stenosis or regurgitation. Cardiac magnetic resonance (CMR) was obtained for further evaluation.

CMR (Figure 2) showed a 2.6 cm lesion in the right ventricular free wall and a 2.4 cm lesion in the left ventricular anteroseptal wall. These lesions demonstrated high T2-weighted signal and isointense T1-weighted signal with postcontrast perfusion, findings compatible with myocardial metastases. Of note, the RV free wall lesion extended superiorly near the base of the tricuspid valve annular region. Balanced cine steady state free precession (bSSFP) images showed abnormal thickening of the anterior tricuspid valve leaflet, and the leaflet did not coapt normally during systole contributing to severe tricuspid regurgitation. The right atrium was moderately dilated.

The patient underwent bioprosthetic tricuspid valve replacement and biopsy and debulking of the myocardial tumors. The myocardial tumors were histologically confirmed as NET metastases. The patient recovered well from

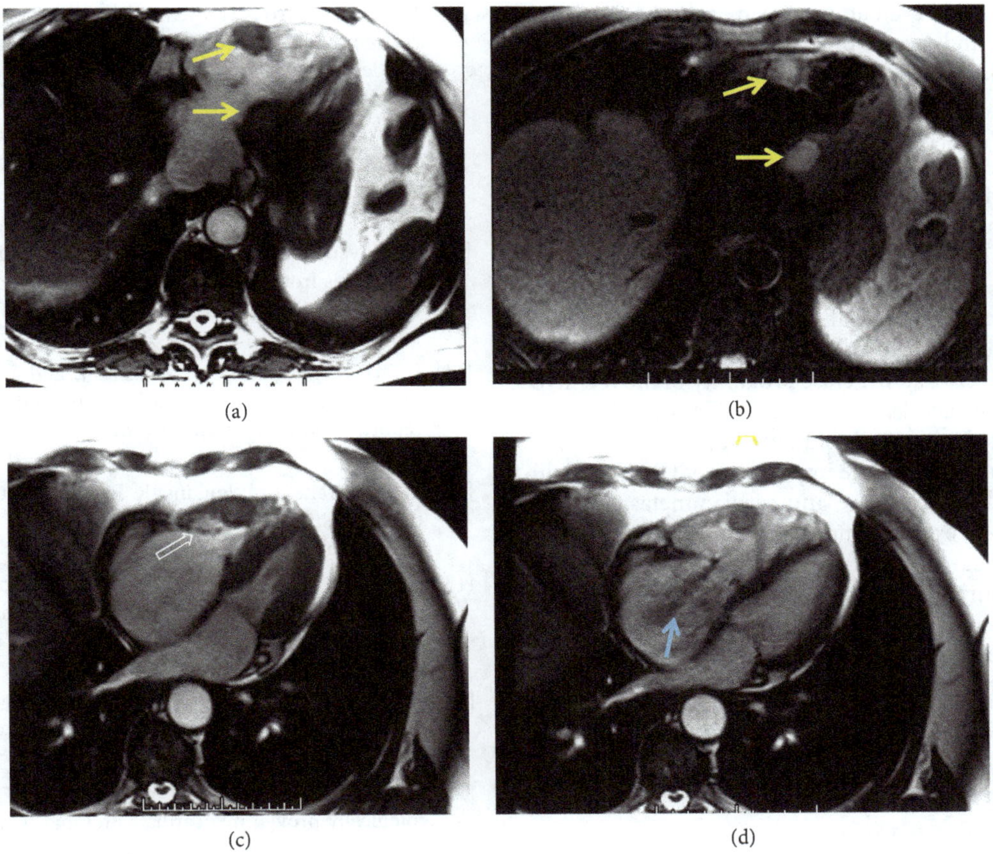

FIGURE 2: (a) Axial bSSFP bright blood image through the right ventricle (RV) shows two masses (yellow arrows) involving the anterior RV wall and basilar interventricular septum. (b) Axial T2 spectral presaturation with inversion recovery dark blood image showing T2 hyperintense signal within the two lesions (yellow arrows). (c) Four-chamber bSSFP bright blood image during late systole shows thickening of the anterior leaflet of the tricuspid valve (open arrow) with an abnormal shortened and retracted configuration near the anterior RV wall mass. (d) Early systole image shows a large low signal tricuspid regurgitant flow jet (blue arrow). Notice the anterior leaflet maintaining an abnormal partially open configuration.

surgery, and follow-up clinical visits demonstrated significant improvement in his carcinoid heart disease. As of the latest visit, the patient has excellent cardiac function with resolution of tricuspid regurgitation. His 9-month postoperative follow-up CT scan showed relatively stable disease, and his urine 5-HIAA was improving. The patient is continuing on octreotide LAR 30 mg.

3. Discussion

We present a unique case of carcinoid heart disease and myocardial metastases both contributing to this patient's severe symptomatic tricuspid regurgitation. The tricuspid valve thickening is a specific finding of carcinoid heart disease, and well-defined lesions with arterial perfusion in the RV and LV walls are specific for metastases. Previous authors have suggested that vasoactive mediators associated with myocardial metastases may accelerate the onset of carcinoid heart disease, which could explain the case described here [12, 16].

Carcinoid heart disease manifests via the accumulation of carcinoid plaque composed of smooth muscle, myofibroblasts, and elastic tissue [3]. Plaque forms a fibrous layer lining the endocardial surface of the valves thus displacing the fibrous tissue on the endocardial surfaces of the heart. Morphologic changes to the heart including dilatation of valve rings can lead to tricuspid or pulmonic valve insufficiency and ultimately right heart failure, while the left heart is involved in less than 10% of cases [3, 13]. When the left heart is involved in carcinoid heart disease, extensive hepatic metastases, bronchial carcinoid, or a patent foramen ovale may be present [17, 18]. Myocardial NET metastases, however, often present as discrete lesions within the right or left ventricular myocardium. In our case, the discrete RV metastasis adjacent to the tricuspid valve annular region likely accelerated carcinoid heart disease due to local tumor release of vasoactive substances including serotonin.

Echocardiography serves as first line screening for cardiac involvement in patients with carcinoid syndrome. Common echocardiographic features of carcinoid heart disease include morphologic changes to the tricuspid valve causing a thick retracted appearance with decreased mobility and enlargement of the right atrium and ventricle related to valvular insufficiency [19]. Surgical valve replacement is considered when patients are symptomatic with severe valvular dysfunction or when RV function significantly declines due to valvular disease [8].

CMR offers more specific evaluation of cardiac lesions to help differentiate benign lesions from metastases compared to echocardiography evaluation which is based on lesion intrinsic signal and perfusion characteristics [20]. While echocardiography allows for excellent real-time myocardial visualization with flow information, the CMR T2-weighted and postcontrast sequences allow for more specific mass characterization [13]. Cardiac metastases can affect the right or the left side of the heart, as well as the ventricular septum, and appear continuous with the affected myocardial wall [3, 11, 16]. CMR images in this case show the right ventricular myocardial tumor in close proximity to the tricuspid valve with markedly abnormal tricuspid valve closing. The anterior tricuspid valve leaflet had a shortened retracted configuration. It is likely that the close proximity of the RV myocardial metastasis accelerated valve leaflet morphological changes associated with carcinoid heart disease.

This case demonstrates the importance of CMR to evaluate for carcinoid heart disease and cardiac metastases. The results of the CMR exam in our case lead to characterization of myocardial metastases and allowed for planning of metastasis resection during the tricuspid valve bioprosthetic surgery. The case also serves as a reminder for providers that while echocardiography may offer first line screening for cardiac involvement when carcinoid heart disease is suspected, CMR may be useful when myocardial metastases are suspected for potential surgical planning.

Supplementary Materials

Figure 3 (supplemental video clip): cine bSSFP 4 chamber imaging demonstrates severe tricuspid regurgitation and abnormal failure of the tricuspid valve to coapt or close during systole. The anterior right ventricular wall metastasis is also noted. *(Supplementary Materials)*

References

[1] B. Oronsky, P. C. Ma, D. Morgensztern, and C. A. Carter, "Nothing but NET: a review of neuroendocrine tumors and carcinomas," *Neoplasia*, vol. 19, no. 12, pp. 991–1002, 2017.

[2] M. J. Calero Rueda, G. Aldamiz-Echevarría, A. A. López et al., "Cardiac metastasis in a patient with a bronchial carcinoid," *Circulation*, vol. 130, no. 1, pp. e1–e3, 2014.

[3] C. C. Caldeira, D. Sayad, J. Strosberg, C. Faber, S. Saouma, and T. Michaud, "Surgical treatment of an isolated metastatic myocardial neuroendocrine tumor," *The Annals of Thoracic Surgery*, vol. 101, no. 2, pp. 747–749, 2016.

[4] A. E. Soyano, M. Kassi, and P. M. Kasi, "Neuroendocrine tumor involving the epicardium," *Case Reports in Oncology*, vol. 10, no. 3, pp. 1144–1149, 2017.

[5] B. G. Taal and O. Visser, "Epidemiology of neuroendocrine tumours," *Neuroendocrinology*, vol. 80, no. 1, pp. 3–7, 2004.

[6] F. M. Watzka, C. Fottner, M. Miederer et al., "Surgical therapy of neuroendocrine neoplasm with hepatic metastasis: patient selection and prognosis," *Langenbeck's Archives of Surgery*, vol. 400, no. 3, pp. 349–358, 2015.

[7] D. J. Fox and R. S. Khattar, "Carcinoid heart disease: presentation, diagnosis, and management," *Heart*, vol. 90, no. 10, pp. 1224–1228, 2004.

[8] K. Khay, S. Arous, T. Bentaoune, A. Drighil, and R. Habbal, "Carcinoid heart disease revealed by cyanosis with both right and left valvular involvement: a case report," *Journal of Medical Case Reports*, vol. 12, no. 1, p. 23, 2018.

[9] Board, PDQATE, "Gastrointestinal carcinoid tumors treatment (PDQ(R)): patient version, in PDQ Cancer Information Summaries," National Cancer Institute (US): Bethesda (MD), 2002.

[10] M. Puvaneswary, D. Thomson, and G. R. Bellamy, "Cardiac metastasis from carcinoid tumour: magnetic resonance imaging findings," *Australasian Radiology*, vol. 48, no. 3, pp. 383-387, 2004.

[11] J. Strosberg, S. Hoffe, T. Hazelton, and L. Kvols, "External beam irradiation of myocardial carcinoid metastases: a case report," *Journal of Medical Case Reports*, vol. 1, no. 1, p. 95, 2007.

[12] W. M. Drake, P. J. Jenkins, R. R. Phillips et al., "Intracardiac metastases from neuroendocrine tumours," *Clinical Endocrinology*, vol. 46, no. 4, pp. 517–522, 1997.

[13] I. Manoly, S. McAnelly, S. Sriskandarajah, and K. McLaughlin, "Prognosis of patients with carcinoid heart disease after valvular surgery," *Interactive Cardiovascular and Thoracic Surgery*, vol. 19, no. 2, pp. 302–305, 2014.

[14] S. Lee, S. P. Lee, and D. W. Sohn, "Diffuse myocardial metastasis of carcinoid tumour," *Heart*, vol. 100, no. 5, pp. 438-439, 2014.

[15] A. A. Studer Bruengger, K. Wechalekar, R. Khattar et al., "Histologically proven myocardial carcinoid metastases: the value of multimodality imaging," *Canadian Journal of Cardiology*, vol. 33, no. 10, pp. 1336.e9–1336.e12, 2017.

[16] U. H. Pandya, P. A. Pellikka, M. Enriquez-Sarano, W. D. Edwards, H. V. Schaff, and H. M. Connolly, "Metastatic carcinoid tumor to the heart: echocardiographic-pathologic study of 11 patients," *Journal of the American College of Cardiology*, vol. 40, no. 7, pp. 1328–1332, 2002.

[17] W. Schweizer, F. Gloor, R. V. Bertrab, and U. C. Dubach, "Carcinoid heart disease with left-sided lesions," *Circulation*, vol. 29, no. 2, pp. 253–257, 1964.

[18] N. E. Strickman, P. A. Rossi, G. A. Massumkhani, and R. J. Hall, "Carcinoid heart disease: a clinical, pathologic, and therapeutic update," *Current Problems in Cardiology*, vol. 6, no. 11, pp. 1–42, 1982.

[19] P. A. Pellikka, A. J. Tajik, B. K. Khandheria et al., "Carcinoid heart disease. Clinical and echocardiographic spectrum in 74 patients," *Circulation*, vol. 87, no. 4, pp. 1188–1196, 1993.

[20] D. Jeong, A. Patel, C. J. Francois, K. L. Gage, and M. G. Fradley, "Cardiac magnetic resonance imaging in oncology," *Cancer Control*, vol. 24, no. 2, pp. 147–160, 2017.

6

Acute Myocardial Infarction due to External Compression of the Left Main Coronary Artery by a Large Pulmonary Artery Aneurysm

H. Sharma,[1] **S. N. Doshi,**[2] **and M. A. Nadir**[2]

[1]*Institute of Cardiovascular Sciences, University of Birmingham, Birmingham, UK*
[2]*Cardiology Department, Queen Elizabeth Hospital, Birmingham, UK*

Correspondence should be addressed to H. Sharma; harish.sharma@nhs.net

Academic Editor: Manabu Shirotani

Background. Although rare, external compression of the left main coronary artery (LMCA) by a pulmonary arterial aneurysm (PAA) as a consequence of pulmonary arterial hypertension causing stable angina pectoris is well described. However, acute myocardial infarction is extremely rare, particularly with a full array of electrocardiographic, biochemical, and echocardiographic features, as in this scenario. *Case.* In this case, a 62-year-old man with a past history of severe fibrotic lung disease was hospitalised with chest pain. The patient had dynamic anterolateral ischaemic changes on electrocardiography and serially elevated high-sensitivity troponin I. Transthoracic echocardiography revealed impaired left ventricular ejection fraction with anterolateral hypokinesis. Coronary angiography with intracoronary imaging revealed external compression of the LMCA. Computer tomography (CT) scans confirmed new PAA, compared to previous scans. The patient was successfully treated by percutaneous coronary stent implantation. *Conclusion.* Progressive dilatation of the pulmonary artery due to pulmonary arterial hypertension can result in acute MI secondary to external compression of the LMCA. Clinicians should be mindful of acute coronary syndromes in patients with long-standing pulmonary hypertension presenting with chest pain.

1. Introduction

Pulmonary arterial hypertension (PAH) is associated with aneurysm of the main pulmonary artery (PA). In normal anatomy, the PA lies adjacent to the left coronary sinus of the aorta. As the left main coronary artery (LMCA) arises from the left coronary sinus, it may be compressed by a PA aneurysm (PAA). Although rare, a small number of case reports have described this phenomenon in the presence [1, 2] and absence of PAH [3]. The most commonly described clinical sequelae of this scenario is stable angina pectoris [4–7].

Myocardial infarction (MI) as a result of external compression of a coronary artery has been previously documented in patients with anomalous coronary origin or course [8] and normal coronary anatomy [9], attributed to PAA (with or without PAH). However, it is rare to see the full gamut of evidence suggesting acute MI, including dynamic electrogram (ECG) changes, elevation of high-sensitivity troponin, and a corresponding regional wall motion abnormality on echocardiography.

2. Case

A 62-year-old man with a past history of severe fibrotic lung disease requiring long-term oxygen therapy was hospitalised with typical angina pain with no resolution despite sublingual glyceryl trinitrate use. ECG demonstrated dynamic anterolateral ST depression with T wave inversion in anterior and lateral leads (Figure 1). High-sensitivity troponin I assays (normal: < 5 ng/L) measured 99 and 250 ng/L. Transthoracic echocardiography revealed a left ventricle ejection fraction of 52% and anterolateral hypokinesis (video 1) with a high likelihood of pulmonary hypertension (estimated systolic PA pressure 110 mmHg), indicating likely group III pulmonary hypertension (secondary to hypoxic lung disease). The main PA diameter was measured at 5.0 cm (Figure 2). Cardiac

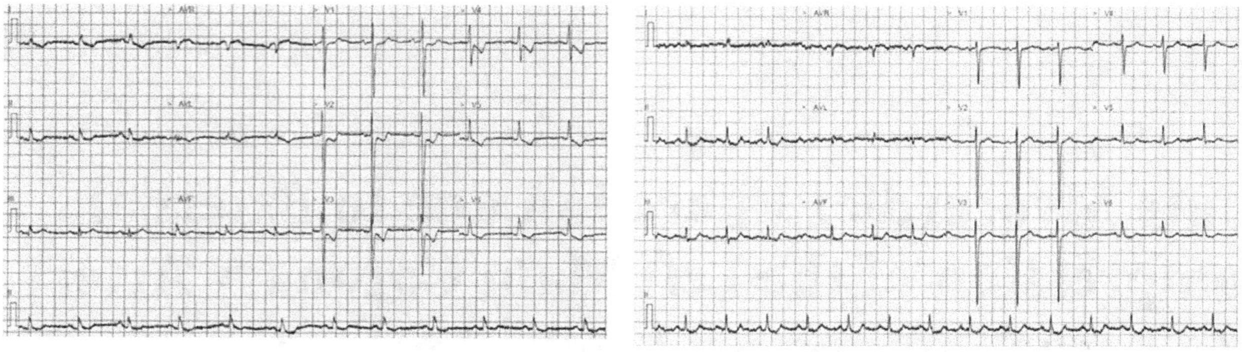

(a) (b)

Figure 1: Electrocardiogram demonstrating (a) anterolateral ischaemic changes (ST depression and T wave inversion); (b) older ECG 6 months earlier.

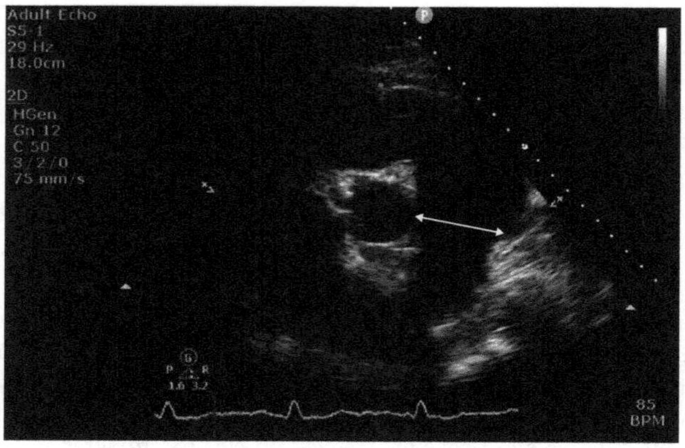

Figure 2: Transthoracic echocardiogram demonstrating significant dilatation of the main pulmonary artery (diameter: 5 cm).

catheterisation assessment as part of a lung transplant work-up 7 years earlier had shown no significant coronary disease (Figure 3(c)) with invasive measurements demonstrating only mild pulmonary hypertension (mean systolic PA pressure 30 mmHg). The differential diagnosis included pulmonary thromboembolism and pulmonary/aortic dissection, although the clinical picture was most consistent with acute MI. The patient was commenced on pharmacological treatment for non-ST elevation myocardial infarction. In view of the significant lung disease, an initial conservative approach was taken, but after continual chest pain despite optimal medical therapy, invasive coronary angiography was necessitated. The transradial coronary angiogram showed a tight narrowing of the LMCA ostium (Figure 3(d)). The smooth tapering appearance (Figure 4(a)) raised the possibility of external compression. This was subsequently confirmed with the use of intravascular ultrasound (IVUS) which showed dynamic external compression of LMCA with a slit-like lumen and absence of atheroma (Figure 4(c), video 2)—suggesting that the patient had developed a type 2 NSTEMI due to demand ischaemia. A gated CT scan confirmed normal origin and course of the LMCA; however, it was compressed by a grossly dilated PA measuring 58 mm (normal ~30 mm) at its maximal diameter (Figure 3(b)), compared to 33 mm 7 years ago (Figure 3(a)).

The patient was not felt to be a suitable candidate for surgery and underwent IVUS-guided percutaneous coronary intervention with a 5 × 20 mm everolimus drug-eluting stent deployed directly without any predilatation. Postdeployment, IVUS confirmed a well-apposed stent (video 3) with resolution of extrinsic compression and restoration of the LMCA lumen (Figures 4(b) and 4(d)). The patient was rendered pain free and discharged home after a short period of observation and remained angina free on subsequent follow-up.

3. Discussion

MI due to external compression of the left main stem can occur by 2 main mechanisms. In normal coronary anatomy, severe PAA can develop following longstanding PAH, resulting in acute compression of the LMCA. In patients with anomalous coronary origin or course interruption of coronary flow, it occurs due to compression of the LMCA between the PA and the high-pressured aorta and can occur without PAA.

In PAH patients who experience LMCA compression by the PA, stable angina pectoris has been the dominant syndrome reported by numerous case reports, but this case demonstrates that acute MI can also occur, and is supported by electrocardiographic, biochemical, and echocardiographic parameters. The LMCA is the vessel most at risk of compression, and due to the significant myocardial territory supplied, occlusion can result in significant or even life-threatening myocardial injury.

Even if the acute MI event is survivable, major infarction of the LMCA territory in PAH patients could significantly impair long-term prognosis. Such patients are likely to have coexisting right ventricular pressure or volume overload, and acute left ventricular infarction may result in biventricular failure. This has the potential to decompensate pulmonary function due to the combination of pre- and postcapillary pulmonary hypertension. Clinicians should therefore be mindful of acute coronary syndromes occurring in PAH patients presenting with chest pain. As demonstrated in this case, such patients can be easily assessed by CT and intracoronary imaging and successfully treated with prompt percutaneous implantation of an intracoronary stent. It is therefore suggested that

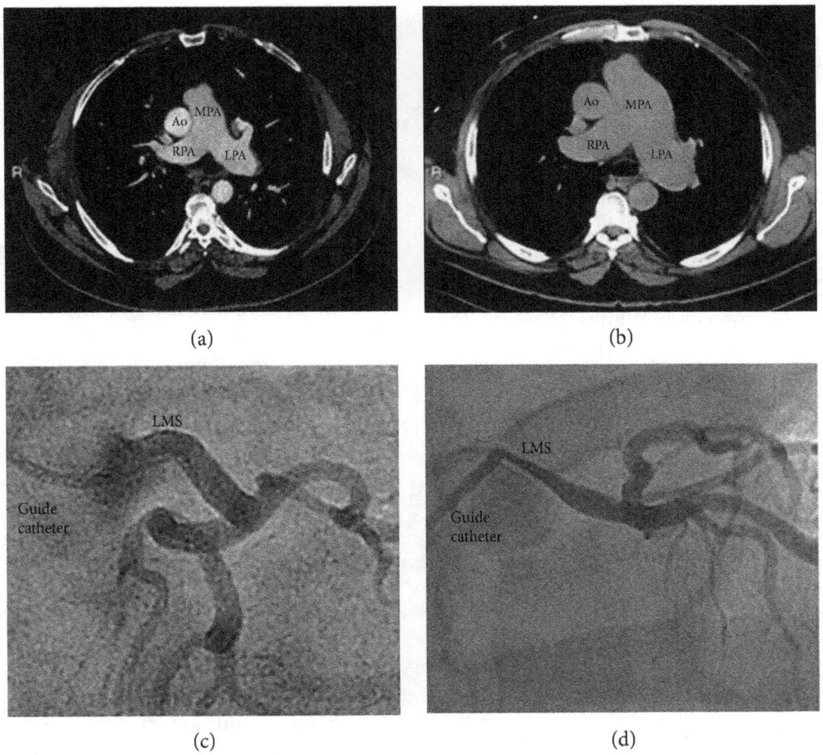

FIGURE 3: (a) CT scan showing main pulmonary artery with a diameter of 33 mm in 2013; (b) CT scan showing main pulmonary artery with a diameter of 58 mm in 2020; (c) normal appearance of LMCA in 2013; (d) severe tapering stenosis of LMCA in 2020. MPA = main pulmonary artery; RPA = right pulmonary artery; LPA = left pulmonary artery; Ao = ascending aorta; LMS = left main stem.

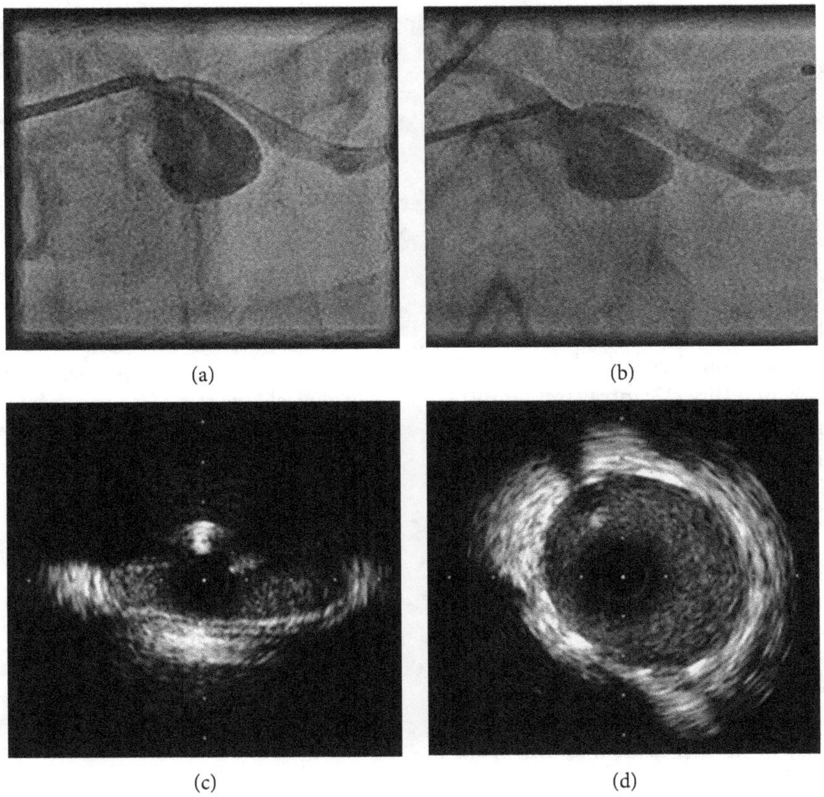

FIGURE 4: (a) Angiography demonstrating severe ostial LMCA stenosis despite intracoronary nitrate and disengaged guide catheter; (b) angiography following deployment of 5×20 mm stent; (c) baseline IVUS with a slit-like lumen of LMCA and distinct lack of atheroma; (d) well-apposed coronary stent and near-circular lumen of LMCA.

extrinsic compression by an aneurysmally dilated PA should be considered in the differential diagnosis of chest pain in patients with severe PAH. Coronary angiography alone can misdiagnose extrinsic LMCA compression, but IVUS can more accurately determine the extent of LMCA stenosis and is associated with lower rates of major clinical events [10].

It is worth noting that because of the slit-like nature of the narrowing, 45° left anterior oblique (LAO) or 30° LAO cranial angulation coronary angiographic planes cross-sectioning the narrow axis of the compressed LMCA best visualise this pathology, whereas other planes crossing the wide axis of the narrowing frequently miss the compression [11]. Shorter stents are often necessary to eliminate the risk of circumflex artery obliteration. Moreover, displacement of the aortic lumina is an important risk during ostial LMCA stenting. Intravascular ultrasound imaging can aid diagnosis (absence of plaque and dynamic external compression) and determine stent size and optimal position of deployment.

Additional Points

Learning Objectives. Longstanding PAH may result in PAA. Patients with known PAA and chest pain should be considered for urgent coronary angiography with IVUS imaging to diagnose and treat possible extrinsic coronary compression. 45° left anterior oblique (LAO) or 30° LAO cranial coronary views are best to visualise the narrowing (other views frequently miss the compression). IVUS can aid diagnosis and determine stent size and optimal position of deployment.

Authors' Contributions

All authors contributed to and approved this manuscript.

Supplementary Materials

Video 1: transthoracic echocardiography demonstrating anterolateral left ventricular hypokinesis. Video 2: intravascular ultrasound examination of the left main coronary artery, demonstrating external compression with a slit-like lumen and absence of atheroma. Video 3: intravascular ultrasound examination of the left main coronary artery, demonstrating resolution of external compression and well-apposed stent. *(Supplementary Materials)*

References

[1] W. Karrowni, G. Sigurdsson, and P. A. Horwitz, "Left main coronary artery compression by an enlarged pulmonary artery," *JACC. Cardiovascular Interventions*, vol. 6, no. 1, pp. e3–e4, 2013.

[2] K. Albadri, J. M. Jensen, E. H. Christiansen, S. Mellemkjær, and J. E. Nielsen-Kudsk, "Left main coronary artery compression in pulmonary arterial hypertension," *Pulmonary Circulation*, vol. 5, no. 4, pp. 734 736, 2016.

[3] B. Miranda-Barrio, E. Garcia-Romero, H. Cuellar-Calabria, and L. Dos-Subira, "Left main coronary artery compression by a large pulmonary artery aneurysm in the absence of pulmonary hypertension: a case report," *European Heart Journal - Case Reports*, vol. 2, no. 4, 2018https://academic.oup.com/ehjcr/article/2/4/yty105/5126422.

[4] N. Galiè, F. Saia, M. Palazzini et al., "Journal of the American College of Cardiology," vol. 69, no. 23, pp. 2808–2817, 2017.

[5] V. A. de Jesus Perez, F. Haddad, R. H. Vagelos, W. Fearon, J. Feinstein, and R. T. Zamanian, "Angina associated with left main coronary artery compression in pulmonary hypertension," *The Journal of Heart and Lung Transplantation*, vol. 28, no. 5, pp. 527–530, 2009.

[6] M. Bijl, J. G. F. Bronzwaer, A. C. van Rossum, and F. W. A. Verheugt, "Angina pectoris due to left main coronary artery compression in Eisenmenger ductus arteriosus," *American Heart Journal*, vol. 125, no. 6, pp. 1767–1771, 1993, https://pubmed.ncbi.nlm.nih.gov/8498323/.

[7] J. F. Patrat, G. Jondeau, O. Dubourg et al., "Left main coronary artery compression during primary pulmonary hypertension," *Chest*, vol. 112, no. 3, pp. 842-843, 1997, https://pubmed.ncbi.nlm.nih.gov/9315824/.

[8] K. Shishido, N. Moriyama, T. Shimizu, and S. Saito, "Anomalous acute left main myocardial infarction due to compression between pulmonary artery and aorta by acute pulmonary thromboembolism," *JACC: Cardiovascular Interventions*, vol. 9, no. 23, pp. e227–e228, 2016, https://interventions.onlinejacc.org/content/9/23/e227.

[9] M. Vaseghi, J. S. Lee, and J. W. Currier, "Acute myocardial infarction secondary to left main coronary artery compression by pulmonary artery aneurysm in pulmonary arterial hypertension," *Journal of Invasive Cardiology*, vol. 19, pp. 375–377, 2009, https://www.invasivecardiology.com/articles/Acute-Myocardial-Infarction-Secondary-Left-Main-Coronary-Artery-Compression-Pulmonary-Arter.

[10] M. Velázquez Martín, J. M. Montero Cabezas, S. Huertas et al., "Clinical relevance of adding intravascular ultrasound to coronary angiography for the diagnosis of extrinsic left main coronary artery compression by a pulmonary artery aneurysm in pulmonary hypertension," *Catheterization and cardiovascular diagnosis*, pp. 1–10, 2020.

[11] O. Y. Akbal, C. Kaymaz, I. H. Tanboga et al., "Extrinsic compression of left main coronary artery by aneurysmal pulmonary artery in severe pulmonary hypertension: its correlates, clinical impact, and management strategies," *European Heart Journal-Cardiovascular Imaging*, vol. 19, no. 11, pp. 1302–1308, 2018, https://academic.oup.com/ehjcimaging/article/19/11/1302/4717459.

7

Fulminant Vasculitis Complicated by ST Elevation Myocardial Infarction and Stroke

Vy A. Pham,[1] Christopher P. Kovach,[2] Karl Gordon Patti,[2] Evan S. Manning,[1] Stephen J. Slade,[3] Rebecca Pollard,[4] Elena Weinstein,[3] Jennifer Simpson,[4] and James E. Carter Jr.[2]

[1]*Department of Medicine, University of Colorado, 12631 E. 17th Ave, Room 8601, Aurora, CO 80045, USA*
[2]*Division of Cardiology, Department of Medicine, University of Colorado, 12631 E. 17th Ave, B130, Aurora, CO 80045, USA*
[3]*Division of Rheumatology, Department of Medicine, University of Colorado, 1775 Aurora Court, B115, Aurora, CO 80045, USA*
[4]*Division of Neurology, Department of Medicine, University of Colorado, 12700 E. 19th Ave, Room 5018, Aurora, CO 80045, USA*

Correspondence should be addressed to Vy A. Pham; vy.2.pham@cuanschutz.edu

Academic Editor: Francesco Nappi

Acute coronary syndrome is a rare complication of vasculitis. We present a case of fulminant medium-vessel vasculitis, most likely PAN, complicated by STEMI and stroke, that was successfully treated with percutaneous revascularization, high-quality stroke care, and immunosuppression. This case highlights the importance of prompt diagnosis and treatment of vasculitis and the recognition of coronary and cerebral ischemia as potentially serious complications.

1. Introduction

Systemic vasculitides are rarely associated with acute myocardial infarction or stroke. Prompt diagnosis and treatment is critical given the increased morbidity and mortality of systemic vasculitis with cardiovascular involvement [1].

2. Case Report

A 30-year-old woman with a one-year history of recurring painful lower extremity skin lesions presented with acute headache, neck pain, and right arm weakness with paresthesia. She was tachycardic but afebrile and normotensive. CT angiography of the head and neck revealed high-grade stenosis of the internal carotids. Subsequently, the patient reported acute chest pain and dyspnea. ECG revealed sinus tachycardia, anterior ST elevation, and reciprocal inferior depression (Figure 1). Labs revealed elevated troponin, serum lactate, and white blood cell count (Table 1). She was given aspirin and intravenous bivalirudin and underwent emergent cardiac catheterization that revealed an acute occlusive thrombus of the proximal left anterior descending (LAD) artery and estimated Fick cardiac index 1.9 L/min/m^2 (Figure 1, Table 1). Aspiration thrombectomy was performed, and a 4.5×30 mm drug-eluting stent was successfully deployed in the proximal LAD. The patient was started on a norepinephrine infusion and transferred to our institution with concern for fulminant medium-vessel vasculitis complicated by ST-elevation myocardial infarction (STEMI), cardiogenic shock, and stroke.

Upon arrival to our hospital, exam demonstrated expressive aphasia, left upper quadrantanopia, and right-sided hemiparesis. Bilateral upper extremity pulses were normal, femoral pulses were reduced, and dorsalis pedis and posterior tibial pulses were absent. A pulmonary arterial catheter was placed (Table 1). Neurology was consulted and urgent head and neck CT angiography revealed high-grade occlusions of the bilateral internal carotid arteries and stigmata of left middle cerebral artery infarct (Figure 1). Brain MRI confirmed evolving left frontal and parietal lobe infarcts (Figure 1). Echocardiogram demonstrated severe left ventricular systolic dysfunction with regional wall motion abnormalities: anterior,

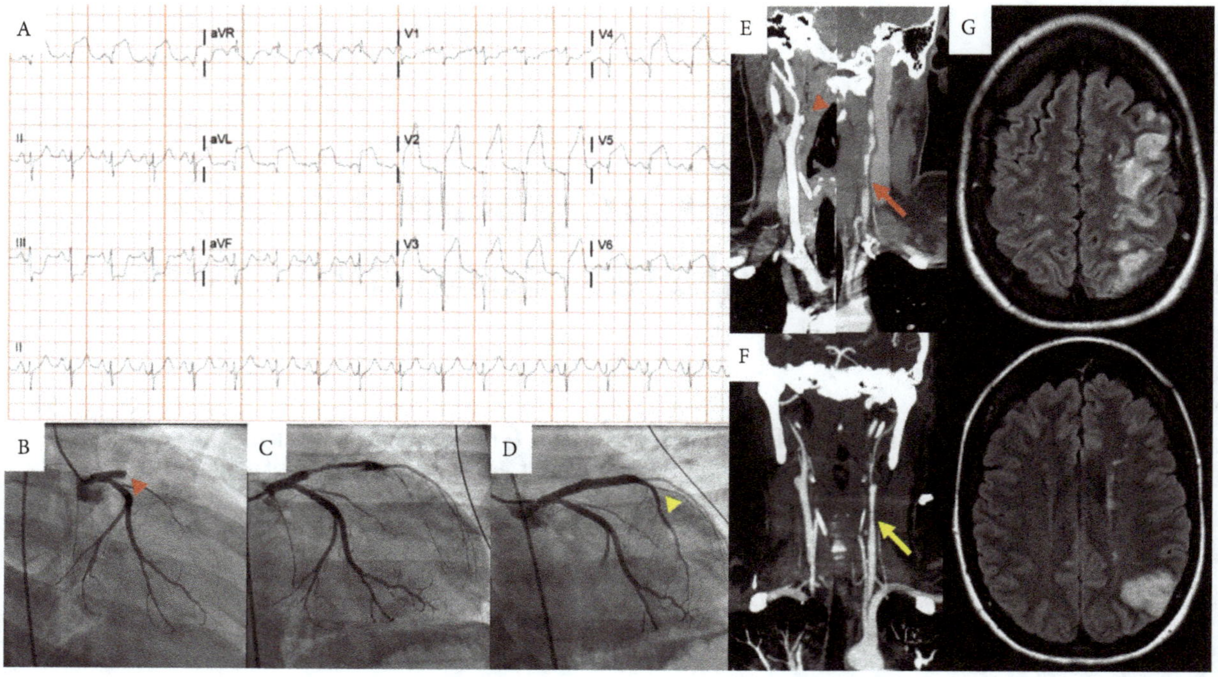

FIGURE 1: Cardiovascular and neurovascular imaging. Electrocardiogram (A) demonstrating anterolateral STEMI. Coronary angiography demonstrated complete occlusion of the LAD (B; red arrowhead) with partial reconstitution of flow following wiring (C) and restoration of normal flow following stent deployment (D; yellow arrowhead). CT angiography (E) demonstrated complete occlusion of the right ICA (red arrowhead) with luminal narrowing and irregularity of the left ICA consistent with dissection and associated thrombus (red arrow). Subsequent CT angiography showed improvement of the left ICA (F, yellow arrow). MRI demonstrated left frontal and parietal lobar multifocal infarction (G).

septal, and apical. CT imaging demonstrated abnormal wall thickening of the thoracic aorta, common iliac arteries, and renal arteries, as well as occlusion of the inferior mesenteric and infratibial arteries. Rheumatology was consulted and a broad serologic evaluation was initiated (Table 1).

2.1. Management. The patient was treated with IV corticosteroids and cyclophosphamide. Shock physiology, likely secondary to myocardial stunning, rapidly resolved. Systemic anticoagulation was discontinued after 48 hours following the determination that arterial occlusions were attributable to vasculitis rather than thrombophilia. Dual antiplatelet therapy with clopidogrel and aspirin was continued.

2.2. Follow-Up. On hospital day 10, the patient was transferred to acute rehabilitation for poststroke care. She was prescribed prednisone, cyclophosphamide, maintenance dual antiplatelet therapy, and a heart failure regimen. Rheumatology recommended outpatient adenosine deaminase 2 (*ADA2*) genetic testing. Three months after discharge, she was doing well on maintenance immunosuppression and following with cardiology for chronic heart failure.

3. Discussion

Cardiac involvement in vasculitis is not uncommon and can include cardiomyopathy, pericarditis, valvular disease, arrythmia, aortic dissection, and coronary complications such as aneurysm, stenosis, thrombosis, or rupture [1]. However, STEMI is an uncommon initial presentation of vasculitis. This report highlights the diagnosis and management of fulminant medium-vessel vasculitis, with features of polyarteritis nodosa (PAN) or adenosine deaminase 2 deficiency (DADA2), presenting as STEMI and acute stroke.

PAN is a systemic medium-vessel necrotizing vasculitis that most frequently involves the skin, kidneys, and peripheral nervous system and is diagnosed by a combination of clinical, angiographic, and pathologic findings [2]. Cardiovascular involvement occurs in only 5-22% of patients and carries a two to threefold higher mortality compared to those without coronary involvement [3]. Coronary involvement in PAN is angiographically characterized by alternating areas of stenosis or occlusion with aneurysm in a "beads on a string" pattern [1, 2]. Treatment involves aggressive immunosuppression, typically with corticosteroids and cyclophosphamide [2]. DADA2 is an autoinflammatory disorder first described in 2014 that clinically resembles PAN and is characterized by vasculitis, dysregulated immune function, and hematologic abnormalities [4, 5]. Pathophysiologically, lack of ADA2 leads to proinflammatory endothelial dysfunction, predisposing patients to systemic vasculitis and recurrent strokes, often beginning in childhood [6]. Significant clinical overlap and lack of commercial enzyme testing makes differentiating ADA2 deficiency from PAN challenging, though genetic testing for *CECR1* mutations can aid in diagnosis. While there is no clearly preferred immunosuppressive therapy for DADA2, tumor necrosis factor inhibitors may be particularly effective [5].

TABLE 1: Clinical, laboratory, and echocardiographic data.

	Day 1	Day 2	Day 4
Vitals			
Temperature, °C	35.6	36.2	36.3
Heart rate, beats/min	150	143	98
Blood pressure, mmHg	120/105	123/87	113/73
Respiratory rate, breaths/min	25	30	22
SpO_2, %	100	98	99
Body mass index, kg/m^2	32	32	32
Laboratories			
Troponin I, ng/L	7.0	—	—
Hs-troponin, ng/L	—	206,452	174,327
NT-proBNP, ng/mL	—	1,059	—
White blood cells, 10^9/L	53	25	16
Hemoglobin, g/dL	16	13	10
Platelets, 10^9/L	460	364	254
Creatinine, mg/dL	0.60	0.80	0.50
Aspartate transaminase, IU/L	1,478	533	113
Alanine aminotransferase, IU/L	158	120	53
International normalized ratio	5.1	2.0	1.1
Lactate, mmol/L	6.2	3.6	1.8
Erythrocyte sedimentation rate, mm/hr	N/A	58	—
C-reactive protein, mg/dL	2.9	125	—
Hemoglobin A1C, %	5.5	5.4	—
Total cholesterol, mg/dL	193	137	—
Triglycerides, mg/dL	224	146	—
HDL cholesterol, mg/dL	44	33	—
LDL cholesterol, mg/dL	104	79	—
Echocardiogram			
LVEDV, mL	115		174
LVESV, mL	89		110
LVEF, %	23		37
Left atrial volume, mL/m^2	15.5		15.3
RVSP, mmHg	—		44.6
Valvular heart disease	None		None
Cardiac hemodynamics			
RA pressure, mmHg	3	5	5
PA mean pressure, mmHg	26	25	27
PCW pressure, mmHg	—	15	—
Cardiac output, L/min	4.1	3.8	5.7
Cardiac index, L/min/m^2	1.9	1.7	2.6
Infectious studies			
HIV			Negative
Hepatitis B DNA PCR			Negative
Hepatitis C			Negative
Blood cultures			Negative
Rheumatologic studies			
ANA titer			1 : 320, speckled
Anti-ds-DNAb			Negative

Table 1: Continued.

	Day 1	Day 2	Day 4
Anti-Smith			Negative
Anti-RNP			Negative
Anti-SSA			Negative
Anti-SSB			Negative
ANCA IgG			Negative
Antimyeloperoxidase			Negative
Antiproteinase 3			Negative
C3			Normal
C4			Normal
Lupus anticoagulant			Negative
Beta-2 glycoprotein-1 IgG/IgM			Negative

Abbreviations: ANA: antinuclear antibody; ANCA: antineutrophil cytoplasmic antibodies; ds-DNA: double stranded DNA; HDL: high-density lipoprotein; HIV: human immunodeficiency virus; Hs: high sensitivity; LDL: low-density lipoprotein; LVEDD: left ventricular end diastolic diameter; LVEDS: left ventricular end systolic dimension; LVEF: left ventricular ejection fraction; MR: mitral regurgitation; RNP: ribonucleoprotein; RVSP: right ventricular systolic pressure; SSA/SSB: Sjogren's syndrome-related antigen A/B.

Takayasu's arteritis (TA) is a large-vessel vasculitis primarily involving the aorta and its major branches that usually affects young women with preexisting cardiac abnormalities [1]. Coronary artery stenosis and occlusions usually occur at the ostia because of the extension of inflammation-induced intimal proliferation and subsequent fibrotic retraction from the ascending aorta [7]. Treatment involves high-dose immunosuppression. TA was felt to be less likely in this patient given the predominantly medium-vessel involvement encompassing multiple vascular territories beyond the aorta.

The patient's clinical presentation, imaging, and laboratory findings were inconsistent with alternative diagnoses such as Behcet's disease, giant cell arteritis, or other systemic rheumatologic conditions.

4. Conclusions

Acute coronary syndrome is a rare complication of vasculitis. Our patient presented with fulminant medium-vessel vasculitis, most likely PAN, complicated by STEMI and stroke, and was successfully treated with percutaneous revascularization, high-quality stroke care, and immunosuppression. This case highlights the importance of prompt diagnosis and treatment of vasculitis and the recognition of coronary and cerebral ischemia as potentially serious complications.

Additional Points

Learning Objectives. (1) Recognize vasculitis as a rare etiology of STEMI. (2) Recognize vasculitis as an uncommon etiology of stroke. (3) Emphasize necessity of early recognition of vasculitis and prompt immunosuppression.

References

[1] L. H. Silveira, "Cardiovascular manifestations of systemic vasculitides," *Current Rheumatology Reports*, vol. 22, no. 10, p. 72, 2020.

[2] A. Hočevar, M. Tomšič, and P. K. Perdan, "Clinical approach to diagnosis and therapy of polyarteritis nodosa," *Current Rheumatology Reports*, vol. 23, no. 3, p. 14, 2021.

[3] D. P. Misra and S. N. Shenoy, "Cardiac involvement in primary systemic vasculitis and potential drug therapies to reduce cardiovascular risk," *Rheumatology International*, vol. 37, no. 1, pp. 151–167, 2017.

[4] P. Navon Elkan, S. B. Pierce, R. Segel et al., "Mutant adenosine deaminase 2 in a polyarteritis nodosa vasculopathy," *The New England Journal of Medicine*, vol. 370, no. 10, pp. 921–931, 2014.

[5] A. Human and C. Pagnoux, "Diagnosis and management of ADA2 deficient polyarteritis nodosa," *International Journal of Rheumatic Diseases*, vol. 22, Suppl 1, pp. 69–77, 2019.

[6] Q. Zhou, D. Yang, A. K. Ombrello et al., "Early-onset stroke and vasculopathy associated with mutations in ADA2," *The New England Journal of Medicine*, vol. 370, no. 10, pp. 911–920, 2014.

[7] M. Endo, Y. Tomizawa, H. Nishida et al., "Angiographic findings and surgical treatments of coronary artery involvement in Takayasu arteritis," *The Journal of Thoracic and Cardiovascular Surgery*, vol. 125, no. 3, pp. 570–577, 2003.

8

Ticagrelor-Induced Torsades de Pointes following Myocardial Infarction

Seong Hyeon Bu[1] **and Sung-Hwan Kim**[2]

[1]*Division of Cardiology, Department of Internal Medicine, Uijeongbu St. Mary's Hospital, College of Medicine, The Catholic University of Korea, Uijeongbu-si, Gyeonggi-do, Republic of Korea*
[2]*Division of Cardiology, Department of Internal Medicine, Seoul St. Mary's Hospital, College of Medicine, The Catholic University of Korea, 222 Banpo-daero, Seocho-gu, Seoul, 06591 Seoul, Republic of Korea*

Correspondence should be addressed to Sung-Hwan Kim; sunghwan@catholic.ac.kr

Academic Editor: Yuli Huang

We report a case of excessive QT prolongation and subsequent torsades de pointes (TdP) following the administration of ticagrelor in a 58-year-old male patient. The patient had no suspected cause of QT prolongation. After cessation of ticagrelor, QT interval was normalized and no further TdP was observed.

1. Introduction

Torsades de pointes (TdP) is caused by bradycardia, drugs, electrolyte imbalance, congenital long QT syndrome, and metabolic diseases [1]. TdP following myocardial infarction (MI) is rare. If polymorphic ventricular tachycardia (VT) occurs in a patient with acute MI, coronary revascularization should be prioritized to resolve ischemia [2]. We encountered a patient that presented with TdP after complete revascularization. After cessation of ticagrelor, QT interval was normalized and no further episode of TdP was observed.

2. Case Description

A 58-year-old man presented to the emergency room one hour after the sudden onset of squeezing chest pain. The initial electrocardiogram (ECG) revealed ST elevations in leads V_1-V_6 and reciprocal changes in leads II, III, and aVF (Figure 1). Emergency coronary angiography was performed, and a loading dose of 180 mg of ticagrelor, 300 mg of aspirin, and 40 mg of atorvastatin were subsequently administered to the patient. His medical history included chronic smoking. His blood pressure was 136/76 mmHg and heart rate 87 beats/min. Chest radiography showed mildly increased pulmonary vascularity. An emergent coronary angiogram (CAG) revealed an acute thrombus completely obstructing the proximal left anterior descending coronary artery (LAD), for which the stent was immediately and successfully deployed. Transthoracic echocardiography demonstrated a left ventricular ejection fraction of 0.45 to 0.49 and a regional wall motion abnormality in the LAD territory. On the fourth hospital day, he was discharged on aspirin, ticagrelor, atorvastatin, and bisoprolol. The ECG revealed no significant QT prolongation (Figure 2).

However, on the third day following discharge, the patient was brought to the emergency room in a state of cardiac arrest. In the morning prior, he was found collapsed in the bathroom. He had ventricular fibrillation. After five cycles of defibrillation, he recovered and was admitted to the emergency room. At the time of admission, ECG showed no ST elevation, his blood pressure was 83/54 mmHg and heart rate 72 beats/min, and he was in a state of stupor. However, his blood pressure gradually improved to 98/55 mmHg and heart rate to 87 beats/min, and he was noted to be confused. CAG showed a patent stent, and optical coherence tomography showed no findings of malapposition, underexpansion, or thrombus in the culprit vessel. However, ECG showed QT prolongation

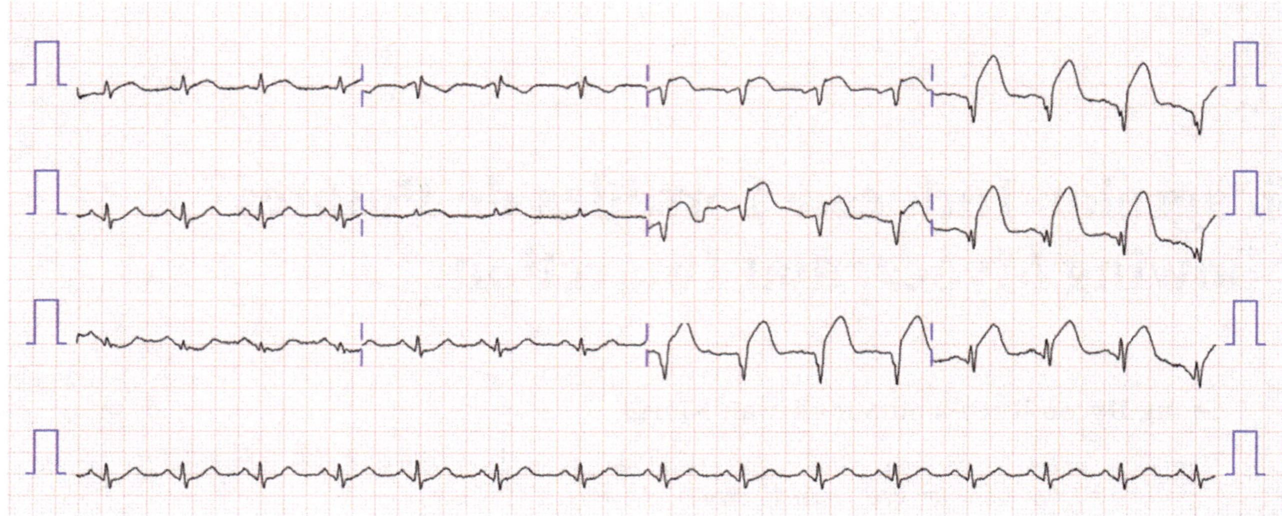

FIGURE 1: Initial ECG of a 58-year-old man in our hospital. This ECG reveals ST elevations in leads V_1-V_6 and reciprocal changes in leads II, III, and aVF. ECG: electrocardiogram.

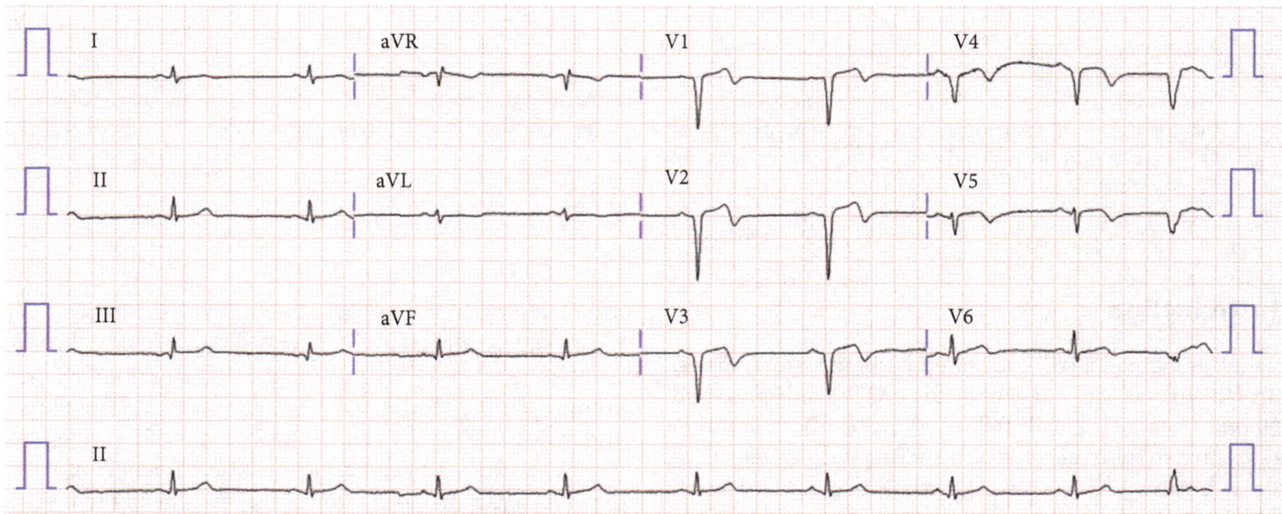

FIGURE 2: On the fourth day of hospital discharge, the ECG reveals no significant QT prolongation.

(Figure 3). Polymorphic VT, which started in a pause-dependent manner with a long-short sequence, was observed frequently (Figures 4(a) and 4(b)). No electrolyte imbalances, including hypokalemia, were observed, and no sedative drugs were prescribed. Intravenous isoproterenol was used to increase the heart rate, and magnesium was administered intravenously. TdP continued for more than 6 days after readmission. We suspected ticagrelor as the cause of QT prolongation and subsequent TdP. Thus, we discontinued ticagrelor and replaced it with clopidogrel. Subsequently, the QT interval was shortened, and no further TdP occurred (Figure 5). After discharge, there were no specific findings for a follow-up period of 3 months.

3. Discussion

When polymorphic VT occurs after MI, three possibilities should be considered: ischemic ventricular fibrillation due to acute ischemia, polymorphic VT with QT prolongation (so-called pseudo-TdP), and true TdP with certain causes of QT prolongation. Ischemic ventricular fibrillation in the setting of acute MI generally occurs during the hyperacute phase, is related to ischemia, and is not associated with QT prolongation. It can be excluded in this case [1]. QT prolongation after MI usually appears within a day or two prior to subsequent normalization [3]. In a case series comparing 8 MI patients with TdP and 100 without TdP, the QT interval in patients without TdP increased significantly on the second day and subsequently returned to normal within the third day after MI [4]. The coupling interval and pause-dependent pattern help discriminate between polymorphic VT that occurs despite QT prolongation (pseudo-TdP) and true TdP with certain causes of QT prolongation. The coupling interval of the ectopic beat triggering the pseudo-TdP was much shorter than that of true TdP.

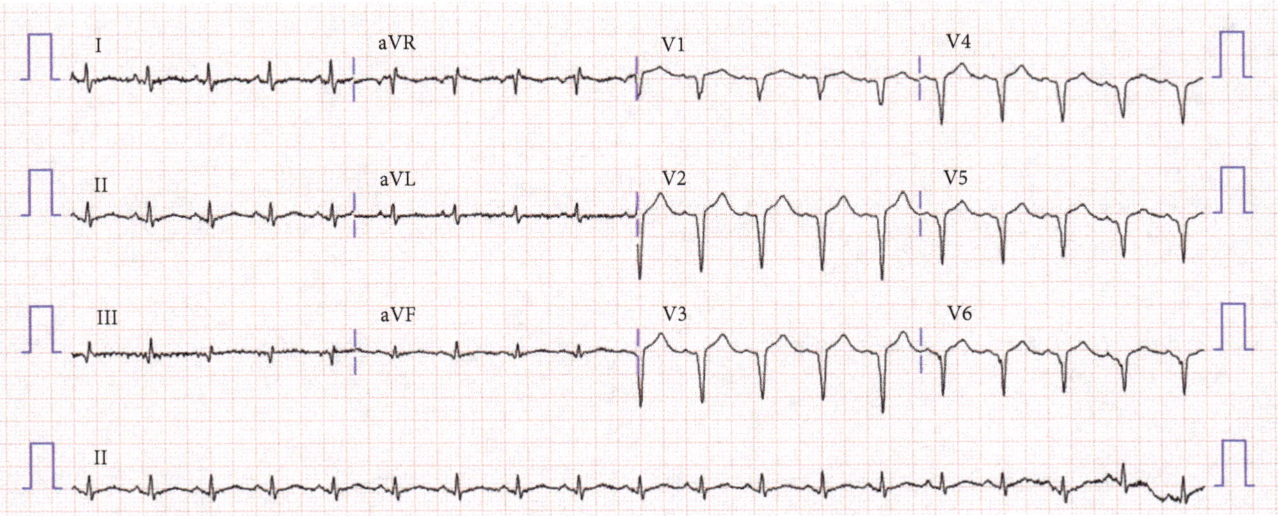

FIGURE 3: A second ECG taken after ROSC following cardiopulmonary arrest. ECG shows QT prolongation. ECG: electrocardiogram; ROSC: return of spontaneous circulation.

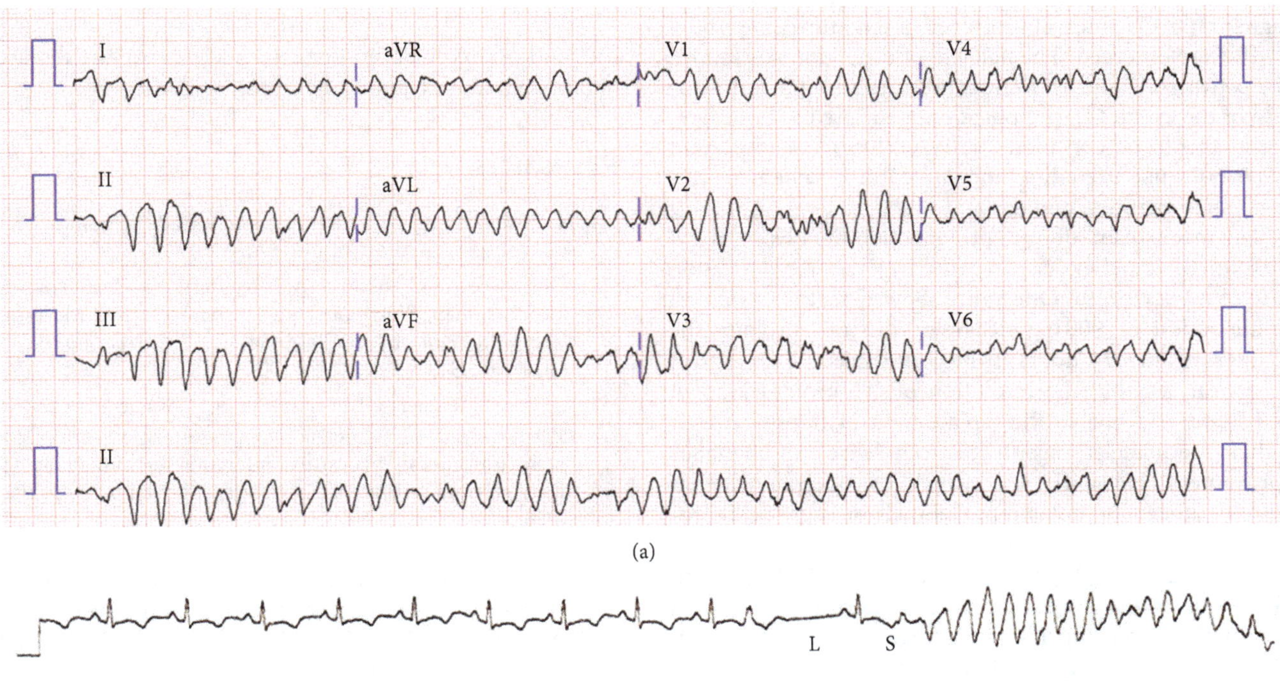

FIGURE 4: Polymorphic VT, (a) which starts in a pause-dependent manner with a long-short sequence and (b) is observed frequently after ROSC. Hence, the initial diagnosis is TdP following an MI. VT: ventricular tachycardia; ROSC: return of spontaneous circulation; TdP: torsades de pointes; MI: myocardial infarction.

The present case showed QT prolongation, polymorphic VT with a pause-dependent, long-short sequence, relatively long coupling interval of triggering TdP, and no acute ischemia. These evidences clearly supported the present TdP which would have a certain cause of QT prolongation rather than acute ischemia. TdP ensued until the sixth day of rehospitalization and did not improve. Therefore, we investigated other potential causes. There was no bradyarrhythmia or electrolyte imbalance. There were no medications administered other than the ones prescribed. A previous study demonstrated that ticagrelor blocks the uptake of adenosine by red blood cells and significantly increases the concentration of adenosine in the blood [5]. There was a report that adenosine induced TdP [6]. Another case report noted an association between prolonged QT and ticagrelor [7]. Based on these literatures, we decided to discontinue

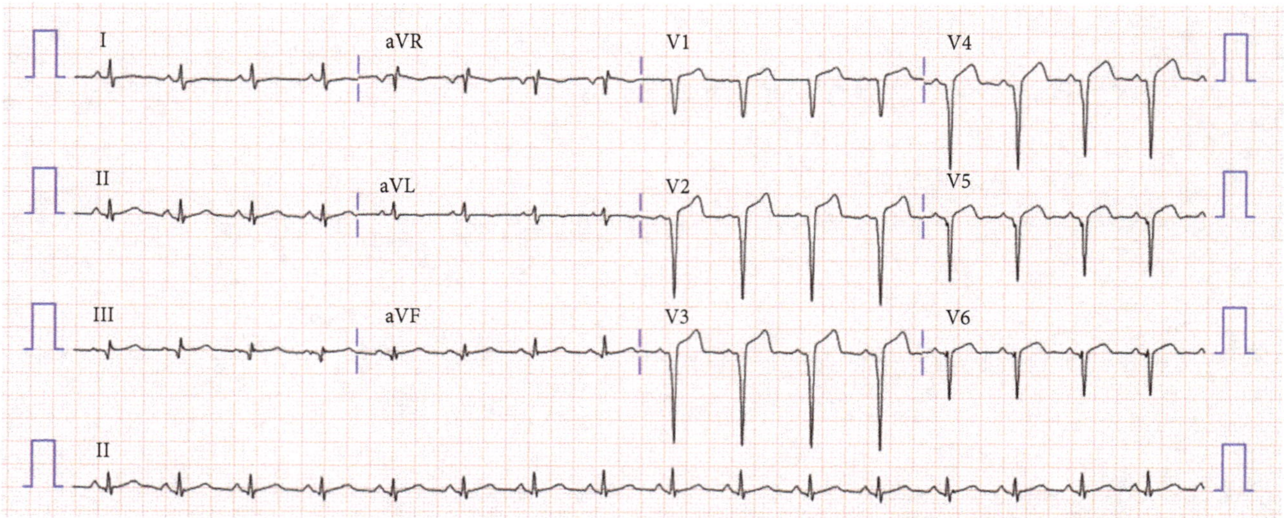

Figure 5: Repeat ECG following discontinuation of ticagrelor. There is shortening of the previously prolonged QT interval. ECG two days after ticagrelor discontinuation. No further cardiac events are sustained in the follow-up period. ECG: electrocardiogram.

ticagrelor. From the evening after the discontinuation of ticagrelor, the QT interval shortened and no further episodes of TdP were observed. The half-life of ticagrelor was known to be between 7.7 and 13.1 hours [8], suggesting that it is the cause of the event. QT prolongation associated with ticagrelor use should be considered after exclusion of important other causes like excluding ongoing cardiac ischemia, electrolyte abnormalities, and drugs.

The mechanism of QT prolongation involves several potassium channel blockades affecting the repolarization phase of myocytes [9]. One study showed that a single oral administration of 900 mg ticagrelor did not prolong the QT interval after 24 hours in healthy subjects [10], and it is not clear whether the resolution of QT prolongation in this patient was due to the replacement of ticagrelor with another antiplatelet agent or otherwise spontaneous improvement. However, it is worth considering whether ticagrelor affects the potassium channels or causes QT prolongation by other mechanisms.

In conclusion, QT prolongation following MI induced TdP in our patient. We were able to identify a temporal and causal relationship between ticagrelor discontinuation and the resolution of QT prolongation.

Ethical Approval

This case was approved by the Institutional Review Board of Uijeongbu St. Mary's Hospital of the Catholic University of Korea (UC15SISI0155).

Consent

The authors received informed consent from the patient.

Disclosure

The authors received no financial support for the research, authorship, and/or publication of this article.

References

[1] S. Viskin, "Long QT syndromes and torsade de pointes," *Lancet*, vol. 354, no. 9190, pp. 1625–1633, 1999.

[2] C. L. Wolfe, C. Nibley, A. Bhandari, K. Chatterjee, and M. Scheinman, "Polymorphous ventricular tachycardia associated with acute myocardial infarction," *Circulation*, vol. 84, no. 4, pp. 1543–1551, 1991.

[3] J. Cinca, J. Figueras, L. Tenorio et al., "Time course and rate dependence of Q-T interval changes during noncomplicated acute transmural myocardial infarction in human beings," *The American Journal of Cardiology*, vol. 48, no. 6, pp. 1023–1028, 1981.

[4] A. Halkin, A. Roth, I. Lurie, R. Fish, B. Belhassen, and S. Viskin, "Pause-dependent torsade de pointes following acute myocardial infarction: a variant of the acquired long QT syndrome," *Journal of the American College of Cardiology*, vol. 38, no. 4, pp. 1168–1174, 2001.

[5] L. Bonello, M. Laine, N. Kipson et al., "Ticagrelor increases adenosine plasma concentration in patients with an acute coronary syndrome," *Journal of the American College of Cardiology*, vol. 63, no. 9, pp. 872–877, 2014.

[6] M. L. Mallet, "Proarrhythmic effects of adenosine: a review of the literature," *Emergency Medicine Journal*, vol. 21, no. 4, pp. 408–410, 2004.

[7] A. Ray, A. Najmi, G. Khandelwal, and B. Sadasivam, "Ticagrelor-induced prolongation of the QTc interval," *Case Reports in Cardiology*, vol. 2019, Article ID 5984847, 4 pages, 2019.

[8] R. Teng, "Ticagrelor: pharmacokinetic, pharmacodynamic and pharmacogenetic profile: an update," *Clinical Pharmacokinetics*, vol. 54, no. 11, pp. 1125–1138, 2015.

[9] M. Li and L. G. Ramos, "Drug-induced QT prolongation and torsades de pointes," *Pharmacy and Therapeutics*, vol. 42, no. 7, pp. 473–477, 2017.

[10] K. Butler, C. Wei, and R. Teng, "Single-dose ticagrelor does not prolong the QT interval in healthy subjects," *International Journal of Clinical Pharmacology and Therapeutics*, vol. 48, no. 10, pp. 643–651, 2010.

9

Conservative Treatment for Right Ventricular Free Wall Rupture in a Patient with Acute Myocardial Infarction

Mohd Al-Baqlish Mohd Firdaus,[1,2] **Nur Syahirah Abdul Rahim**,[2] **Nurtasneem Rusdi**,[2] **Nor Saadah Idris**,[3] **Mohd Ridzuan Mohd Said**,[2] **and Imran Zainal Abidin**[1]

[1]*Division of Cardiology, Department of Medicine, University Malaya Medical Centre, 59100 Kuala Lumpur, Malaysia*
[2]*Department of Internal Medicine, Kulliyyah of Medicine, International Islamic University Malaysia, 25200 Kuantan, Pahang, Malaysia*
[3]*Department of Radiology, University Malaya Medical Centre, 59100 Kuala Lumpur, Malaysia*

Correspondence should be addressed to Mohd Al-Baqlish Mohd Firdaus; baqlish@gmail.com

Academic Editor: Marcio Barros

Ventricular wall rupture possesses a high mortality rate in patients with acute myocardial infarction. We presented a case of a ninety-year-old gentleman who presented with acute inferolateral myocardial infarction in cardiogenic shock and right ventricular free wall rupture. He was treated conservatively and survived.

1. Introduction

Cardiac rupture is a major complication following acute myocardial infarction (AMI) apart from ventricular fibrillation and cardiogenic shock [1]. Although the incidence was reduced with the practice of reperfusion therapy, yet it still carries a high mortality rate of more than 50% [2]. Cardiac rupture may involve free wall of ventricles, the interventricular septum, and atrium or papillary muscles, in which cases of free wall rupture (FWR) are approximately ten times less frequent compared to the septal and papillary muscle rupture [2–4]. Left ventricular rupture accounts for the majority of ventricular rupture cases reported, while isolated right ventricular free wall rupture (RVFWR) is a rare entity with very few cases reported previously [3]. Here, we presented a case of RVFWR in cardiogenic shock secondary to AMI, treated conservatively and survived.

2. Case Report

A ninety-year-old gentleman with underlying dementia and hypertension was presented with a sudden onset of central chest pain while watching television. Upon arrival at the emergency department, he was in severe pain and sweaty. Initial blood pressure was 90/50 mmHg with a heart rate of 110 beats per minute. ECG showed acute inferolateral myocardial infarction. On cardiovascular examination, there was no clinical sign of cardiac tamponade, and the auscultation of the lung was clear. Bedsides, echocardiography was performed showing pericardial effusion with a maximum diameter of 1.3 cm over the apex with no features of cardiac tamponade. The inferior lateral wall was hypokinesia, and the right ventricle wall was akinetic. Given the ECG and echocardiographic findings, and the patient was in severe pain, we decided to proceed with CT aortogram to rule out aortic dissection. The CT scan showed no evidence of aortic dissection; however, there was a presence of hemopericardium (Figure 1). We decided to proceed with a primary percutaneous coronary angiogram (Figure 2).

The patient was persistently hypotensive and did not respond to fluid resuscitation and inotropic support. We decided to abundant the angioplasty procedure and proceeded with emergency pericardial tapping (Figure 3). 350 ml of blood was drained from the pericardium. The

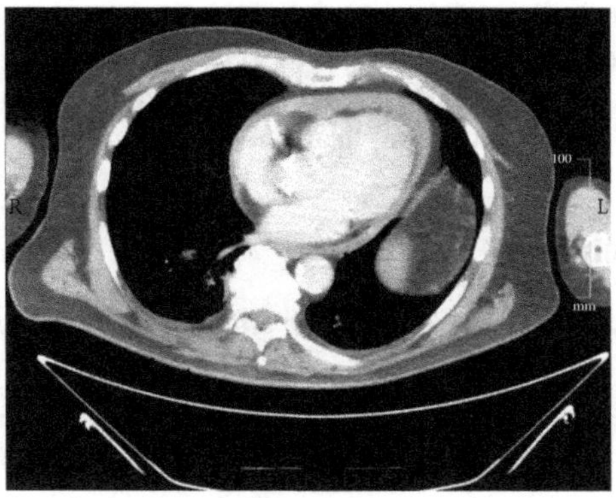

FIGURE 1: CT scan showed the presence of global pericardial effusion.

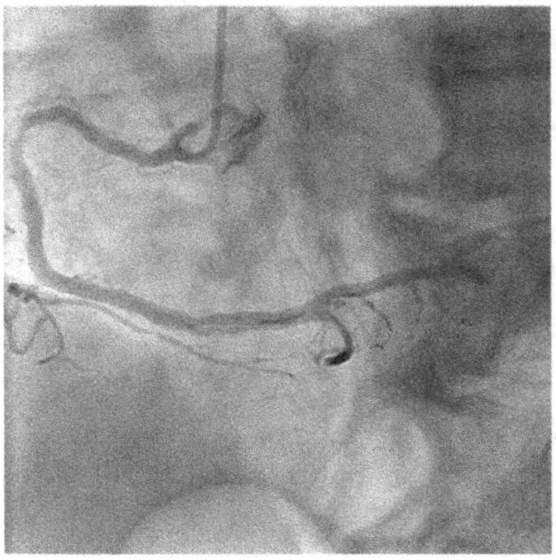

FIGURE 2: Presence of ulcerated plaque at the proximal right coronary artery with total occlusion of the posterior descending artery and posterolateral branch artery.

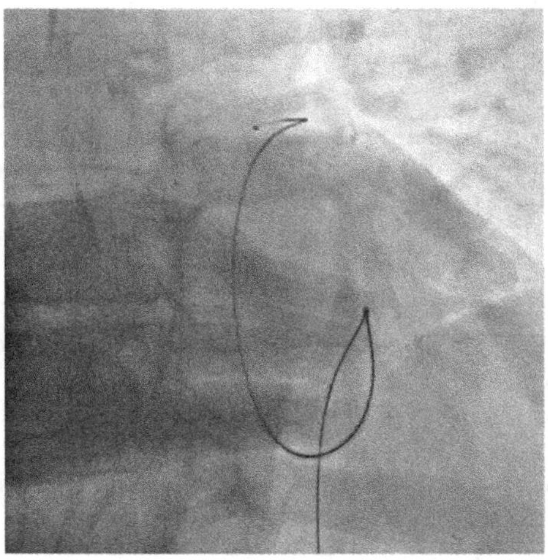

FIGURE 3: A guidewire was being inserted into the pericardium.

hypotension resolved after the procedure, and we were able to off the inotropic infusion. The pericardial drainage was in situ for three days and drained haemoserous fluid. After removal of the pericardial drainage, there was a reaccumulation of pericardial effusion. We referred the patient to the cardiothoracic surgeon, but the patient and family opted for conservative treatment and refused for any invasive or surgical intervention. The patient was not given heparin throughout the hospital stay and discharged home with a single antiplatelet. The proximal right coronary artery was stented three months later. He was last seen in our clinic in December 2019 and is currently doing well. The echocardiogram was repeated, and it illustrates mild left ventricular dysfunction with an ejection fraction of 47%. There was no significant residual pericardial effusion. The right ventricular function was normal.

3. Discussion and Literature Review

Ventricular rupture is a rare but fatal mechanical complication of AMI. Most cases were associated with death following cardiac tamponade and cardiogenic shock [5, 6]. The incidence of ventricular rupture secondary to AMI was reported between 2 and 4% and responsible for 10-15% of hospital death [2, 4, 6]. Data from the SHOCK registry showed that the incidence of ventricular wall rupture presented as a cardiogenic shock was 3.9% and the mortality rate was 87.3% [7]. About 80-90% of cases involved the left ventricle, while cases of isolated postinfarction RVFWR appeared to be extremely rare since most literature was referring the cases as an extension of ventricular septal rupture [2, 3, 8]. Isolated RVFWR is mainly caused by inferolateral MI and right coronary artery occlusion [9, 10]. It was postulated that very low incidence of RVFWR was due to lower pressure effect over the right ventricle and it rarely undergoes transmural infarction [3, 6].

Previous literatures demonstrated that patients with advanced age, female, and concomitant hypertension had a higher risk of cardiac rupture [2, 3, 5, 6]. Some authors found that patients with the first episode of AMI, especially involving the massive infarction of anterior or lateral wall with high ST elevation, tend to develop this complication [2, 3, 9]. On the other side, any delay in the administration of treatment after the onset of the symptom was identified as one of the major risk factors of cardiac rupture along with the thinned ventricle wall, less collateral circulation, and disfiguration of elastic tissue after transmural MI [9, 10].

Early detection and management were crucial to reduce patients' mortality. Physicians need to be aware regarding the signs and symptoms of ventricular rupture or impending rupture in patients with AMI. Generally, it includes loss of consciousness, facial cyanosis, bradycardia, and hypotension following pericardial haemorrhage. Such patients may also complain of chest pain which is resistant even to opiates, agitation, and recurrent emesis. These may also be associated with muffled heart sound, pericardial rub, pulsus paradoxus, cardiac tamponade, shock, or asystole [2, 5]. A review done by Bajaj et al. [11] showed that 70% of cases of acute ventricular free wall rupture presented with sudden cardiac death. In contrast, in a few cases, it can be a gradual or incomplete rupture with slow or recurrent bleeding into the pericardium, causing progressive or recurrent cardiac tamponade, which is termed as subacute ventricular free wall rupture. In such cases, they usually presented with hypotension with or without cardiogenic shock, and urgent intervention may be life-saving [2, 11]. Apart from that, a higher survival chance may be expected if a small rupture limits the haemorrhage, a tortuous tract of dissection within the ventricular muscle, or the formation of a seal by fibrin clots or pericardial tissue [5]. Referring to our case, it is an acute isolated RVFWR, and it can be speculated that a small-sized rupture and formation of thrombus limit the amount of blood extravasated into the pericardium, hence making the free wall rupture without surgical repair compatible with long-term survival [10].

The findings of electromechanical dissociation and echocardiographic or radiological evidence of pericardial haemorrhage favour the diagnosis of ventricular free wall rupture [12]. In clinically suspected rupture, transthoracic echocardiography is a fast and sensitive test to confirm the diagnosis. However, there might be some limitations in evaluating the right ventricle because of its crescent shape, substernal location, and the presence of a large amount of artefact [6, 9]. Fortunately, in our case, the echocardiographic finding of pericardial effusion and the evidence of right coronary artery occlusion and its branches on primary percutaneous coronary angiogram brought us to the diagnosis of RVFWR after excluding aortic dissection by CT aortogram. Previously cited by Bajaj et al. [11], the presence of echocardiographic finding of pericardial effusion greater than 5 mm with intrapericardial echoes in a hypotensive patient carries 90.9% sensitivity for cardiac rupture, and it is associated with 43% of 30-day mortality.

In managing ventricular rupture, available treatment options include conservative measures and salvageable surgery. However, currently, there are no specific guidelines available in determining patient criteria and specific timing for surgical intervention [13]. Conservatively, patients were treated to achieve hemodynamic stability, and this includes fluid management, inotrope support, and reperfusion therapy. As cited by Dandeniyaarachci et al. [3] and Bajaj et al. [11], the incidence of cardiac rupture can be reduced with reperfusion therapy; however, the risk increases if thrombolysis is being done after 14 hours of symptom onset. The rationale behind treating patients is conservatively mainly due to the tamponade effect created by the thrombus that previously formed from extravasating blood in which only applicable for a small-sized rupture [10].

Some authors reported that surgery is the only salvageable procedure and superior to conservative measures once hemopericardium is confirmed [1, 2]. Most of the salvaged cases reported have been treated only by closure of the rupture site [14]. Few techniques have been described, including direct compression, suturing with pledgets, and sutureless patch glue [3]. With early surgical treatment, it reduced mortality with the survival rate of 85% after a successful repair [3, 7].

With regard to our case, an initial referral was made for surgical intervention. However, upon the patient's request, he was treated conservatively, and surprisingly, he survived and well. A similar case was being reported by Sherer et al. [10], and this remote phenomenal can be explained by quick resolution of the thrombus along with the small myocardial defect that later became impermeable to the blood. However, the recurrent rate of right ventricular rupture was not well established previously; therefore, regular follow-up with the timely echocardiogram is essential in detecting any recurrence or presence of complications.

4. Conclusion

Postinfarction RVFWR is a rare entity with a fatal outcome. Therefore, early detection and prompt interventions are life-saving and crucial in reducing the mortality rate.

Acknowledgments

We would like to thank all the doctor and staff at the University Malaya Medical Centre who were involved directly or indirectly during the management of this patient.

References

[1] M. Dellborg, H. L. Blom, A. Stadelmann, and A. Vedin, "Heart rupture in myocardial infarction," *Läkartidningen*, vol. 81, no. 46, pp. 4296–4303, 1984.

[2] K. K. Goyal, S. Rajasekharan, and C. G. S. Kader Muneer, "De Winter sign: a masquerading eletrocardiogram in ST-elevation myocardial infarction," *Hear India*, vol. 5, no. 1, pp. 17–23, 2017.

[3] S. D. Arachchi and R. Ruwanpura, "A rare case of post-infarction right ventricular rupture," *Cardiovascular Pathology*, vol. 47, p. 107203, 2020.

[4] M. S. Ülgen, Ö. Öztürk, M. Kayrak, A. Soylu, M. A. Düzenli, and F. Koç, "A lethal but treatable complication: free wall rupture after acute myocardial infarction," *Electronic Journal of General Medicine*, vol. 3, no. 1, pp. 41–44, 2006.

[5] T. Bashour, S. S. Kabbani, D. G. Ellertson, J. Crew, and E. S. Hanna, "Surgical salvage of heart rupture: report of two cases and review of the literature," *The Annals of Thoracic Surgery*, vol. 36, no. 2, pp. 209–213, 1983.

[6] D. Ueno, T. Nomura, K. Ono et al., "Fatal right ventricular free wall rupture during percutaneous coronary intervention for inferior acute myocardial infarction," *American Journal of Case Reports*, vol. 20, pp. 1155–1158, 2019.

[7] J. S. Hochman, C. E. Buller, L. A. Sleeper et al., "Cardiogenic shock complicating acute myocardial infarction—etiologies, management and outcome: a report from the SHOCK Trial Registry," *Journal of the American College of Cardiology*, vol. 36, no. 3, pp. 1063–1070, 2000.

[8] L. de Gennaro, N. D. Brunetti, G. Ramunni et al., "Septal rupture with right ventricular wall dissecting haematoma communicating with left ventricle after inferior myocardial infarction," *European Heart Journal - Cardiovascular Imaging*, vol. 11, no. 6, pp. 477–481, 2010.

[9] M. Akcay, E. B. Senkaya, M. Bilge, E. Yeter, M. Kurt, and V. Davutoglu, "Rare mechanical complication of myocardial infarction: isolated right ventricle free wall rupture," *Singapore Medical Journal*, vol. 52, no. 1, pp. 7–9, 2011.

[10] Y. Sherer, Y. Levy, L. Leibovich, Y. Shoenfeld, A. Shahar, and E. Konen, "Survival without surgical repair of acute rupture of the right ventricular free wall," *Clinical Cardiology*, vol. 22, no. 4, pp. 319-320, 1999.

[11] A. Bajaj, A. Sethi, P. Rathor, N. Suppogu, and A. Sethi, "Acute complications of myocardial infarction in the current era," *Journal of Investigative Medicine*, vol. 63, no. 7, pp. 844–855, 2015.

[12] J. M. Calcino Cuela, F. Ramírez Calderón, and R. Vásquez Alva, "Reconocimiento de rotura miocárdica en emergencia: reporte de caso," *Revista de la Facultad de Medicina Humana*, vol. 19, no. 2, pp. 113–117, 2019.

[13] (MOH) MOHM, "Malaysia A of M of. Clinical practice guidelines management of acute St segment elevation myocardial infarction (Stemi) 2019," *Society*, vol. 14, 2019.

[14] A. B. Woldow, S. J. Mattleman, S. G. G. Abkza, and F. K. Nakhjavan, "Isolated rupture off the right ventricle in a patient with acute inferior wall MI," *Chest*, vol. 98, no. 2, pp. 484-485, 1990.

10

Acute Coronary Syndrome (ACS) due to Coronary Artery Embolism in a Patient with Atrial Fibrillation

Hussein Daoud,[1] **Ashraf Abugroun**,[1] **Shruti Erramilli**,[1] **and Surender Kumar**[2]

[1]*Department of Internal Medicine, Advocate Illinois Masonic Medical Center, 836 W Wellington Ave., Chicago, IL 60657, USA*
[2]*Department of Cardiology, Advocate Illinois Masonic Medical Center, 836 W Wellington Ave., Chicago, IL 60657, USA*

Correspondence should be addressed to Hussein Daoud; hussein.daoud@advocatehealth.com

Academic Editor: Aiden Abidov

Acute coronary syndrome (ACS) secondary to a coronary embolism is an unusual occurrence, yet an important consideration given the difficult diagnosis. We report a case of a 69-year-old male with a medical history of paroxysmal atrial fibrillation who presented with chest pain and shortness of breath. A coronary angiogram was significant for three focal transluminal and translucent areas in the ostial, mid, and distal circumflex artery consistent with embolic disease. The patient was subsequently managed medically with anticoagulation. Despite being a relatively rare entity, thromboembolism into the coronary arteries can provoke an acute myocardial infarction, with atrial fibrillation being the most common risk factor. Treatment modalities for ACS secondary to thromboembolism include stent placement, intracoronary thrombolysis, and thrombus aspiration.

1. Introduction

Acute myocardial infarction secondary to a coronary embolism was first reported in 1856 by the famous German physician Rudolf Virchow [1]. Approximately 3% of acute coronary syndromes (ACS) are caused by a coronary embolism. Coronary emboli can arise through various mechanisms including a left atrial appendage thrombus due to atrial fibrillation, valve vegetations secondary to infective or autoimmune endocarditis, deep venous thrombi embolizing paradoxically through a patent foramen ovale (PFO), or iatrogenic secondary to coronary interventions [2]. Of these, atrial fibrillation is thought to be the most common etiology of coronary emboli, though there are few cases reported in the literature. Particularly, a non-ST-segment elevation myocardial infarction (NSTEMI) caused by embolic occlusion of a coronary artery in the setting of atrial fibrillation is a rare entity. The clinical presentation is like ACS of any cause. In this report, we discuss a case of a 69-year-old male with a history of paroxysmal atrial fibrillation who presented with chest pain and exertional dyspnea. The coronary angiogram demonstrated three lesions in the ostial, mid, and distal circumflex artery consistent with emboli.

2. Case Report

A 69-year-old male presented to the emergency department complaining of chest pain and shortness of breath. His medical history was significant for paroxysmal atrial fibrillation on warfarin, coronary artery disease (CAD) with a proximal left anterior descending artery (LAD) stent, balloon valvuloplasty for severe aortic stenosis, and end-stage renal disease (ESRD) treated with peritoneal dialysis. The patient reported intermittent chest tightness that worsened with exertion and that was associated with progressive shortness of breath for one week before hospital arrival.

On admission, his heart rate was 104 beats per minute, blood pressure was 104/67 mmHg, respiratory rate was 22 breaths per minute, and the patient's oxygen saturation was above 94% on ambient air. The physical exam revealed a grade II/VI systolic ejection murmur over the aortic valve area. Labs showed a potassium of 5.8, BUN of 65 mg/dL, creatinine of 12.47 mg/dL (unknown baseline), hemoglobin of 8.4 g/dL, and a troponin I of 2.76 ng/dL (normal < 0.05) that peaked on repeat at 3.79 ng/dL. His international normalized ratio (INR) on admission was 2.0, though his compliance with anticoagulation and the INR in the weeks leading up

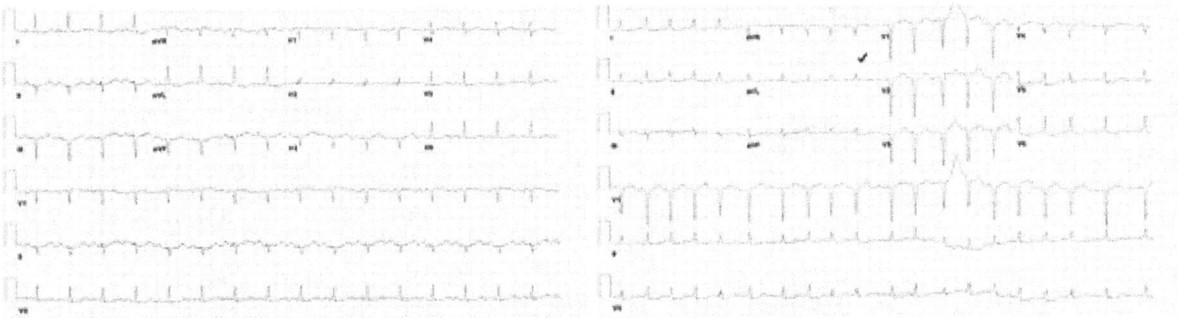

FIGURE 1: Admission electrocardiogram (ECG) on the left with a normal sinus rhythm and ECG on the right taken during the hospital stay showing atrial fibrillation with a rapid ventricular response.

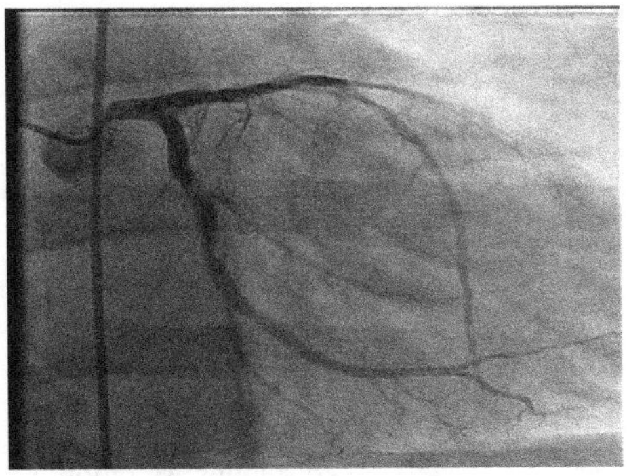

FIGURE 2: Left heart catheterization showing three focal transluminal and translucent areas in the ostial, mid, and distal circumflex artery that was mobile and hazy appearing—concerning for emboli.

to his admission was unknown. A chest X-ray was remarkable for mild cardiomegaly, interstitial pulmonary edema, and trace bilateral pleural effusions. An electrocardiogram (ECG) showed a normal sinus rhythm with an old apical infarct, and a transthoracic echocardiogram (TTE) revealed an ejection fraction of 15-20% with grade two diastolic dysfunction and "possible" severe aortic valve stenosis (Figure 1).

The patient was diagnosed with a non-ST-segment elevation myocardial infarction (NSTEMI) and underwent both a right- and left-sided heart catheterization. The coronary angiogram revealed three focal transluminal and translucent areas in the ostial, mid, and distal circumflex artery consistent with coronary emboli (Figure 2). The left circumflex artery was otherwise angiographically normal. Given the patient's low ejection fraction and history of severe aortic stenosis, the interventional cardiologist recommended medical management with anticoagulation, instead of potential thrombolysis or thrombus aspiration, as he would be high risk for any coronary intervention.

A transesophageal echocardiogram (TEE) with agitated saline was subsequently ordered and did not reveal a patent foramen ovale (PFO), atrial septal defect (ASD), evidence of an embolic source (in the left atrial appendage or left ventricle), or any valve vegetation. The patient denied any episodes of chest pain or dyspnea during his hospital stay. He was deemed a poor candidate for aortic valve surgery by cardiothoracic surgery and was ultimately discharged on his home doses of aspirin, carvedilol, amiodarone, and warfarin with a follow-up for continued evaluation for a transcatheter aortic valve replacement (TAVR) procedure as his prior balloon valvuloplasty was completed as a bridging intervention.

3. Discussion

Individuals with atrial fibrillation are at an increased risk of thrombus formation in the left atrium, particularly in the left atrial appendage, through Virchow's triad of blood stasis, endothelial damage, and hypercoagulable state. They may also develop nonleft atrial appendage thrombi due to the overall diseased state of the atrium (atriopathy). This subsequently puts this population at an increased risk of thromboembolic events of the systemic circulation. Thromboembolism most often occurs during episodes of fibrillation or within the first ten days following cardioversion back to sinus rhythm. Sites of systemic embolism include the brain, splenic artery, renal artery, mesenteric artery, and limbs [3].

Myocardial infarction has been known to cause atrial fibrillation through multiple mechanisms, including ventricular ischemia/infarction and subsequent atrial stretching or directly through atrial ischemia [4]. Conversely, atrial fibrillation has been linked to myocardial infarction through its association with multiple atherosclerotic risk factors including diabetes, hypertension, and dyslipidemia. Additionally, atrial fibrillation is associated with inflammation that may promote a prothrombotic state and subsequent myocardial infarction. When these two conditions coincide, clinical management becomes more complex given the higher risk of bleeding when combining anticoagulant and antiplatelet medications [5].

The phenomenon of thromboembolism into the coronary arteries is rare with an unknown prevalence given its difficult diagnosis. Acute myocardial infarction secondary to a coronary embolism was first reported in 1856 by the famous German physician Rudolf Virchow [1]. In patients with myocardial infarction, 4-7% are found to not have atherosclerotic vascular disease [6]. In an autopsy study of 419 patients, 55 (13%) were found to have an embolic infarct in their coronary arteries [7]. A study by Shibata et al. looked at new-onset acute myocardial infarctions between 2001 and 2013, and 1776 consecutive cases were analyzed with a focus on coronary embolism (CE) diagnosis through angiography, histology, and imaging. In that study, 52 patients were acknowledged to have CE (2.9%) and the most common

Table 1: Reported cases of coronary artery embolism with embolus location and outcomes.

Author	Patient age	Patient gender	History of atrial fibrillation or flutter	Peak troponin	Embolus location	Outcomes	References
Antoine et al.	58	M	Yes.	Troponin I 9.56 (unknown units).	Distal left circumflex artery (LCX).	NSTEMI managed by embolectomy.	[12]
Camaro et al.	66	F	Yes, new-onset.	Unknown.	Distal right coronary artery (RCA).	STEMI managed conservatively with anticoagulation after failed PCI.	[13]
Diaz et al.	52	M	Yes, new-onset.	Troponin I 0.6 ng/mL (normal < 0.024).	Proximal left anterior descending artery (LAD).	NSTEMI managed by thrombectomy.	[14]
Everett et al.	30	M	No.	Unknown.	Distal LAD.	Acute coronary syndrome managed by thrombectomy and anticoagulation.	[9]
Garg et al.	53	F	New-onset atrial fibrillation.	Troponin T 5.0 ng/mL (normal < 0.10 ng/mL).	Posterolateral branch of the LCX.	NSTEMI managed with anticoagulation.	[15]
Kotooka et al.	88	F	Yes.	Unknown.	Proximal RCA.	STEMI managed by thrombectomy.	[16]
	50	M	No.	Unknown.	Ostium of RCA.	STEMI treated by thrombus aspiration.	
	85	M	Yes.	Unknown.	Left main coronary artery (LCA).	STEMI complicated by cardiogenic shock, managed by dobutamine and an intra-aortic balloon pump and subsequently a thrombectomy and stent placement.	
Koutsampasopoulos et al.	69	F	Yes.	High sensitivity troponin T 5.33 ng/L (N < 0.014).	Midsegment of LAD.	STEMI managed with thrombectomy.	[17]
Nakano et al.	82	F	Yes.	Troponin I 0.65 ng/mL.	Unclear. ECG showed atrial fibrillation, an inverted T wave in V1-V3, an abnormal Q wave in V1 -V4, and ST-segment elevation in V3 and V4.	The patient was too unstable for an angiogram, thus was treated with intravenous heparin but died within 24 hours (diagnosis suspected by criteria proposed by Shibata et al.).	[11]
OSullivan et al.	70	M	Perioperative atrial fibrillation after noncardiac surgery with subsequent embolization.	High sensitivity troponin T 0.540 μg/L (normal < 0.014).	Complete occlusion of RCA up to ostium.	STEMI managed with thrombectomy.	[18]
Sakai et al.	72	M	Yes.	Unknown, CKMB peaked at 2929 IU/L (normal < 180).	Proximal RCA.	STEMI managed by thrombectomy.	[19]

Table 1: Continued.

Author	Patient age	Patient gender	History of atrial fibrillation or flutter	Peak troponin	Embolus location	Outcomes	References
Takenaka et al.	65	F	Yes.	Unknown.	Distal LAD.	STEMI managed by balloon angioplasty and thrombolysis.	[20]
Van de Walle et al.	64	M	Yes.	Unknown.	Midsegment of LAD.	STEMI managed by stenting.	[1]
Zakaria et al.	65	F	New-onset atrial flutter.	Unknown.	Origin of LCX.	NSTEMI managed by thrombectomy.	[21]

etiologies were atrial fibrillation, cardiomyopathy, and valvular heart disease with a prevalence of 73%, 25%, and 15%, respectively [8].

Therefore, even though atrial fibrillation is thought to be the most common risk factor, other potential sources for coronary embolization exist. These include a left ventricular mural thrombus from a prior myocardial infarction, thromboemboli from the trabeculated myocardium in noncompaction cardiomyopathy, or intrapulmonary shunting through arteriovenous malformations or fistulae [9, 10]. However, cardiac magnetic resonance imaging (MRI), computed tomography angiography (CTA) chest, or ventilation-perfusion (VQ) studies, which could identify some of these other potential causes, were not pursued in this patient.

Coronary embolisms can manifest as a non-ST-segment elevation myocardial infarction (NSTEMI) like in our patient or an ST-segment elevation myocardial infarction (STEMI) as seen in other case reports (Table 1). The condition has also been seen in the setting of a concomitant stroke and diffuse systemic embolization [11]. The National Cerebral and Cardiovascular Center (NCVC) criteria for the clinical diagnosis of coronary artery embolism (CE) was proposed by Shibata et al. and uses combinations of major and minor criteria to categorize the diagnosis of CE into definite or probable [8] (Table 2). In that study, out of the 52 patients, 32 met the definitive criteria and 20 the probable criteria. Based on the proposed criteria, our patient would fall under the category of "probable" CE given the angiographic findings and risk factor of atrial fibrillation (one major and one minor criterion). Although no embolic source was found on echocardiography, the absence does not rule out CE.

In our case report, the patient was managed medically with anticoagulation given his high risk for coronary intervention, but additional therapeutic options exist that are consistent with other causes of ACS including stent placement, intracoronary thrombolysis, and thrombus aspiration—which is generally favored because of the decreased risk of distal embolization [1].

Table 2: Proposed National Cerebral and Cardiovascular Center (NCVC) criteria for the clinical diagnosis of coronary artery embolism (CE) [1].

Major criteria
Angiographic evidence of CE and thrombosis without atherosclerotic components
Concomitant coronary artery embolization at multiple sites[a]
Concomitant systemic embolization without left ventricular thrombus attributable to acute myocardial infarction
Minor criteria
<25% stenosis on coronary angiography, except for the culprit lesion
Evidence of an embolic source based on transthoracic echocardiography transesophageal echocardiography, computed tomography, or magnetic resonance imaging
Presence of embolic risk factors: atrial fibrillation, cardiomyopathy, rheumatic valve disease, prosthetic heart valve, patent foramen ovale, atrial septal defect, history of cardiac surgery, infective endocarditis, or hypercoagulable state
Definite CE
Two or more major criteria, or
One major criterion plus ≥ 2 minor criterion, or
Three minor criteria
Probable CE
One major criterion plus 1 minor criterion, or
Two minor criteria
A diagnosis of CE should not be made if there is
Pathological evidence of atherosclerotic thrombus
History of coronary revascularization
Coronary artery ectasia
Plaque disruption or erosion detected by intravascular ultrasound or optic coherence tomography in the proximal part of the culprit lesion

The present proposed diagnostic criteria for CE include three major and three minor criteria. Weighted scoring of the criteria is used to differentiate between definite and probable CE in patients with acute myocardial infarction. [a]Multiple vessel within one coronary artery territory or multiple vessels in the coronary tree. Note: this table is reproduced from Nakano H, Yamagami H, Ofuchi H. A case report of systemic embolic events associated with atrial fibrillation. Acute Medicine & Surgery 2017;4:12730. doi:10.1002/ams2.235.

4. Conclusion

Coronary embolism is an unusual and therefore likely an underreported etiology of ACS. Patients often have varying levels of concurrent atherosclerosis which can further confound the picture. Distinctions can, however, be made angiographically. Management is the same for both: anticoagulation, thrombolysis, and percutaneous coronary intervention (PCI). Thrombus aspiration may be considered in patients with a heavy thrombus burden. However, following initial management, it is vital to further investigate the source of emboli in these patients. It is important to contemplate atrial fibrillation not only as a consequence of ACS but also as a cause of it. Additionally, it is important to consider bleeding risks given the need for both anticoagulation and antiplatelet therapy in these groups of patients.

References

[1] S. Van de Walle and K. Dujardin, "A case of coronary embolism in a patient with paroxysmal atrial fibrillation receiving tamoxifen," *International Journal of Cardiology*, vol. 123, no. 1, pp. 66–68, 2007.

[2] C. E. Raphael, J. A. Heit, G. S. Reeder et al., "Coronary embolus," *JACC: Cardiovascular Interventions*, vol. 11, no. 2, pp. 172–180, 2018.

[3] J. Menke, L. Lüthje, A. Kastrup, and J. Larsen, "Thromboembolism in atrial fibrillation," *The American Journal of Cardiology*, vol. 105, no. 4, pp. 502–510, 2010.

[4] M. Alasady, N. J. Shipp, A. G. Brooks et al., "Myocardial infarction and atrial fibrillation: importance of atrial ischemia," *Circulation: Arrhythmia and Electrophysiology*, vol. 6, no. 4, pp. 738–745, 2013.

[5] F. Violi, E. Z. Soliman, P. Pignatelli, and D. Pastori, "Atrial fibrillation and myocardial infarction: a systematic review and appraisal of pathophysiologic mechanisms," *Journal of the American Heart Association*, vol. 5, no. 5, 2016.

[6] B. Waller, B. F. Waller, E. T. A. Fry, J. B. Hermiller, T. Peters, and J. D. Slack, "Nonatherosclerotic causes of coronary artery narrowing—part II," *Clinical Cardiology*, vol. 19, no. 7, pp. 587–591, 1996.

[7] K. R. Prizel, "Coronary artery embolism and myocardial infarction: a clinicopathologic study of 55 patients," *Annals of Internal Medicine*, vol. 88, no. 2, pp. 155–161, 1978.

[8] T. Shibata, S. Kawakami, T. Noguchi et al., "Prevalence, clinical features, and prognosis of acute myocardial infarction attributable to coronary artery embolism," *Circulation*, vol. 132, no. 4, pp. 241–250, 2015.

[9] M. E. Everett, J. N. Kirkpatrick, and R. M. Lang, "Noncompaction of the myocardium complicated by coronary artery embolism," *Journal of the American Society of Echocardiography*, vol. 18, no. 2, pp. 194–196, 2005.

[10] S. Windecker, S. Stortecky, and B. Meier, "Paradoxical embolism," *Journal of the American College of Cardiology*, vol. 64, no. 4, pp. 403–415, 2014.

[11] H. Nakano, H. Yamagami, and H. Ofuchi, "A case report of systemic embolic events associated with atrial fibrillation," *Acute Medicine & Surgery*, vol. 4, no. 1, pp. 127–130, 2017.

[12] S. Antoine, D. Lowe, K. Jessamy, O. Anozie, and V. Frechette, "Myocardial infarction caused by coronary artery thromboembolism in a atrial fibrillation patient on rivaroxaban," *Chest*, vol. 150, no. 4, article 100A, 2016.

[13] C. Camaro and W. R. M. Aengevaeren, "Acute myocardial infarction due to coronary artery embolism in a patient with atrial fibrillation," *Netherlands Heart Journal*, vol. 17, no. 8, pp. 297 299, 2009.

[14] J. C. Díaz, D. Weir, W. Uribe et al., "Acute myocardial infarction due to coronary embolism in atrial fibrillation: case presentation and systematic review," *Revista Mexicana de Cardiolog*, vol. 27, no. 4, pp. 171–180, 2016.

[15] R. K. Garg and N. Jolly, "Acute myocardial infarction secondary to thromboembolism in a patient with atrial fibrillation," *International Journal of Cardiology*, vol. 123, no. 1, pp. e18–e20, 2007.

[16] N. Kotooka, Y. Otsuka, S. Yasuda, I. Morii, A. Kawamura, and S. Miyazaki, "Three cases of acute myocardial infarction due to coronary embolism: treatment using a thrombus aspiration device," *Japanese Heart Journal*, vol. 45, no. 5, pp. 861–866, 2004.

[17] K. Koutsampasopoulos, A. Datsios, S. Grigoriadis, and I. Vogiatzis, "Atrial fibrillation causing ST elevation myocardial infarction due to coronary embolism: case report and review of the literature," *Hippokratia*, vol. 20, no. 2, pp. 160–162, 2016.

[18] C. J. OSullivan, M. Sprenger, D. Tueller, and F. R. Eberli, "Case report: coronary thromboembolic acute myocardial infarction due to paroxysmal atrial fibrillation occurring after non-cardiac surgery," *BMJ Case Reports*, vol. 2015, 2015.

[19] K. Sakai, K. Inoue, and M. Nobuyoshi, "Aspiration thrombectomy of a massive thrombotic embolus in acute myocardial infarction caused by coronary embolism," *International Heart Journal*, vol. 48, no. 3, pp. 387–392, 2007.

[20] T. Takenaka, M. Horimoto, K. Igarashi, H. Yoshie, I. Tsujino, and M. Morihira, "Multiple coronary thromboemboli complicating valvular heart disease and atrial fibrillation," *American Heart Journal*, vol. 131, no. 1, pp. 194–196, 1996.

[21] A. Zakaria, B. A. Share, G. Kaspar, and D. Small, "A fluttering coronary event," *Journal of Family Medicine and Primary Care*, vol. 7, no. 2, pp. 468–470, 2018.

11

The Challenges of ST Elevation Myocardial Infarction in COVID-19 Patients

Ju Young Bae,[1] **Khalil Ian Hussein**,[1] **Christopher John Howes**,[1,2] **and John Francis Setaro**[1,2]

[1]*Department of Medicine, Greenwich Hospital, Yale-New Haven Health System, 5 Perryridge Road, Greenwich, CT 06830, USA*
[2]*Section of Cardiovascular Medicine, Department of Internal Medicine, Yale University School of Medicine, 333 Cedar St, New Haven, CT 06510, USA*

Correspondence should be addressed to John Francis Setaro; john.setaro@yale.edu

Academic Editor: Vincenzo Russo

By July 2021, the United States had over 34.4 million confirmed COVID-19 cases. Various cardiovascular manifestations of COVID-19 have been reported including ST-elevation myocardial infarction (STEMI), and there is concern that SARS-CoV-2 may be associated with a higher thrombus burden. We performed a retrospective chart review of 535 adult patients with COVID-19 admitted at Yale-New Haven Health Greenwich Hospital from February 1, 2020, to May 13, 2020. All admitted patients had undergone testing for serum troponin I and various inflammatory markers, and we identified three patients who were diagnosed with acute STEMI. Data was collected via manual chart review and included patient demographics, comorbidities, laboratory tests, electrocardiogram (ECG) results, echocardiography results, diagnoses during hospitalization, inpatient therapies, and outcomes including length of hospital stay, revascularization results, and mortality. Three of our patients had obstructive coronary artery disease confirmed via angiography. One subject was noted to display vasospasm in addition to coronary atherosclerotic obstruction and refractory thrombus formation. Among our patients with COVID-19 and STEMI, presentations were variable in terms of timing of onset of ECG changes, age, gender, race, comorbidities, symptomology, and outcomes.

1. Introduction

As of July 2021, the United States has over 34.4 million confirmed cases of COVID-19, which is an infectious disease caused by severe acute respiratory syndrome coronavirus 2 (SARS-CoV-2) [1]. SARS-CoV-2 infection has variable manifestations in humans, and there are reported cases of patients with COVID-19 presenting with a broad spectrum of cardiovascular manifestations including acute coronary syndrome, arrhythmia, myopericarditis mimicking ST-elevation myocardial infarction (STEMI), ischemic and stress-induced cardiomyopathy, coronary vasospasm, and pericardial effusion [2–4].

2. Case Presentation

We performed a single-center retrospective chart review of 535 adult patients with COVID-19 admitted to our suburban community hospital, Yale-New Haven Health Greenwich Hospital, from February 1, 2020, to May 13, 2020, and we identified three cases of acute STEMI who underwent coronary angiography. These patients diagnosed with COVID-19 had a positive result on polymerase chain reaction (PCR) testing of a nasopharyngeal sample. After being granted Institutional Review Board approval, subjects were identified by requesting access to a list of all hospitalized patients with COVID-19 from our Infection Control department.

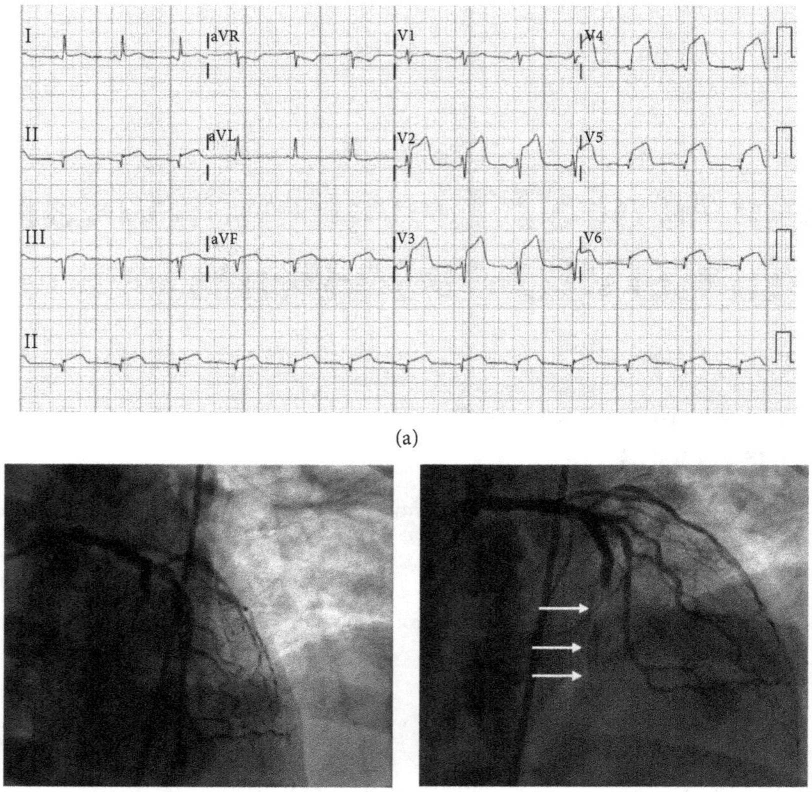

(a) (b) (c)

Figure 1: ECG on admission and LHC findings. (a) ECG showing ST elevations in anterior leads. (b) Initial coronary angiography. (c) Coronary angiography after PCI. Arrows indicate the course of LAD.

3. Case 1

A 59-year-old Caucasian male was admitted for hypoxia in the setting of COVID-19. His past medical history was notable for type 2 diabetes mellitus, hyperlipidemia, and overweight BMI, and he took aspirin 81 mg daily for primary prevention. On admission, blood pressure (BP) was 148/79 mmHg, respiratory rate was 24, and oxygen saturation was 89% on room air. There were no notable findings on the physical exam. Chest X-ray (CXR) showed patchy bilateral pulmonary infiltrates. Hospitalization was complicated by acute chest pain on hospital day five with ECG showing anterior wall STEMI (Figure 1(a)). He was intubated and left heart catheterization (LHC) revealed 40% stenosis of distal left main artery (LM), 100% stenosis of midleft anterior descending artery (LAD), normal left circumflex (LCx), 80% stenosis of proximal right coronary artery (RCA), and proximal posterior descending artery (Figure 1(b)). The procedure was complicated by heavy thrombus burden in LAD and "no-reflow" phenomenon despite the use of rescue thrombectomy, multiple intracoronary vasodilators, and 3 drug-eluting stent (DES) placement; flow was not reestablished to the apex (Figure 1(c)), which was concerning for stent thrombosis. Troponin I peaked at 105.0 ng/mL (normal <0.015). Postcatheterization transthoracic echocardiogram (TTE) showed a left ventricular ejection fraction of 41-45% and distal anterior and apical akinesis. Treatment was started with ticagrelor, aspirin, atorvastatin, and metoprolol tartrate. Course was further complicated by elevated D-dimer of 33.35 mg/L FEU for which he was started on heparin drip, new atrial flutter, and septic shock in setting of prolonged ventilator requirement. He received digoxin 62.5 mcg daily, metoprolol tartrate 37.5 mg every 6 hours, and amiodarone loading dose followed by maintenance at 200 mg daily for atrial flutter. He eventually required the initiation of norepinephrine for blood pressure support, which also optimized the patient's heart rate, so metoprolol was discontinued. For management of COVID-19, the patient received a 5-day course of azithromycin, a 9-day course of hydroxychloroquine, one dose of tocilizumab, and a 5-day course of Lopinavir-Ritonavir, as was recommended by the Yale-New Haven Health system's treatment guidelines at the time. The patient expired on day 30 of hospitalization after the family opted to transition to comfort care.

4. Case 2

A 47-year-old Hispanic male presented with a 2-week history of intermittent substernal chest pain with exertion and dyspnea. He had completed a 5-day course of azithromycin as an outpatient. His past medical history was notable for prediabetes, hypertension treated with amlodipine 5 mg daily, and class I obesity. Admission vital signs included BP 105/54 mmHg, pulse of 90 bpm, respiratory rate of 28, and oxygen saturation of 95% on room air. Physical exam was notable for bilateral rales. Labwork was pertinent for WBC

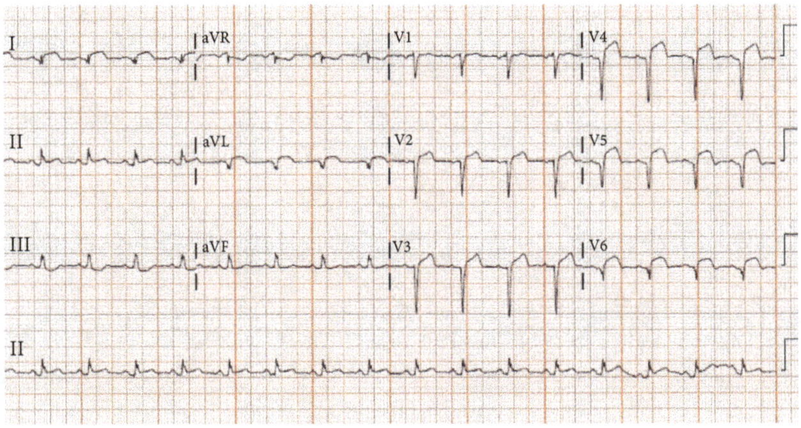

(a)

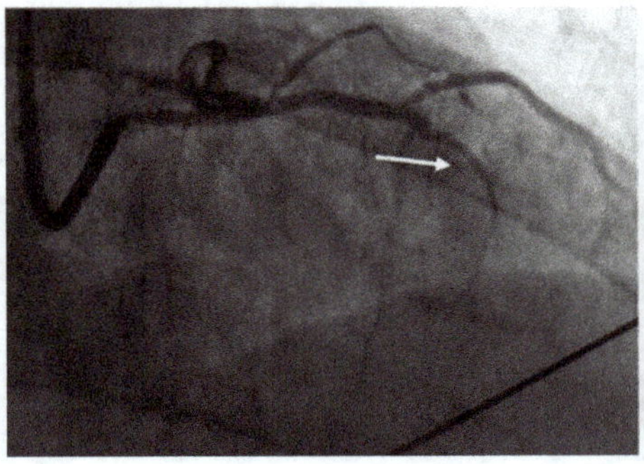

(b)

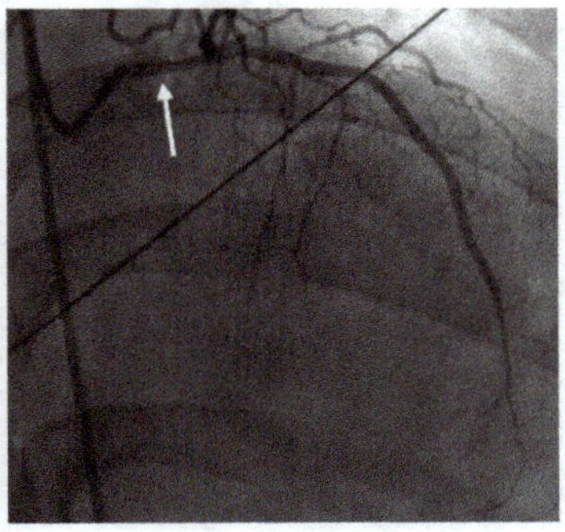

(c)

FIGURE 2: ECG on admission and LHC findings. (a) ECG showing ST elevations in anterolateral leads. (b) Initial coronary angiography with arrow showing occluded LAD. (c) Coronary angiography after PCI with arrow showing coronary vasospasm in distal LM.

of 15.3 ×1000/μL, Troponin I of 72.4 ng/mL, pro-BNP of 1,184 pg/mL, and total CK of 3,549 U/L. COVID-19 PCR was positive. CXR showed mild heterogeneous bilateral ground-glass opacities. ECG demonstrated ST-elevation over anterolateral wall distribution (Figure 2(a)). The patient was electively intubated, and LHC revealed late presenting anterior wall MI with 30% stenosis of distal LM, 100% stenosis of LAD, normal LCx, and normal RCA. Left ventricular (LV) filling pressures were moderately elevated at 18 mmHg (Figure 2(b)). Coronary vasospasm was noted and was treated using intracoronary vasodilators. Two DES were placed in the proximal and distal LAD, but no reflow was observed with noteworthy thrombus burden likely from stent thrombosis (Figure 2(c)). Troponin I peaked at 131.2 ng/mL. Postprocedure TTE showed reduced LVEF of 35-40%, mild MR and TR, mild LVH, anterior, antero-apical akinesis-dyskinesis, and spontaneous echo-contrast in the LV apex. With rising D-dimer that peaked at 2.29 mg/L FEU, the patient was started on warfarin with enoxaparin bridge. The patient was extubated successfully one day after LHC, and he was started on metoprolol, atorvastatin, lisinopril, aspirin, and ticagrelor. He also required treatment with nitroglycerin drip for vasospasm. For management of COVID-19, he received a 5-day course of hydroxychloroquine. The patient was discharged home on room air after a 9-day hospitalization with recommendation to remain on oral anticoagulation for one month due to elevated D-dimer without any proven venous thromboembolism.

5. Case 3

A 75-year-old African American female presented with acute nausea, diaphoresis, and weakness while climbing stairs. Past medical history was notable for hypertension treated with amlodipine 10 mg and hydrochlorothiazide 25 mg daily, overweight BMI, and illness four weeks prior to this admission that was suspected to be COVID-19. CXR showed diffuse interstitial changes. ECG performed by EMS showed atrial fibrillation with ST segment elevation. Vitals on presentation included HR 58 bpm, RR 22, BP 99/56mmHg, and SpO2 of 100% on room air. Physical exam was noncontributory. Laboratory work showed WBC 12.7 ×1000/μL, D-dimer 0.6 mg/L, Troponin I <0.015 ng/mL (peaked 2.27 ng/mL), and positive COVID-19 PCR test. Repeat ECG in the ED demonstrated inferolateral ST-elevation (Figure 3(a)). Treatment of atrial fibrillation with rate-controlling medications was deferred to heart rate between 50 and 60 beats per minute and borderline low blood pressure. Coronary angiography revealed 99% ostial stenosis of the RCA with TIMI-2 flow, mid-RCA 40% stenosis, distal RCA 60% stenosis, 40% proximal lesion in LAD, and LCX without obstruction (Figure 3(b)). DES was placed to ostial RCA with good flow (Figure 3(c)). Post-PCI echocardiogram showed LVEF of 45-50%, basal inferior hypokinesis, mild to moderate MR, and left atrial enlargement. Systemic anticoagulation was not initiated due to the patient's spontaneous conversion to normal sinus rhythm after successful PCI.

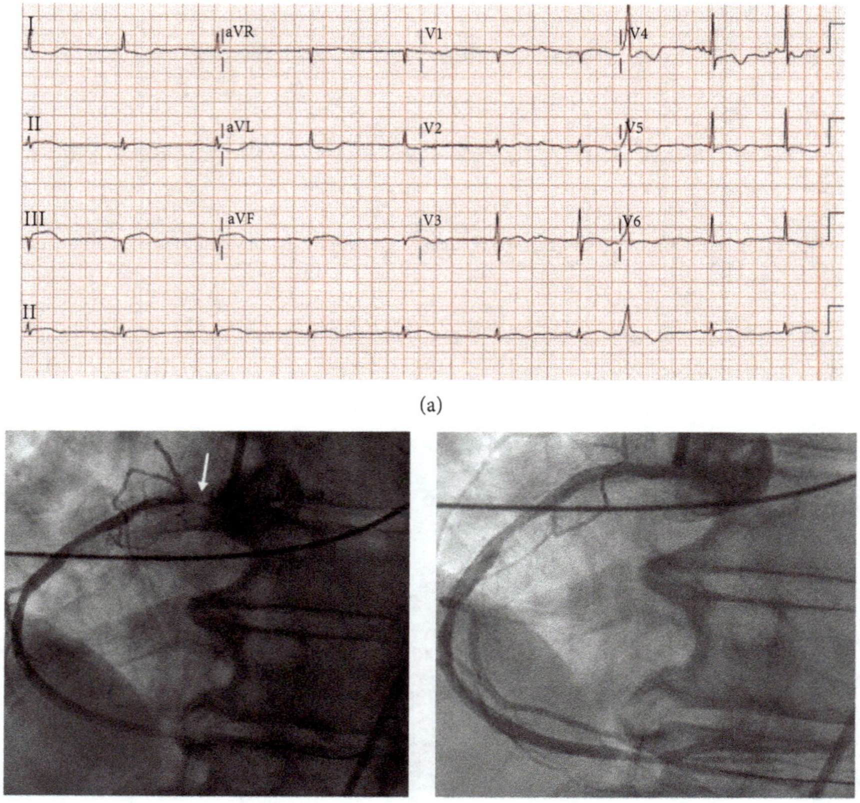

(a)

(b) (c)

Figure 3: ECG on admission and LHC findings. (a) ECG showing ST elevations in inferolateral leads. (b) Initial coronary angiography with arrow showing RCA ostium. (c) Coronary angiography after PCI.

The patient's hospital course was eventful for development of bilateral neck swelling and angioedema without airway compromise considered to be an atypical presentation of angioedema from ticagrelor use. These symptoms were treated with intravenous methylprednisone. The patient was discharged home after six-day hospitalization. She was comfortable on room air throughout this hospitalization, and Yale-New Haven Health system's COVID-19 treatment protocols did not recommend specific treatments for COVID-19 in patients who did not require supplemental oxygen.

6. Discussion

Key characteristics of each case varied including the timing of presentation, age, gender, race, and symptomology. However, all three patients had risk factors for CVD, including hypertension, hyperlipidemia, diabetes mellitus, and/or overweight or obese BMI. One patient expired during their hospitalization, and yet our two cases that presented with delayed symptom onset both survived. One subject displayed vasospasm in addition to coronary atherosclerotic obstruction and refractory thrombus formation. In addition, we noted signs of hypercoagulability such as flow not being reestablished fully in two cases as well as all three cases having elevated D-dimer, which is nonspecific but may signify that our patients were experiencing undetected thrombotic events or tendencies. None had prior history of venous thromboembolism, atrial fibrillation, or atrial flutter, so they were not on any oral anticoagulation therapy prior to hospitalization. Ultimately, two patients were started on anticoagulation due to new atrial flutter or significantly elevated D-dimer worrisome for venous thromboembolism. This highlights the need for clinicians to consider the role of oral anticoagulation started before or during hospital admission for COVID-19 patients. A recent retrospective study found that clinical outcomes were no better for COVID-19 patients who were previously on oral anticoagulation prior to hospital admission compared to those not on any anticoagulation, even after balancing for confounders such as differences in age and chronic disease burden [5]. While some of the most feared complications of COVID-19 are managed with anticoagulation, anticoagulation does not offer proven benefit for other serious complications of COVID-19 such as acute respiratory distress syndrome, and anticoagulation therapy carries risks. Therefore, we do not recommend therapeutic anticoagulation for COVID-19 patients in the absence of well-established indications.

A case series by Bangalore et al. reported a total of 18 cases of STEMI in patients with COVID-19 [6]. Of the 18 subjects, 9 underwent invasive intervention with angiography, but only two-thirds of those procedures confirmed obstructive coronary disease. That finding suggested that in addition to obstructive disease, there were nonobstructive cardiovascular diseases associated with COVID-19, which may represent perimyocarditis, ischemic/stress cardiomyopathy, or coronary vasospasm. There are numerous hypotheses regarding the mechanism of myocardial injury caused by SARS-CoV-2 infection. These include roles for (i) SARS-CoV-2 binding of angiotensin enzyme 2, which is found on myocytes and type 2 pneumocytes and which can directly cause toxicity to myocardial cells [7]; (ii) oxygen supply versus demand mismatch created secondary to hypoxemic respiratory failure arising from COVID-19-induced lung injury, which then causes type 2 myocardial infarction [8]; and (iii) COVID-19 induction of a prothrombotic effect related to cytokine-mediated inflammation and endotheliopathy, which can then lead to plaque instability, vasospasm, and rupture [9]. A recent case report describes the autopsy results of a patient with suspected STEMI and COVID-19, which found "extensive microvascular thrombosis in the absence of epicardial coronary obstruction despite no detectable virus in several sections of myocardial tissue [10]".

The unprecedented nature of the COVID-19 pandemic justifies a reevaluation of standard of care for treating patients with STEMI. Recent commentary written by experts reveals an openness to debate the use of fibrinolytic therapy versus PCI as the primary intervention [11]. In a recent multicenter case series by Hamadeh et al., 21% of subjects with COVID-19 and STEMI treated with PCI experienced stent thrombosis, and overall in-hospital mortality risk was 12% [12]. An observational study by Choudry et al., which compared outcomes between STEMI patients with COVID-19 to those without the disease, also demonstrated increased thrombus burden in those who were infected [13]. This phenomenon correlated with what was observed in our group of STEMI patients. Given the evidence that COVID-19 patients with STEMI are at increased risk of stent thrombosis and potentially are more difficult revascularize, interventional strategies for these patients should be revisited in light of the fact that fibrinolytic therapy can be an effective treatment and exposes healthcare workers to lower theoretical risk of COVID-19 transmission.

There are several domains of investigation that are needed, including (i) determining the relative risk of STEMI and other myocardial injury in patients with COVID-19 compared to those without active infection, (ii) etiologies to explain any potential increase in relative risk so that focused therapies can be developed, and (iii) relative effectiveness of fibrinolytic therapy versus PCI, given that complications from COVID-19 may hamper the effectiveness of PCI.

Consent

No written consent has been obtained from the patients as there is no patient identifiable data included in this case report.

Acknowledgments

We offer our very sincere thanks to Donna Belcinski, Greenwich Hospital medical librarian, for her assistance in finding relative literature and acquiring articles.

References

[1] C. Disease, *(COVID-19) Weekly Epidemiological Situation Report*, 2019, https://www.who.int/publications/m/item/weekly-epidemiological-update-on-covid-19—20-july-2021.

[2] E. Mahmud, H. L. Dauerman, W. FGP et al., "Management of Acute Myocardial Infarction During the COVID-19 Pandemic: A Position Statement From the Society for Cardiovascular Angiography and Interventions (SCAI), the American College of Cardiology (ACC), and the American College of Emergency Physicians (ACEP)," *Journal of the American College of Cardiology*, vol. 76, no. 11, pp. 1375–1384, 2020.

[3] V. Russo, R. Bottino, A. Carbone et al., "COVID-19 and heart: from clinical features to pharmacological implications," *Journal of Clinical Medicine*, vol. 9, no. 6, 2020.

[4] V. Russo, A. Rago, A. Carbone et al., "Atrial fibrillation in COVID-19: from epidemiological association to pharmacological implications," *Journal of Cardiovascular Pharmacology*, vol. 76, no. 2, pp. 138–145, 2020.

[5] V. Russo, R. Bottino, A. D'Andrea et al., "Chronic oral anticoagulation and clinical outcome in hospitalized COVID-19 patients," *Cardiovascular Drugs and Therapy*, pp. 1–8, 2021.

[6] S. Bangalore, A. Sharma, A. Slotwiner et al., "ST-segment elevation in patients with Covid-19 - a case series," *New England Journal of Medicine*, vol. 382, no. 25, pp. 2478–2480, 2020.

[7] M. Hoffmann, H. Kleine-Weber, S. Schroeder et al., "SARS-CoV-2 cell entry depends on ACE2 and TMPRSS2 and is blocked by a clinically proven protease inhibitor," *Cell*, vol. 181, no. 2, 2020.

[8] F. Castagna, R. Cerrud-Rodriguez, M. A. Villela, and A. E. Bortnick, "SARS-COV-2 infection presenting as ST-elevation myocardial infarction," *Catheterization and Cardiovascular Interventions*, vol. 97, 2020.

[9] F. A. Klok, M. J. H. A. Kruip, N. J. M. van der Meer et al., "Incidence of thrombotic complications in critically ill ICU patients with COVID-19," *Thrombosis Research*, vol. 191, pp. 145–147, 2020.

[10] G. Guagliumi, A. Sonzogni, I. Pescetelli, D. Pellegrini, and A. V. Finn, "Microthrombi and ST-segment-elevation myocardial infarction in COVID-19," *Circulation*, vol. 142, no. 8, pp. 804–809, 2020.

[11] M. J. Daniels, M. G. Cohen, A. A. Bavry, and D. J. Kumbhani, "Reperfusion of ST-segment-elevation myocardial infarction in the COVID-19 era: business as usual?," *Circulation*, vol. 141, no. 24, pp. 1948–1950, 2020.

[12] A. Hamadeh, A. Aldujeli, K. Briedis et al., "Characteristics and Outcomes in Patients Presenting With COVID-19 and ST-Segment Elevation Myocardial Infarction," *The American Journal of Cardiology*, vol. 131, pp. 1–6, 2020.

[13] F. A. Choudry, S. M. Hamshere, K. S. Rathod et al., "High Thrombus burden in patients with COVID-19 presenting with ST-segment elevation myocardial infarction," *Journal of the American College of Cardiology*, vol. 76, no. 10, pp. 1168–1176, 2020.

12

Acupuncture-Induced Tension Pneumothorax Presenting as Acute Heart Failure

Alia Arif Hussain,[1] Jeppe Nygaard,[2] Kasper Kofod Pedersen,[3] Celi Anne Schoenike,[2] Erik Kovacs,[1] and Steen Hylgaard Jørgensen[4]

[1]*Emergency Department, North Denmark Regional Hospital, Denmark*
[2]*Department of Abdominal Surgery, North Denmark Regional Hospital, Denmark*
[3]*Department of Radiology, North Denmark Regional Hospital, Denmark*
[4]*Department of Cardiology, North Denmark Regional Hospital, Denmark*

Correspondence should be addressed to Alia Arif Hussain; alia.arif.hussain@gmail.com

Academic Editor: Dirk Bandorski

Takotsubo syndrome (TSS) is a reversible, acute cardiomyopathy with transient heart failure, often secondary to other disorders. A 64-year-old woman, with no history of ischemic heart disease, was admitted to the emergency department after developing sudden-onset dyspnea after a planned acupuncture treatment for back pain. Acute echocardiography showed decreased left ventricular function with basal hypercontraction and apical akinesia and was interpreted, and treated, as acute heart failure. When the attending cardiologist arrived, the patient still had dyspnea with a declining blood pressure (97/65 mmHg) and tachycardia (111/minute). The cardiologist suspected a tension pneumothorax induced by the penetration of an acupuncture needle to the apex of the lung, as well as secondary TSS cardiomyopathy. An acute chest X-ray was performed, which showed a large left-sided rim pneumothorax. The attending surgeon placed a chest tube in the left 6th intercostal space in the midaxillary line, and the patient reported immediate pain relief and improvement in her dyspnea. The patient's clinical condition improved, and a control X-ray showed that the lung was fully expanded. The chest tube was removed, but after a few minutes, the patient developed a massive subcutaneous emphysema in the upper chest and in the face and her clinical condition deteriorated rapidly. A new chest tube was inserted, and the patient's tachycardia diminished, with her clinical condition improving immediately. The patient remained hospitalized for the next seven days. After three continuous days without any escaped air in the chest tube, the tube was removed, and the patient was observed for another 48 hours. This time, the removal was without any complications and within two days, the patient was ready for discharge. The follow-up echocardiography showed complete recovery of left ventricular function.

1. Introduction

Takotsubo syndrome (TSS) is a reversible, acute cardiomyopathy with transient heart failure, often secondary to other disorders [1, 2]. The word "takotsubo" is Japanese and translates to "octopus trap", because when affected by TSS, the left ventricle of the heart takes on a shape resembling an octopus trap. Recently, a systematic review and meta-analysis reported that 36% of patients had experienced physical stress prior to TSS. Chest pain and dyspnea were reported in an additional 64% and 26%, respectively [3]. Acupuncture is associated with rare but serious complications including pneumothorax, subarachnoid hemorrhage and cardiac tamponade [4–6]. This case report describes a case of acupuncture-triggered tension pneumothorax with secondary takotsubo.

2. Case Report

A 64-year-old woman, with a history of mild chronic obstructive pulmonary disease (COPD) and with no history of ischemic heart disease, was admitted to the emergency

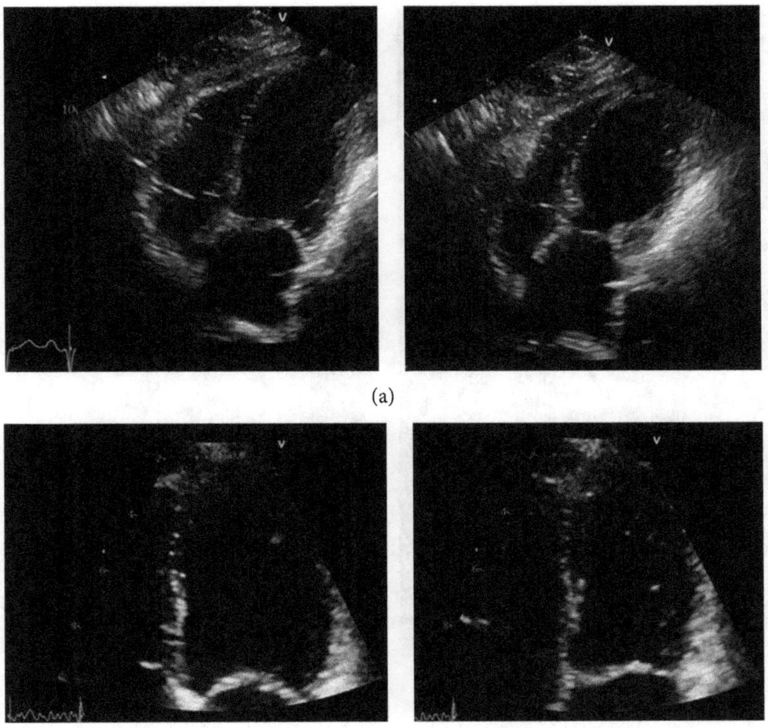

(a)

(b)

FIGURE 1: (a) Echocardiography in the acute phase. The first echocardiography showing modified 4 ch view of end-diastolic and end-systolic left ventricular volume. Basal hypercontraction and apical ballooning is evident, interpreted as acute heart failure/takotsubo cardiomyopathy. (b) Echocardiography after remission of tension pneumothorax and subcutaneous emphysema. Follow-up echocardiography showing 4 ch view of end-diastolic and end-systolic left ventricular volume 1 month later. Left ventricular ejection fraction (LVEF) has normalized.

department (ED) at North Denmark Regional Hospital. The patient reported severe, sudden-onset shortness of breath and chest pain, starting ten minutes after the patient had left her general practitioner for a planned acupuncture appointment. In the ambulance, the patient was treated with inhalations of salbutamol, which reduced her chest pain. Sublingual administration of nitroglycerin and aspirin did not further ameliorate symptoms. Upon arrival to the ED, the patient had dyspnea while speaking and was sitting up in bed, using axillary respiratory muscles; peripheral oxygen saturation (SpO_2) was 80% without oxygen therapy; respiratory rate was 25/minute; heart rate (HR) was 127 bpm; and blood pressure was 116/83 mmHg. The SpO_2 increased to 96% with nasal oxygen therapy set to 10 liters/minute. Auscultation of the lungs revealed vesicular respiration with normal breath sounds, possibly with slightly decreased breath sounds over the base of the left lung. Chest-wall palpation did not evoke pain nor did the patient have leg edema. The ECG showed sinus tachycardia without signs of ischemia, and blood tests were normal. The arterial blood gas (ABG) indicated a metabolic acidosis without respiratory compensation (pH 7.27, pO_2 7.8 kPa and pCO_2 5.5 kPa) with elevated lactate of 3.7 mmol/L. An echocardiography (Figure 1(a)) performed in the ED showed decreased left ventricular ejection fraction (LVEF) with basal hypercontraction and apical akinesia, which was interpreted as acute heart failure. The patient was transferred to an in-patient department with the suspicion of a cardiac cause to her symptoms. Thus, the attending cardiologist was summoned. When the cardiologist arrived, the patient still had dyspnea with a declining blood pressure (97/65 mmHg) and tachycardia (111/minute). Auscultation of the lungs revealed reduced breath sounds on the left side with hyperresonance/hypertympanism over the left hemithorax as compared to the right. The cardiologist suspected a tension pneumothorax induced by the penetration of an acupuncture needle to the apex of the lung, as well as secondary TSS cardiomyopathy. The patient's blood pressure remained low but unchanged, and therefore, an acute chest X-ray was performed (Figure 2(a)), which showed a large left-sided rim pneumothorax, extending along the entire lateral border of the lung from the base to the apex. The attending surgeon placed a 24-French chest tube left at the 6th intercostal space in the midaxillary line. The patient reported immediate pain relief and improvement in her dyspnea. A chest X-ray confirmed that the chest tube was placed correctly. The patient was transferred to the general surgery ward for observation and pain management. Two days later, the patient's clinical condition had improved, and a control X-ray showed that the lung was fully expanded except for a small 1 cm section in the apical part of the left pleural cavity. The chest tube was removed, but after a few minutes, the patient developed a massive subcutaneous emphysema in the upper chest and in the face and her clinical condition deteriorated rapidly. The patient had tachycardia

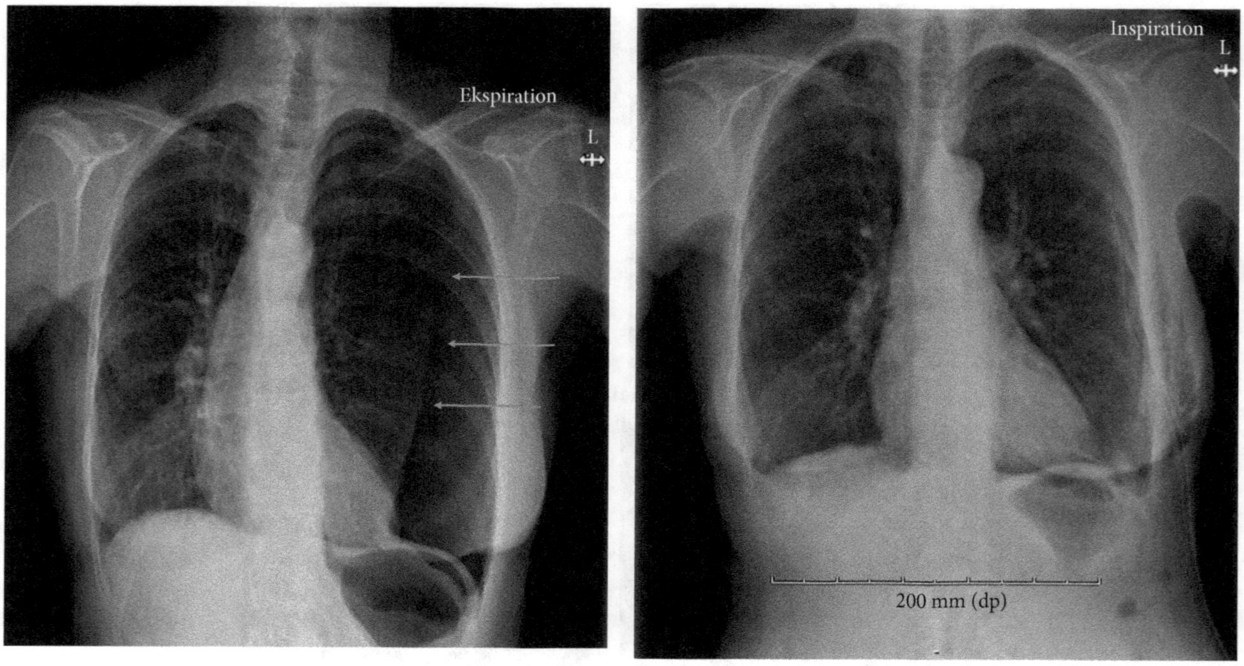

(a) (b)

FIGURE 2: (a) Chest X-ray showing tension pneumothorax of the left lung. The first chest X-ray showed a large left-sided rim pneumothorax, extending along the entire lateral border of the lung, from the base to the apex, and with a maximal width of 6 cm at the base of the left lung. (b) Chest X-ray showing subcutaneous emphysema. A postintervention chest X-ray showed an intercostal drain placed at about the 8th intercostal space on the left side. A near complete regression of the pneumothorax is seen, with the lung parenchyma again extending to the borders the left hemithorax and a smaller residual rim apicolaterally measuring 12 mm. In the soft tissues at the puncture point, multiple diffuse hypodense areas are seen, resembling subcutaneous emphysema.

and dyspnea and was unable to open her eyes due to the massive subcutaneous emphysema (Figure 2(b)). A new chest tube was inserted, and the patient's tachycardia diminished, with her clinical condition that improved immediately. Seven days later, no air was seen escaping via the chest tube and a chest X-ray showed an improvement in the subcutaneous emphysema with only a small pneumothorax (1 cm) remaining in the apical part of the lung. Once again, the drain was removed, and four hours later, the patient again developed dyspnea and massive subcutaneous emphysema with a pulse rate of 150 bpm, blood pressure of 172/97 mmHg, and an SpO_2 of 97% on 15 liters of oxygen/minute. A new chest tube was inserted, and the effect was immediate, as made apparent by reduction in the patient's dyspnea, as well as a stabilization of her vital signs.

The patient remained hospitalized for the next seven days. Thoracic surgeons were consulted, but they found no evidence of pleural bullae on the chest CT. After three continuous days without any escaped air in the chest tube, the tube was removed, and the patient was observed for another 48 hours. This time, the removal was without any complications and within two days, the patient was ready for discharge. The follow-up echocardiography showed complete recovery of left ventricular function (Figure 1(b)).

3. Discussion

In the presented case, a 64-year-old woman, with no history of ischemic heart disease, developed severe sudden-onset dyspnea after a planned acupuncture treatment for back pain by her general practitioner. Echocardiography showed decreased LVEF with basal hypercontraction and apical akinesia and was interpreted as acute heart failure. When the attending cardiologist arrived, the patient's blood pressure had decreased (to 97/65 mmHg), and auscultation of the lungs revealed reduced breath sounds on the left side. Tension pneumothorax was suspected and confirmed by an acute chest X-ray. The tension pneumothorax was presumably induced by an acupuncture needle penetrating the apex of the lung, resulting in subsequent secondary takotsubo cardiomyopathy. In the present case, we had no information about the general practitioner's experience with acupuncture.

TSS, also known as stress cardiomyopathy, is characterized by a temporary weakening of the left ventricle most probably caused by an increase in catecholamine concentration triggered by significant physical stress.

Tension pneumothorax is a rare but serious and potentially fatal complication of acupuncture. A history of thoracic surgery, chronic bronchitis, emphysema, pneumonia, tuberculosis, and lung cancer may increase the postacupuncture risk of iatrogenic pneumothorax [7]. In the present case report, TSS temporarily concealed the underlying tension pneumothorax. However, TSS was secondary to the physical stress of the tension pneumothorax but due to fast, bedside ultrasound diagnostics, the patient's symptoms were treated assuming a cardiac origin.

To our knowledge, this is the first reported case of TSS secondary to an acupuncture-induced tension pneumothorax

[8–12]. This case illustrates that TSS is often caused by a physical or emotional stressor, which should be diagnosed and treated immediately. Furthermore, both the patient and acupuncturist should be informed and aware of complications related to acupuncture in the thoracic region, especially the possibility of injuries to internal organs and the early symptoms of pneumothorax. In high-risk patients, an observation period of 15 minutes after acupuncture in the thoracic region could ensure earlier detection of fatal complications such as tension pneumothorax.

Consent

Written informed consent has been obtained.

References

[1] K. Kato, A. R. Lyon, J.-R. Ghadri, and C. Templin, "Takotsubo syndrome: aetiology, presentation and treatment," *Heart*, vol. 103, no. 18, pp. 1461–1469, 2017.

[2] G. Parodi, B. Bellandi, S. del Pace et al., "Natural history of tako-tsubo cardiomyopathy," *Chest*, vol. 139, no. 4, pp. 887–892, 2011.

[3] F. Pelliccia, V. Pasceri, G. Patti et al., "Long-term prognosis and outcome predictors in Takotsubo syndrome: a systematic review and meta-regression study," *JACC: Heart Failure*, vol. 7, no. 2, pp. 143–154, 2019.

[4] H. J. Lee, Y. J. Kim, and W. Y. Kim, "Safety concerns with thoracoabdominal acupuncture: experience at a tertiary-care emergency department," *Pain Medicine*, vol. 18, no. 12, pp. 2504–2508, 2017.

[5] C. M. Witt, D. Pach, B. Brinkhaus et al., "Safety of acupuncture: results of a prospective observational study with 229,230 patients and introduction of a medical information and consent form," *Forschende Komplementärmedizin*, vol. 16, no. 2, pp. 91–97, 2009.

[6] J. Zhang, H. Shang, X. Gao, and E. Ernst, "Acupuncture-related adverse events: a systematic review of the Chinese literature," *Bulletin of the World Health Organization*, vol. 88, no. 12, pp. 915-921C, 2010.

[7] S. K. Lin, J. M. Liu, R. J. Hsu, H. C. Chuang, Y. X. Wang, and P. H. Lin, "Incidence of iatrogenic pneumothorax following acupuncture treatments in Taiwan," *Acupuncture in Medicine*, vol. 37, no. 6, pp. 332–339, 2019.

[8] M. Abu Ghanimeh, B. Bhardwaj, A. Aly, and P. Baweja, "Takotsubo cardiomyopathy secondary to spontaneous right-sided pneumothorax," *BMJ case reports*, vol. 2017, article bcr2017219384, 2017.

[9] Y. J. Akashi, M. Sakakibara, and F. Miyake, "Reversible left ventricular dysfunction "takotsubo" cardiomyopathy associated with pneumothorax," *Heart*, vol. 87, no. 2, article E1, 2002.

[10] W. S. Chen and M. J. Hung, "Tension pneumothorax-induced Takotsubo syndrome: a case report," *Medicine (Baltimore)*, vol. 98, no. 16, article e15190, 2019.

[11] M. Gale, P. Loarte, B. Mirrer et al., "Takotsubo cardiomyopathy in the setting of tension pneumothorax," *Case Reports in Critical Care*, vol. 2015, Article ID 536931, 5 pages, 2015.

[12] A. Kumar, S. Padala, D. C. Morales, and H. Swales, "Broken lung and broken heart: a case of right pneumothorax resulting in Takotsubo cardiomyopathy," *Connecticut Medicine*, vol. 77, no. 2, pp. 99–102, 2013.

13

Isolated Cardiac Sarcoidosis with High-Grade Heart Block: Utilization of New Diagnostic Guidelines

Matthew R. Petersen,[1] **Christopher Perry**,[2] **and Rachel Nickels**[3]

[1]*Department of Internal Medicine, University of Florida, USA*
[2]*Department of Cardiology, University of Florida, USA*
[3]*United States Department of Veterans Affairs, North Florida South Georgia VA Hospital, USA*

Correspondence should be addressed to Matthew R. Petersen; matthew.petersen@medicine.ufl.edu

Academic Editor: Ertugrul Ercan

Cardiac sarcoidosis can present with heart failure and conduction disease. This is a case of a 58-year-old male who presented for dyspnea, edema, and varying degrees of heart block. Using new updated diagnostic guidelines and multimodal cardiac imaging, he was diagnosed with isolated cardiac sarcoidosis.

1. History of Present Illness

A 58-year-old male presented to the emergency room with bradycardia and lower extremity edema. A few weeks prior, he originally presented to a neighboring hospital for new onset dyspnea on exertion and lower extremity edema. On arrival, ECG showed baseline atrial fibrillation with junctional escape rhythm at a rate of 35-40 beats per minute. He was normotensive, and his only complaints were lower extremity edema and subacute fatigue.

Physical exam revealed an obese middle-aged male in no acute distress. His was mildly tachypneic, was sitting upright on the edge of the bed, and his lung exam revealed bibasilar crackles. His heart rate was slowed but was in a regular rhythm. He had 2+ bilateral lower extremity edema, and his extremities were warm. Initial labs revealed hemoglobin of 13.4 g/dL, hematocrit 42.2%, and platelets 143 k/cmm with normal differential. Metabolic panel revealed electrolytes within normal limits; serum creatinine was 1.4 mg/dL which was slightly above the patients baseline of 1.2 mg/dL. Albumin, calcium, transaminases, and bilirubin were within normal limits. High sensitivity troponin was 32 ng/L with no change on serial repeat tests, and NT pro BNP was 3018 pg/mL.

2. Past Medical History

The patient had a past medical history of obesity and asymptomatic bradycardia first reported several years prior to presentation. He recently had been diagnosed with heart failure with preserved ejection fraction (EF) a few weeks prior at a neighboring hospital.

2.1. Differential Diagnosis. Due to the presentation of a middle age, normotensive black male with heart failure and bradycardia, there was suspicion for an infiltrative cardiomyopathy such as amyloidosis, both light chain and transthyretin types, as well as sarcoidosis with cardiac involvement.

2.2. Investigations. Serial ECGs showed several different bradycardic rhythms (Figure 1). He was noted to have intermittent second-degree Mobitz type 1 atrioventricular block (AVB) but also periods of high-grade AVB. Transthoracic echocardiogram revealed asymmetric left ventricular hypertrophy, normal systolic function (EF estimated at 55%), normal wall motion, and grade 1 diastolic dysfunction. There was no evidence of outflow tract obstruction, and ventricular filling pressures were estimated to be normal. He underwent

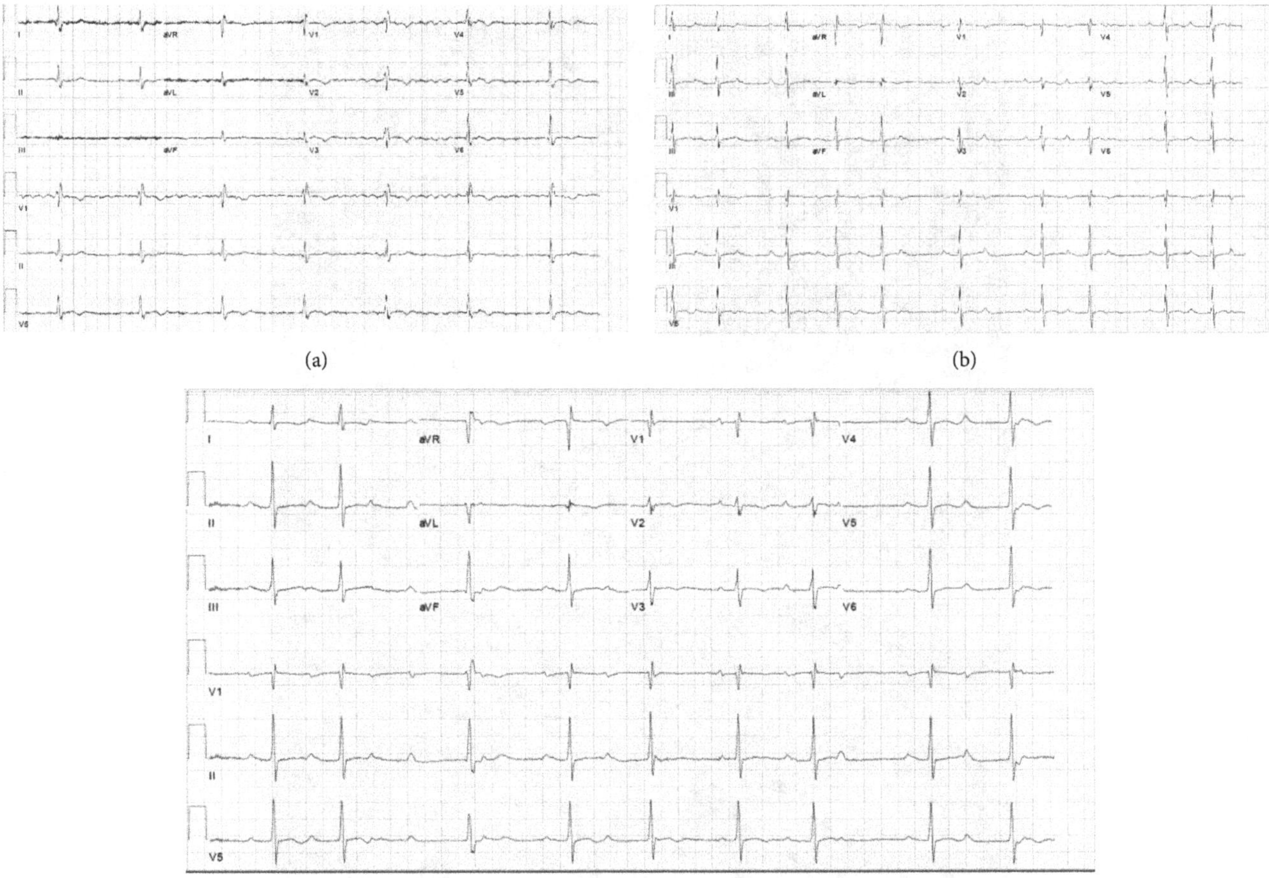

(a) (b) (c)

Figure 1: ECG of variable heart block in a patient with cardiac sarcoidosis: (a) baseline atrial fibrillation with junctional escape rhythm; (b) second-degree Mobitz type 1 AV block; (c) high grade AV block.

a treadmill stress test, demonstrating chronotropic competency without evidence of ischemia. Cardiac magnetic resonance (CMR) imaging revealed asymmetric hypertrophy of the ventricular septum with patchy myocardial late gadolinium enhancement involving the mid- to basal septum with heterogeneous uptake in the apex. Labs revealed a normal protein electrophoresis making light chain amyloidosis unlikely. The patient underwent a CT scan of the chest to examine for evidence of pulmonary sarcoidosis; however, this was unremarkable. A technetium-pyrophosphate scan was obtained for assessment of transthyretin amyloid; however, this was negative as well.

The patient was scheduled for follow-up Fluorodeoxyglucose Positron Emission Tomography-Computed Tomography (FDG PET CT) scan. When he obtained the scan, it was positive for FDG uptake in the left ventricular myocardium as well as the apical inferior wall, with no abnormal extracardiac FDG uptake (see Figure 2). These findings were consistent with active isolated cardiac sarcoidosis primarily involving the mid- to basal myocardium.

2.3. Management. During his hospitalization, the patient was administered intravenous loop diuretics for his volume overload. He underwent dual chamber pacemaker implantation, as well as empiric implantable cardiac defibrillator (ICD) placement for primary prevention against ventricular arrhythmias. ICD placement was felt appropriate despite not yet obtaining a definitive diagnosis of cardiac sarcoidosis (CS) for two reasons: (1) the patient's existing need for a pacemaker for treatment of bradycardia and high-grade AVB and (2) the high suspicion for CS. The team did not want to delay primary prevention therapy due to risk of sudden cardiac death in patients with CS and heart block. The patient's cardiac device was set to DDD (dual chamber paced, dual sensed, and dual inhibited) settings given his high degree of block as well as underlying paroxysmal atrial fibrillation. Upon follow-up interrogation of the device, the patient was paced from the right atrial lead 54% of the time and from the right ventricular lead 100% of the time and was in atrial fibrillation 28% of the time, showing his high-grade heart block and underlying bradycardia. He has not had any ventricular arrhythmias to date.

3. Discussion

Sarcoidosis is a granulomatous disorder of unknown etiology that can affect multiple organ systems. The histopathologic hallmark of sarcoidosis is the presence of noncaseating granulomas in affected organs. An estimated 5-25% of patients with sarcoidosis have cardiac involvement [1]. CS can cause

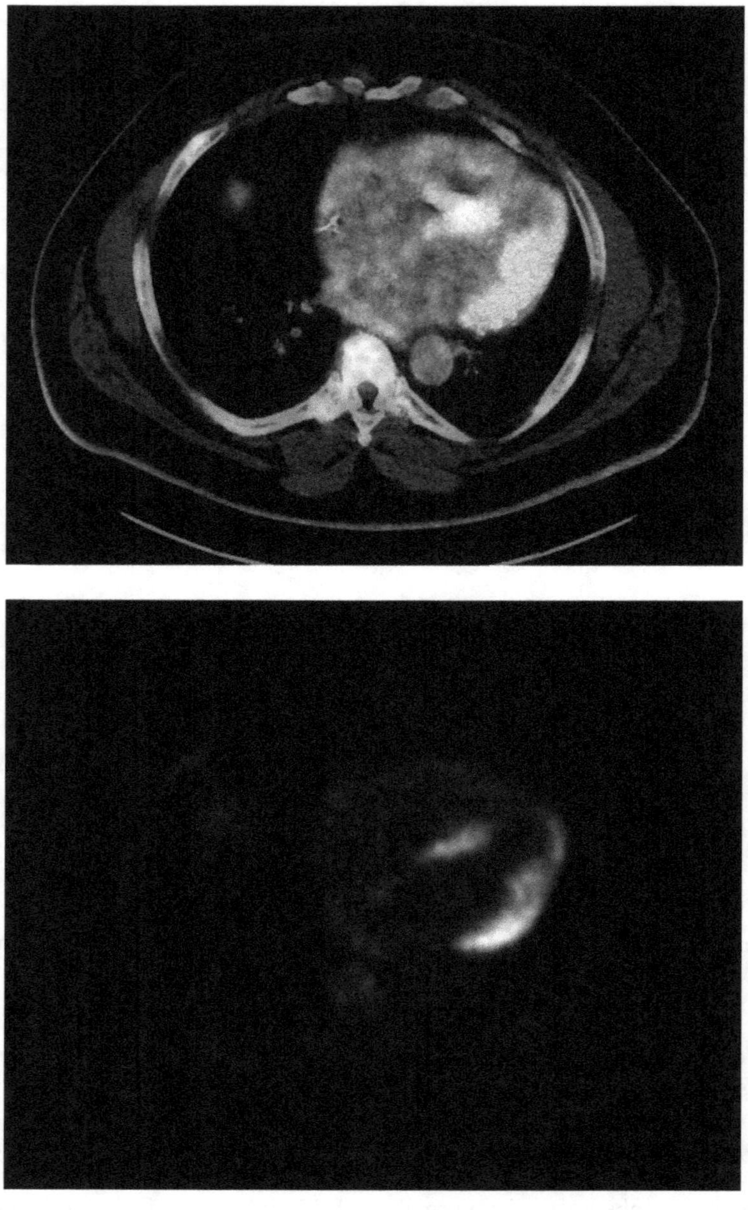

Figure 2: Active sarcoid seen in myocardium on FDG PET CT. FDG PET CT showing abnormal uptake in the myocardium as well as apical inferior wall with sparing of the apex with no extracardiac FDR uptake.

a variety of cardiac problems, including heart failure and conduction disease. In a European registry of sarcoidosis patients, high-grade atrioventricular blocks were the most common presentation of those affected, seen in about 44% of CS patients [2]. Those with CS have increased risk of arrhythmias, particularly ventricular arrhythmias. One cohort study found that the 5-year incidence of VT was 56% in those with EF below 25% and 25% in those with normal EF [2]. There is also an increased risk of sudden cardiac death in CS patients ranging from 9% in those with normal EF and no history of VT to 34% in those with EF below 25% and prior history of VT [2]. Given these risks, diagnosing cardiac sarcoidosis early is imperative.

Previous guidelines for diagnosis required biopsy-proven disease either of the cardiac tissue or extracardiac tissue with other signs of cardiac involvement [3]. These and other European and American diagnostic guidelines have been too reliant on biopsy data, which has poor diagnostic yields, [4] and does not take into account recent advancements in cardiac imaging. New Japanese diagnostic guidelines for CS and isolated cardiac sarcoidosis (ICS) were published in 2017. These new guidelines proposed the diagnosis of CS via major and minor criteria to classify cardiac involvement that includes analysis of ECG, ECHO, CMR, and FDG PET findings (Table 1) [5]. These guidelines have been shown to capture more patients with CS and ICS, allowing them to proceed to recommended therapies such as steroid treatment and cardiac devices for primary prevention [6].

This patient was diagnosed with ICS based on these guidelines as he had FDG-PET data consistent with cardiac

TABLE 1: Summary of "New Guidelines for Diagnosis of Cardiac Sarcoidosis in Japan" by Terasaki and Yoshinaga (2017).

(a)

	Cardiac sarcoidosis	Isolated cardiac sarcoidosis
Histological diagnosis group	(i) Endomyocardial biopsy or surgical specimens confirm noncaseating granulomatous tissue	(i) Prerequisite required+ (ii) Endomyocardial biopsy or surgical specimens confirm noncaseating granulomatous tissue
Clinical diagnosis group	(i) Patient diagnosed with sarcoidosis via tissue biopsy diagnosis of noncardiac site and (ii) Signs of cardiac involvement*	(i) Prerequisite required+ (ii) F-FDG PET reveals abnormally high accumulation of radiotracer in cardiac tissue and (iii) 3/4 of the other major criteria for cardiac involvement* are met

(b)

*Cardiac involvement Requires 2/5 major criteria or 1/5 major criteria and 2/3 minor criteria	(i) Major criteria (a) High-grade AV block (b) Abnormal ventricular wall anatomy (c) LVEF < 50% (d) F-FDG PET with increased tracer uptake in cardiac tissue (e) Cardiac MRI with delayed gadolinium enhancement in myocardium (ii) Minor criteria (a) Abnormal ECG findings (b) Perfusion defects on myocardial perfusion scintigraphy (c) Cardiac biopsy with monocyte infiltration or fibrosis
+Prerequisite required for ICS	(i) No clinical findings of sarcoidosis in extracardiac organs and no signs of hilar or mediastinal lymphadenopathy (ii) F-FDG PET with no uptake accumulation in extracardiac organs

involvement without extracardiac involvement, high-grade AVB, abnormal ventricular wall anatomy, and late gadolinium enhancement seen on CMR.

Treatment with immunosuppression has little high-level data, and most recommendations are driven by expert consensus. One review that discusses induction of steroids for improvement of both ejection fraction and conduction disease described a modest improvement in conduction disease in those treated with steroids, as well as improvement in ejection fraction in those with initial EF below 35%, however no significant improvement in those with moderately reduced EFs [7]. One systematic review examining the benefits of steroid treatments in CS patients concluded that treatment with exogenous corticosteroids improved conduction disease in about 50% of those treated; however, there was too little data to support recommendations in steroids to treat ventricular arrhythmia burden or mortality [8].

3.1. Follow-Up. The patient followed up with outpatient cardiology after discharge. He continues on diuretics and rivaroxaban for anticoagulation given his atrial fibrillation. Follow-up ECHO 6 months after initial diagnosis showed reduced ejection fraction at 25%, and the patient was started on guideline-directed medical therapy for heart failure with reduced ejection fraction with betablocker, RAAS inhibition, and Aldactone. He underwent eye exam and thorough pulmonology workup, which was again negative for extracardiac manifestations of sarcoidosis, and the patient just recently was initiated on systemic corticosteroids at 40 mg daily for three months, with tapering dose to 5-15 mg daily thereafter. A repeat echocardiogram will be obtained in 3 months, and repeat cardiac device interrogation to examine for progression or improvement on conduction disease will occur at one-year follow-up.

4. Conclusion

This case of suspected CS with variable high-grade conduction blocks highlights the utilization of recently updated diagnostic guidelines for CS. This case illustrates the need to continue to develop progressive diagnostic guidelines in line with available technology. This can lead to more accurate and earlier diagnosis, which allows for more CS patients to benefit from cardiac device and steroid treatment for arrhythmias and primary prevention of sudden cardiac death.

Additional Points

Learning Objectives. (i) Cardiac sarcoidosis can present as heart failure or conduction disease such as high-degree AVB or ventricular arrhythmias. (ii) New Japan diagnostic guidelines allows for use of advanced cardiac imaging for diagnosis of CS and ICS, addressing the problems of poor diagnostic yield with endomyocardial biopsies and taking advantage of new medical technologies. (iii) Patients with

CS, particularly those with reduced EF, are at high risk for ventricular arrhythmias and sudden cardiac death. These can be treated with ICD placement and systemic corticosteroids.

References

[1] D. H. Birnie, P. B. Nery, A. C. Ha, and R. S. B. Beanlands, "Cardiac sarcoidosis," *Journal of the American College of Cardiology*, vol. 68, no. 4, pp. 411–421, 2016.

[2] H. K. Nordenswan, J. Lehtonen, K. Ekström et al., "Outcome of cardiac sarcoidosis presenting with high-grade atrioventricular block," *Circulation. Arrhythmia and Electrophysiology*, vol. 11, no. 8, p. e006145, 2018.

[3] T. Tachibana and K. Iwai TT, *Study on the cause of death in patients with sarcoidosis in Japan*, Presented at: XII World Congress on Sarcoidosis, Kyoto, Japan, 1991.

[4] M. K. Bennett, N. A. Gilotra, C. Harrington et al., "Evaluation of the role of endomyocardial biopsy in 851 patients with unexplained heart failure from 2000-2009," *Circulation: Heart Failure*, vol. 6, no. 4, pp. 676–684, 2013.

[5] F. Terasaki and K. Yoshinaga, "New guidelines for diagnosis of cardiac sarcoidosis in Japan," *Ann Nucl Cardiol*, vol. 3, no. 1, pp. 42–45, 2017.

[6] H. Kawai, M. Sarai, Y. Kato et al., "Diagnosis of isolated cardiac sarcoidosis based on new guidelines," *ESC Hear Fail*, vol. 7, no. 5, pp. 2662–2671, 2020.

[7] D. H. Birnie, R. Kandolin, P. B. Nery, and M. Kupari, "Cardiac manifestations of sarcoidosis: diagnosis and management," *European Heart Journal*, vol. 38, no. 35, pp. 2663–2670, 2016.

[8] M. M. Sadek, D. Yung, D. H. Birnie, R. S. Beanlands, and P. B. Nery, "Corticosteroid therapy for cardiac sarcoidosis: a systematic review," *The Canadian Journal of Cardiology*, vol. 29, no. 9, pp. 1034–1041, 2013.

14

Relapsed Brucellosis Manifested as Endocarditis with Vegetation on the Implantable Cardioverter Defibrillator Lead

Bisher Sawaf,[1] Wael Kanjo,[1] Yasir Alabbas,[1] Ahmad Hatim,[1] Unus K. Bedardeen,[2] and Wafer A. Dabdoob[2]

[1]*Internal Medicine, Department of Medical Education, Hamad Medical Corporation, Doha, Qatar*
[2]*Department of Cardiology, Heart Hospital, Hamad Medical Corporation, Doha, Qatar*

Correspondence should be addressed to Wafer A. Dabdoob; wdabdoob@hamad.qa

Academic Editor: Francesco Nappi

Implantable cardioverter defibrillator lead endocarditis due to Brucella melitensis is a rare and life-threatening complication of brucellosis. Successful management requires a combination of medical treatment and device extraction. We present a case of relapsing brucellosis manifested as infective endocarditis colonizing the lead of the implantable cardioverter defibrillator with formation of vegetation on the lead. A 63-year-old male presented to the rehabilitation unit with hypotension. No other signs of infection were noted. The patient had a history of drinking unpasteurized milk since childhood and a previous episode of Brucella infective endocarditis. A transthoracic echocardiography showed an oscillating vegetation on the lead of the tip of the right atrial ICD, and the blood cultures were positive for Brucella melitensis. Surgical removal of the device was infeasible, and medical management was the only feasible option in this case.

1. Introduction

Brucellosis is one of the most encountered endemic zoonoses in many developing regions including the Middle East (ME), sub-Saharan Africa, South Asia, and South America [1]. This disease is caused by Brucella melitensis, a gram-negative, nonencapsulated, nonmotile, facultative intracellular coccobacillus [2, 3]. The mode of transmission of this infection is from infected animals to humans through either direct contact such as cut and aerosol inhalation or indirect contact such as ingestion of unpasteurized dairy products, urine, tissues, and products of conception (placenta) [4, 5]. Consumption of unpasteurized dairy products from contaminated milk is the main pathway of spread globally, especially in the Middle East [6].

Brucellosis presents with a broad spectrum of clinical manifestations including fever, arthralgia, myalgia, and back pain, and it is sometimes complicated with endocarditis, neurobrucellosis, and epididymo-orchitis [7]. Cardiovascular involvement is prevalent in 1% of brucellosis patients, with endocarditis being the most serious form and leading to brucellosis-related mortality [7, 8]. Although endocarditis caused by infection of a prosthetic device or implant is a rare complication of brucellosis, the most suitable therapeutic approach in this scenario is to remove the device. However, oftentimes the presence of multiple comorbidities and other factors, such as age, renders surgical management an infeasible approach, and the only option is to retain the device and place the patient on a prolonged antimicrobial treatment [9]. Due to the low number of reported cases of brucella infective endocarditis with device colonization, there is lack of consensus on the most appropriate approach for the management of these patients who are not candidates for surgery [10, 11].

A review of the literature revealed that about 25% of the reported cases of Cardiac Device-Related Brucella Endocarditis (CDRBrE) were in the Middle East [11–16]. In this report, we aim to describe the first case of recurrent brucellosis manifested as infective endocarditis colonizing the lead of the implanted cardioverter defibrillator (ICD) with formation of vegetation on the lead. To the best of our knowledge, this is also the first study to provide a comprehensive summary of CDRBrE cases reported in the literature.

2. Case Presentation

A 64-year-old Egyptian gentleman residing in Qatar, he has a long-standing history of hypertension, atrial fibrillation, and idiopathic dilated cardiomyopathy with a low ejection fraction (LV EF 26%), underwent implantation of a cardiac resynchronization therapy device (CRT-D) in 2013. Two years later, the CRT-D was downgraded to ICD.

On February 11th, 2020, the patient suffered from an ischemic stroke in the right middle cerebral artery for which he required decompressive craniectomy. Shortly after the procedure, his hospital stay was complicated with fever and malaise. Ingestion of partially boiled cow's milk was noted from the history. Blood cultures were positive for Streptococcus pneumoniae and Brucella melitensis. Based on these results, he was diagnosed with pneumonia and brucellosis, and antibiotics were commenced for treatment. As a result of the stroke, the patient suffered from hemiplegia which left him bed-bound and shifted to a rehabilitation centre for continuity of care. There, the patient showed only minor improvements in speech, but none in mobility. Nevertheless, the family refused to transfer him to a multispecialty hospital that provides medical, surgical, and long-term care.

On November 20th, 2020, while the patient was still in the rehabilitation centre, his health started to deteriorate. He was found to be hypotensive with a blood pressure of 80/40, but afebrile with an oral temperature of 37.0°C. His heart rate and respiratory rate were 93 beats/minute and 18 breaths/minute, respectively. Physical examination revealed no skin changes over the ICD pocket, no cardiac murmurs on auscultation, and no apparent localized signs of infection. Blood tests revealed a normal white blood cell count (5 × 103 cells/mm^3) and high C-reactive protein level (77 mg/L). Blood cultures were positive for Brucella melitensis. These tests were followed with transthoracic echocardiography which showed a single oscillating mass measuring 0.8 × 0.4 cm attached to the tip of the right atrial lead of the ICD suggestive of vegetation (Figure 1).

The patient was then transferred to the Heart Hospital as a case of relapsing brucellosis with brucella endocarditis and ICD-lead colonization. The Infectious Disease Team was consulted, and three-drug regimen was commenced including rifampicin (600 mg/day), gentamicin (5 mg/kg/day), and doxycycline (200 mg/day). Gentamicin was then increased to 7 mg/kg/day as the postdose peak levels were low, and trimethoprim/sulfamethoxazole (960 mg/12 h) was added to the treatment, with a recommendation to remove the ICD. A transesophageal echocardiography (TEE) was tried but was technically difficult to conduct due to the restricted neck movements and limited jaw mobility of the patient, which rendered the TEE probe impossible to insert. Therefore, a positron emission tomography (PET) scan was performed to confirm the nature of the vegetation, yet the results were being inconclusive.

The case was discussed in a multidisciplinary team (MDT) meeting, and all possibilities to deal with this infected ICD wires were explored. Due to the unavailability of laser-assisted lead extraction, surgery was proposed as an option; however, because of the patient's general condition, surgical removal was considered a high-risk procedure, and the final decision was to keep the ICD in place and to treat him conservatively with antibiotics. Another PET scan was requested that was also inconclusive, and a repeated echocardiogram revealed a slight increase in vegetative size (0.8 × 0.6 cm). Eventually, Gentamicin was stopped due to renal impairment.

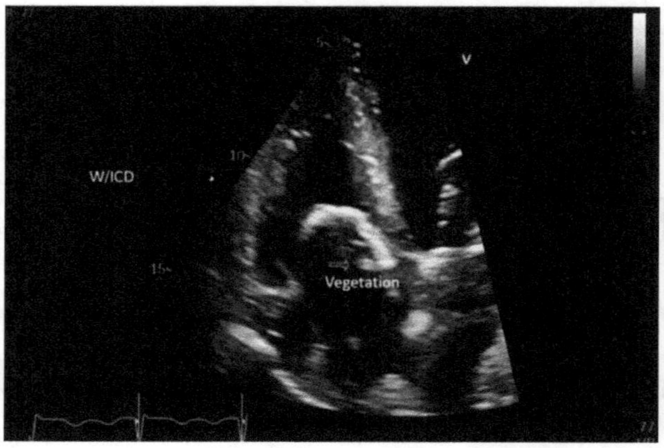

FIGURE 1: Vegetationson top of ICD lead. Transthoracic echocardiography, apical four-chamber view showing a large vegetation on the top of ICD atrial lead in a case of brucella endocarditis.

On December 17th, 2020, the patient was medically fit for discharge and was sent home with oral antibiotics for 6 weeks.

On March 29th, 2021, the patient was doing well and still on oral antibiotics.

3. Discussion

Brucella infective endocarditis is a rare and life-threatening complication of brucellosis. A systematic review assessing the clinical manifestations of brucellosis revealed brucellosis-associated endocarditis was prevalent in an overall 1% of patients [7]. Another study found that 1 in 23 CDRIE cases was caused by Brucella melitensis [15]. Nevertheless, despite its low prevalence and insidious progression, infective endocarditis is a very severe complication of brucellosis, and it has been reported in a few of Cardiac Device-Related Infective Endocarditis (CDRIE) cases. In our review of 14 published CDRBrE cases, we found that 11 patients were males, two were females, and one was unidentified, none of them with involvement of the device lead. Moreover, their ages ranged between 38 and 82 years old (Table 1).

Diagnosing brucellosis begins with an assessment of epidemiological factors. Our patient mentioned a history of drinking unpasteurized milk since childhood. A history of contact with animals (sheep and goats), consumption of dairy products, or consumption of uncooked meat was noted in several studies as a common trait of the majority of brucellosis patients [11, 12, 16–19]. An assay of blood, bone marrow, or other body fluids or tissue cultures are considered the gold standards for the diagnosis of brucellosis.

However, it is imperative to underscore that Brucella is a fastidious bacteria requires special culture media with a

Table 1: Case reports of brucellosis involving pacemakers and cardiac devices.

Study/year	Country	Gender	Age (years)	Type of device	Brucella relapse	Brucella blood culture	Miscellaneous cultures	Device and leads removed	Antibiotics	Treatment duration
de la Fuente et al. [28]	Spain	Male	63	Chamber end cavitary pacemaker	Yes	No	Pacemaker, leads, pus, necrotic tissue	Yes	Doxycycline Rifampin Streptomycin	45 days 45 days 21 days
Francia et al. [29]	Spain	Male	71	Pacemaker	Yes	No	Pacemaker and leads. Negative TEE	Yes	Doxycycline Rifampin	6 weeks 8 weeks
Ulkar et al. [12]	Turkey	Male	68	Pacemaker	No	Yes	Abscess culture	Yes	Doxycycline Rifampin	6 weeks 6 weeks
Miragliotta et al. [10]	Italy	Female	70	Single-chamber pacemaker	Yes	Yes	Cutaneous swab from fresh wound of recent removal and replacement of pacemaker	No	Rifampicin Ciprofloxacin Minocycline	6 weeks 6 weeks 6 weeks
Dourakis et al. [17]	Greece	Male	70	ICD	Yes	Yes	TEE showed mass on tricuspid, pacemaker, and leads had vegetation	Yes	Doxycycline Ciprofloxacin Rifampin	12 months 12 months 12 months
Al-Majid [13]	Saudi Arabia	Male	38	Pacemaker	Yes	Yes	Leads	Yes	Doxycycline Rifampin	6 weeks 6 weeks
Gungor et al. [14]	Turkey	Male	61	Pacemaker	No	Yes	Ultrasonography revealed an abscess and a fistula. Cultures from sputum samples, drained materials from the abscess, and the pacemaker pocket	Yes	Doxycycline Rifampin	6 weeks 6 weeks
Osmonov et al. [15]	Turkey	N/A	N/A	Pacemaker	N/A	Yes	Lead culture TEE showed vegetation	Yes	N/A	6 weeks
Elmardi et al. [16]	Saudi Arabia	Female	54	ICD	No	No	TEE showed large masses attached to all leads. Culture from pocket fluid and tissues	Yes	N/A	N/A
	Saudi Arabia	Male	52	Single-chamber ICD	Yes	No	Culture from pocket tissue	Yes	Cotrimoxazole Doxycycline Gentamicin	N/A
Al-Adsani and Al-Mousa [11]	Kuwaiti	Male	70	Pacemaker	No	Yes	Transthoracic echo showed calcification and thickening of the aortic valve with two mobile masses attached to the aortic valve. TEE was unremarkable.	No	Doxycycline Rifampin Cotrimoxazole Gentamicin	3 months 3 months 3 months 2 weeks
Dhand and Ross [18]	United States	Male	66	ICD	No	No	Cultures from superficial specimen, tissue from the pocket, ICD, and leads	Yes	Gentamicin Ciprofloxacin Doxycycline	6 weeks 6 weeks
Enjalbert et al. [30]	France	Male	65	ICD	N/A	No	Culture from device	Yes	N/A	N/A
Kanji and Saxinger [19]	Canada	Male	82	Pacemaker	No	No	Cultures from leads and ventricular tissue	Yes	Gentamicin Doxycycline Rifampin	12 weeks 12 weeks

variable and more prolonged incubation period, which could justify why only seven patients had positive blood cultures (Table 1). There are multiple serological tests used to diagnose brucellosis, with the most common being the serum agglutination test. In general, agglutination titres ≥ 1 : 160 are considered diagnostic, although a titre of ≥1 : 320 is considered diagnostic in endemic areas. Enzyme-linked immunosorbent assay (ELISA) is another popular serological method used to diagnose brucellosis. ELISA detects total Brucella immune-specific IgM, IgA, and IgG immunoglobulins [20–22].

Optimal management of CDRIE should include removal of the whole device and prolonged antibiotic therapy to eradicate the pathogen from the body, especially in the presence of unusual organisms such as Brucella melitensis. This treatment is also recommended when CDRIE is suspected in the case of occult infections without any known source of disease [9]. Considering the inherent risk of an open surgical operation, our patient was deemed a high-risk candidate for surgical device removal and medical management was adopted in place [23]. The same approach was reported in two other studies on brucella CDRIE with good outcomes. In both studies, the patients had an implanted pacemaker which was not removed, while they received medical treatment for brucellosis. Follow-up examination revealed that they were both in good condition without any remaining signs of infection, and no recurrence of the illness was reported (Table 1) [10, 11]. On the other hand, other studies show that medical therapy alone is associated with high risk of disease recurrence and mortality [24]. It remains to be seen in the near future whether our patient and the patients in the previous studies will remain disease-free [10, 11]. In most cases of brucella CDRIE, device removal and lead extraction followed by extended antibiotic therapy are required for the effective treatment of this disease (Table 1).

Nuclear studies such as positron emission tomography (PET) scan and single photon emission computed tomography (SPECT) are used in the diagnosis of the difficult cases of device-related endocarditis [25]; however, in our patient, the result of PET scan was inconclusive because of the intense physiologic left ventricular myocardial uptake, and the area of the right ventricle lead could not be evaluated.

The proposed therapy for brucellosis endocarditis by the European Society of Cardiology (ESC) includes doxycycline (200 mg/24 h), cotrimoxazole (trimethoprim and sulfamethoxazole) (960 mg/12 h), and rifampin (300–600/24 h) for 3–6 months, with some recommending gentamicin to be added for the first 3 weeks, while the addition of streptomycin (15 mg/kg/24 h in 2 doses) for the first few weeks is optional [9]. An alternative regimen includes doxycycline and rifampin for a total of 6 weeks, but this regimen shows a higher failure rate, and it is not recommended for osteoarticular disease [25]. The relapse rate in patients treated with the latter is 14.4% and 22.6% [26, 27]. In our case, we followed the recommendations of ESC and used a combination of rifampicin (600 mg/day), doxycycline (200 mg/day), septrin (trimethoprim and sulfamethoxazole) (960 mg/12 h), and gentamicin (7 mg/kg/day); the latter administered at a low dose for fear of renal impairment. Only one study adopted this medical management and reported good outcomes with no relapse up to date [11]. A study that reported multiple relapses used rifampicin (600 mg/day) and minocycline (100 mg bd), for 12 weeks; rifampicin (600 mg/day) and ciprofloxacin (500 mg bd), for 6 weeks; rifampicin (600 mg/day), trimethoprim-sulfamethoxazole (2 g intravenous bd), and minocycline (100 mg bd); rifampicin, ciprofloxacin, and minocycline, for 6 weeks, on 4 separate occasions for treatment [10].

Interestingly, brucella CDRIE can occur practically at any time after device implantation, where relapse of brucella CDRIE was noted in six cases as well as in our patient (Table 1) [10, 13, 16, 17, 28, 29]. Routine follow-ups should be a requirement in cases of systemic brucella infection to avoid overlooking the rare complication of relapsing infective endocarditis. This must be implemented in the care plan of our patient and any future patients when surgical intervention is impractical.

4. Conclusion

The present case report highlights the possibility of brucella being an agent that can complicate the placement of an ICD. A high degree of awareness of the possibility of colonization of implanted devices with brucella in patients residing in endemic regions is fundamental for early laboratory recognition of this virulent pathogen to ameliorate the course of the disease. Routine follow-ups must be conducted on patients with ICD recovering from brucellosis who are not good candidates for surgical management.

Abbreviations

ME: Middle East
CDRIE: Cardiac Device-Related Infective Endocarditis
ICD: Implantation of cardioverter defibrillator
CRT-D: Cardiac resynchronization therapy device
TEE: Transesophageal echocardiography
PET: Positron emission tomography
ESC: European Society of Cardiology.

Consent

Written consent was obtained from the patient.

Acknowledgments

We are thankful to the management of Hamad Medical Corporation for the support.

References

[1] K. A. Franc, R. C. Krecek, B. N. Häsler, and A. M. Arenas-Gamboa, "Brucellosis remains a neglected disease in the developing world: a call for interdisciplinary action," *BMC Public Health*, vol. 18, no. 1, p. 125, 2018.

[2] H. Wyatt, "Lessons from the history of brucellosis," *Revue Scientifique et Technique de l'OIE*, vol. 32, no. 1, pp. 17–25, 2013.

[3] F. George, "Update on laboratory diagnosis of human brucellosis," *International Journal of Antimicrobial Agents*, vol. 36, Supplemnt 1, pp. S12–S17, 2010.

[4] B. Mantur, S. Amarnath, and R. J. Shinde, "Review of clinical and laboratory features of human brucellosis," *Indian Journal of Medical Microbiology*, vol. 25, no. 3, pp. 188–202, 2007.

[5] D. L. Heymann, *Control of communicable diseases manual: an official report of the American Public Health Association*, World Health Organization/American Public Health Association, Washington DC, 18th edition, 2004.

[6] F. María Pía, M. Maximilian, R. Gilman, and H. J. L. I. D. Smits, "Human brucellosis," *The Lancet*, vol. 7, no. 12, pp. 775–786, 2007.

[7] A. S. Dean, L. Crump, H. Greter, J. Hattendorf, E. Schelling, and J. J. P. N. T. D. Zinsstag, "Clinical manifestations of human brucellosis: a systematic review and meta-analysis," *PLoS Neglected Tropical Diseases*, vol. 6, no. 12, article e1929, 2012.

[8] G. Pappas, N. Akritidis, M. Bosilkovski, and E. Tsianos, "Brucellosis," *The New England Journal of Medicine*, vol. 352, no. 22, pp. 2325–2336, 2005.

[9] G. Habib, P. Lancellotti, M. J. Antunes et al., "2015 ESC guidelines for the management of infective endocarditis," *European Heart Journal*, vol. 36, no. 44, pp. 3075–3128, 2015.

[10] G. Miragliotta, A. Mosca, G. Tantimonaco, R. De Nittis, R. Antonetti, and A. J. I. H. J. Di Taranto, "Relapsing brucellosis related to pacemaker infection," *Italian Heart Journal*, vol. 6, no. 7, pp. 612-613, 2005.

[11] W. al-Adsani, A. Ahmad, and M. al-Mousa, "A case of *Brucella melitensis* endocarditis in a patient with cardiovascular implantable electronic device," *Infection and drug resistance*, vol. 11, pp. 387–390, 2018.

[12] U. G. Ulkar, T. Demiray, H. Aydoğan, Z. Dansuk, C. Kocakavak, and A. Mert, "Pacemaker infection due to Brucella melitensis: a case report," *Archives of internal medicine*, vol. 161, no. 15, pp. 1910-1911, 2001.

[13] F. M. Al-Majid, "Pacemaker lead endocarditis due to Brucellosis," *Saudi Medical Journal*, vol. 31, no. 4, pp. 448–450, 2010.

[14] O. Gungor, M. Yalcin, E. Ozel, K. Biberoglu, and K. Topal, "Pacemaker infection due to Brucella melitensis," *Hippokratia*, vol. 16, no. 4, pp. 390-391, 2012.

[15] D. Osmonov, K. S. Ozcan, I. Erdinler et al., "Cardiac device-related endocarditis: 31-years' experience," *Journal of Cardiology*, vol. 61, no. 2, pp. 175–180, 2013.

[16] M. Elmardi, Y. al Hebaishi, S. al Kassab et al., "Implantable cardioverter device infection due to *Brucella melitensis* in two patients," *Hellenic Journal of Cardiology*, vol. 57, no. 4, pp. 271-272, 2016.

[17] S. Dourakis, H. Sambatakou, D. Tsiachris, N. Kittou, A. Alexopoulou, and A. J. Archimandritis, "A 70-year-old stock-breeder with tricuspid valve and defibrillator lead brucella endocarditis," *International Journal of Cardiology*, vol. 126, no. 3, pp. e47–e49, 2008.

[18] A. Dhand and J. J. Ross, "Implantable cardioverter-defibrillator infection due to Brucella melitensis: case report and review of brucellosis of cardiac devices," *Clinical Infectious Diseases*, vol. 44, no. 4, pp. e37–e39, 2007.

[19] J. N. Kanji and L. J. C. Saxinger, "*Brucella* infection at cardiac pacemaker site in a patient who had consumed raw caribou meat in Northern Canada," *CMAJ*, vol. 190, no. 37, pp. E1108–E1110, 2018.

[20] M. P. Franco, M. Mulder, R. H. Gilman, and H. G. Smits, "Human brucellosis," *The Lancet*, vol. 7, no. 12, pp. 775–786, 2007.

[21] D. Kasper and A. Fauci, "Harrison's Infectious Diseases," *McGraw-Hill Education*, pp. 560–564, 2017, 3rd edition.

[22] A. del Río, I. Anguera, J. M. Miró et al., "Surgical treatment of pacemaker and defibrillator lead endocarditis: the impact of electrode lead extraction on outcome," *Chest*, vol. 124, no. 4, pp. 1451–1459, 2003.

[23] T. M. Peery and L. F. Belter, "Brucellosis and heart disease: II. Fatal brucellosis: a review of the literature and report of new cases," *The American Journal of Pathology*, vol. 36, no. 6, pp. 673–697, 1960.

[24] J. Solís García del Pozo and J. Solera, "Systematic review and meta-analysis of randomized clinical trials in the treatment of human brucellosis," *PLoS One*, vol. 7, no. 2, article e32090, 2012.

[25] P. A. Erba, P. Lancellotti, I. Vilacosta et al., "Recommendations on nuclear and multimodality imaging in IE and CIED infections," *European Journal of Nuclear Medicine and Molecular Imaging*, vol. 45, no. 10, pp. 1795–1815, 2018.

[26] O. Karabay, I. Sencan, D. Kayas, and I. Şahin, "Ofloxacin plus rifampicin versus doxycycline plus rifampicin in the treatment of brucellosis: a randomized clinical trial [ISRCTN11871179]," *BMC Infectious Diseases*, vol. 4, no. 1, p. 18, 2004.

[27] A. Hasanain, R. Mahdy, A. Mohamed, and M. Ali, "A randomized, comparative study of dual therapy (doxycycline-rifampin) versus triple therapy (doxycycline-rifampin-levofloxacin) for treating acute/subacute brucellosis," *The Brazilian Journal of Infectious Diseases*, vol. 20, no. 3, pp. 250–254, 2016.

[28] A. de la Fuente, J. R. Sanchez, J. Uriz, J. Reparaz, J. L. Lopez-Coronado, and I. J. T. H. I. J. Moriones, "Infection of a pacemaker by Brucella melitensis," *Texas Heart Institute Journal*, vol. 24, no. 2, pp. 129-130, 1997.

[29] E. Francia, P. Domingo, M. A. Sambeat et al., "Pacemaker infection by Brucella melitensis: a rare cause of relapsing brucellosis," *Archives of Internal Medicine*, vol. 160, no. 21, pp. 3327-3328, 2000.

[30] L. Enjalbert, N. Moatti, G. Chabanon, P. Castany, and P. Gaurand, "The cardiac pacemaker and melitococcus," *La Nouvelle Presse Médicale*, vol. 6, no. 4, p. 277, 1977.

15

Out-of-Hospital Cardiac Arrest due to Coronary Spasm with Recurrent Ventricular Fibrillation

Vrijraj Sinhji Rathod, Tanmay Kanitkar, and Grigoris Karamasis

Essex Cardiothoracic Centre, Basildon University Hospital, Nethermayne, Basildon, UK SS16 5NL

Correspondence should be addressed to Vrijraj Sinhji Rathod; vrijraj.rathod@btuh.nhs.uk, Tanmay Kanitkar; tkanitkar@gmail.com, and Grigoris Karamasis; grigoris.karamasis@btuh.nhs.uk

Academic Editor: Antonio de Padua Mansur

We present a case of ventricular fibrillation (VF) secondary to ischaemia induced by coronary artery spasm. An 82-year-old man initially presented with an out-of-hospital VF arrest. On return of spontaneous circulation (ROSC), he was found to be in fast atrial fibrillation (AF); an invasive coronary angiogram revealed unobstructed coronary arteries. During his hospital stay, he developed chest pain, with concomitant ST elevation on ECG (electrocardiogram), which spontaneously resolved. A repeat coronary angiography revealed coronary spasm. Later, he had further ST elevation resulting in ventricular fibrillation. It became clear his initial presentation was most likely due to coronary vasospasm rather than a plaque-rupture or ventricular scar-related event, and he was thus successfully treated with multiple vasodilators and an implantable cardiac defibrillator. This case report highlights how conventional imaging modalities may not always lead to a diagnosis.

1. Introduction

Coronary artery spasm resulting in arrhythmia is a rare but recognised cause of syncope and sudden cardiac death [1]. However, if the coronary artery spasm does not cause chest pain, the diagnosis and management are very difficult. Diagnosis of the silent coronary artery spasm is possible if the attack occurs under ECG monitoring; however, it may not occur during ambulatory monitoring or during exercise testing. Long-term surveillance such as repeated ambulatory Holter ECGs or an implantable loop recording may be needed to establish the diagnosis. Since calcium channel blockers (CCB) do not eliminate the risk of further events, combination therapy with CCB and an implantable cardioverter defibrillator (ICD) may be appropriate.

2. Case Report

An 82-year-old man presented with an out-of-hospital VF arrest. He reportedly felt very unwell whilst in a supermarket, before suffering from angina and collapsing. He was promptly attended by an ambulance crew who found he was initially in fast AF whilst conscious, before descending into VF, requiring cardiac pulmonary resuscitation (CPR) and subsequent DC cardioversion (DCCV). ROSC was achieved after 10 minutes, where he was found to be in fast AF with anterior ST elevation on ECG, resulting in a HEMS (Helicopter Emergency Medicine Service) transfer for possible primary percutaneous coronary intervention. His cardiovascular risk factors included hypertension, possible previously untreated MI, type 2 diabetes mellitus, previous smoker, and poor compliance with all medication whilst also suffering longstanding chronic obstructive pulmonary disease (COPD). On angiography, he was found to have non-flow limiting moderate plaque disease in the left anterior descending artery (LAD), with no significant atheroma in the other coronary arteries. He was thus returned to the ward, clinically stable and without any coronary intervention. Furthermore, his troponin T results suggested he had not suffered a myocardial infarction, rising from an initial 44 to just 48 units (3 and 6 hours, normal < 14 units), which could be explained by fast AF, CPR, or DCCV—in combination or alone. His resting ECG (electrocardiogram) showed T wave inversion in the anterior leads suggesting previous

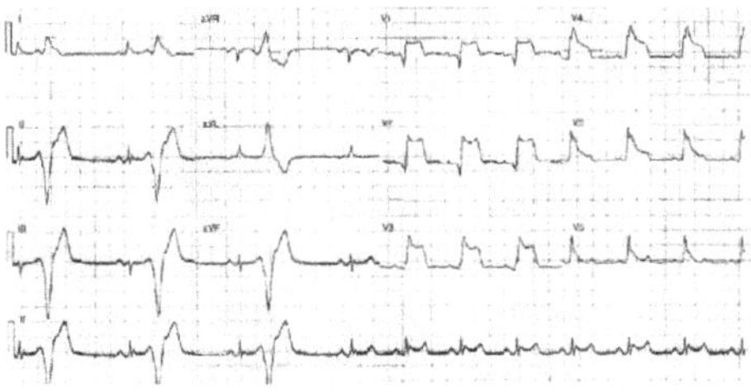

FIGURE 1: ECG showing ST elevation in the anterior leads while the patient was experiencing chest pain.

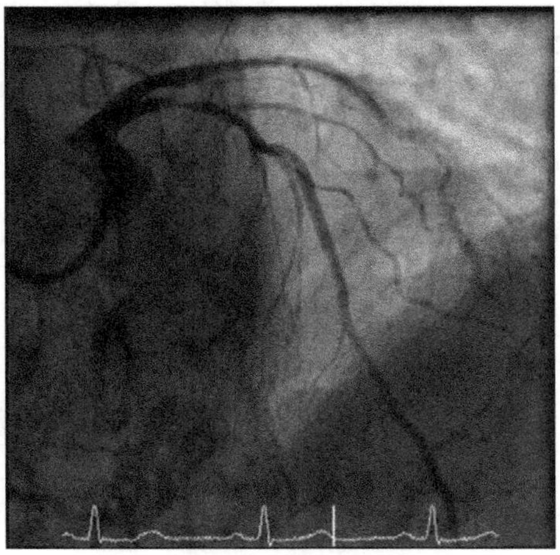

FIGURE 2: Coronary angiogram illustrating spasm in the LAD.

myocardial insult. His electrolytes were all within range, with a potassium of 4.1 mmol/l, sodium of 137 mmol/l, and magnesium of 0.9 mmol/l. His Creatinine was 100 μmol/l and glucose was 7.1 mmol/l. A cardiac MRI was carried out, which identified a left ventricle scar that can be a plausible explanation for his initial VF arrest, with MI unlikely due to a lack of surrounding oedema and reasonable LV contractility. During his stay in the ward, he had further chest pain and ST elevation (Figure 1) in the anterior leads which self-resolved. On subsequent review of his angiographic images, the consensus was he should have a further coronary angiogram with a pressure wire study to the LAD. During the angiogram, the LAD went into coronary spasm (Figure 2) which was associated with further chest pain and ST elevation, which resolved once IV nitrates were administrated through the coronary catheter (Figure 3). He was clinically stable throughout the procedure and returned to the ward for a provisional plan to implant an ICD. He suffered three further VF arrests that same night, which made clear the diagnosis. Each episode of VF was preceded by both chest pain and significant ST elevation in anterior leads before descending into VF (Figure 4), which was terminated by prompt DCCV. The following morning, an ICD was inserted with concomitant vasodilator therapy started. He received a combination of diltiazem and bisoprolol, which he tolerated well and remained stable on. He was discharged soon after, with no shocks delivered by his ICD and no further episodes of chest pain in the ward.

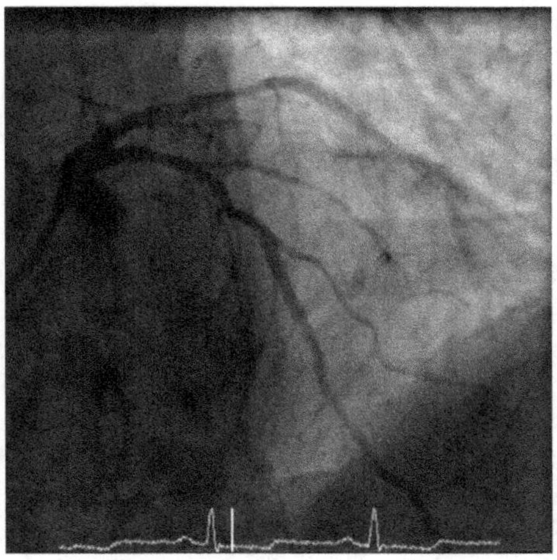

FIGURE 3: After administration of IV nitrates and resolution of the narrowing in the LAD.

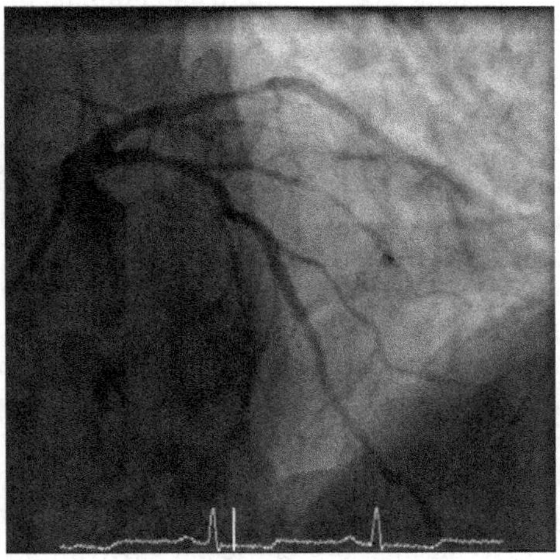

FIGURE 4: Ventricular fibrillation.

3. Discussion

Cardiac ischaemia secondary to coronary spasm is a well-known pathology, but risk of developing ventricular arrhythmia from the sequela is still rare. Like our patient, who was initially admitted with VF and subsequently had mild coronary artery disease on an angiogram and no structural heart disease on imaging, it can be challenging to establish coronary spasm as the underlying substrate for ventricular arrhythmia. Conventionally, these patients have a low recurrence rate; hence, these patients are given a presumed diagnosis on clinical suspicion or misdiagnosed to a have small thromboembolic phenomenon that leads to the event. Fortunately, this patient had a recurrence of his symptoms during his admission, and we were able to identify the underlying aetiology on a repeat coronary angiogram. Even though this case has been described before, this case gave us a rare opportunity to correlate the clinical features of coronary spasm to angiography findings.

An observation study of patients with ICD implants because of out-of-hospital cardiac arrests secondary to coronary spasm had no events in the 5-year follow-up [2].

Kobayashi et al. have previously published that vasogenic coronary spasm was the precipitant of ventricular arrhythmia in 7% of patients suffering from out hospital cardiac arrests [3]. Matsue et al. followed 23 patients who had out-of-hospital VF/VT arrests and then underwent an ICD implant. These patients had no structural heart disease or obstructive coronary disease but did have coronary spasm with acetylcholine change. After a follow-up of nearly 3 years, 4 patients had experienced a further episode of VF which activated their device and prevented sudden death [4]. Interestingly, the median time to first appropriate shock was 2.9 years.

A Japanese registry consisting of 1429 patients with coronary spasms included 35 patients with VF as a primary manifestation of their coronary spasm, 14 patients had an ICD implant, and 2 patients from the ICD implant group had appropriate shock. They also discovered that patients who had their medication discontinued or reduced were more at risk of sudden cardiac death and nonfatal myocardial infarction [5].

The above data corroborates the risk of further ventricular arrhythmias in this group of patients. Currently, calcium channel blockers and smoking cessation are main forms of therapy for coronary spasm and angina episodes [6]. There is no randomised multicentre trial which has compared the ICD implant with medical therapy versus medical therapy alone. Aoki et al. reported a 0.6% per year rate of cardiac arrest in patients only receiving medical therapy for coronary spasm [7]. The above data constructs an overwhelming case of significant risk of cardiac arrest in this cohort of patients; therefore, a clinical trial consisting of an arm receiving only medical therapy would be deemed unethical. We have retrospective cohort studies which have emphasised the high degree of reoccurrence of ventricular arrhythmia patients with coronary spasm, but these events occur after 12 months of the primary event. Our case is unique because the patient had multiple episodes of spasm within a short period of time and gave us the opportunity of capturing the aetiology on angiography.

Additional Points

Learning Points. (i) Coronary spasm is not a benign pathology, and patients should be assessed for reoccurrence and risk for sudden cardiac death. (ii) Medical therapy plays a vital role in preventing further cardiac arrhythmias, but an ICD should be considered. (iii) Coronary spasm should be considered as a differential diagnosis for VF in individuals with unobstructed coronary arteries.

References

[1] C. Meune, L. M. Joly, J. D. Chiche et al., "Diagnosis and management of out-of-hospital cardiac arrest secondary to coronary artery spasm," *Resuscitation*, vol. 58, no. 2, pp. 145–152, 2003.

[2] Y. Yamashina, T. Yagi, A. Namekawa et al., "Favorable outcomes of patients with vasospastic angina associated with cardiac arrest," *Journal of Cardiology*, vol. 63, no. 1, pp. 41–45, 2014.

[3] N. Kobayashi, N. Hata, T. Shimura et al., "Characteristics of patients with cardiac arrest caused by coronary vasospasm," *Circulation Journal*, vol. 77, no. 3, pp. 673–678, 2013.

[4] Y. Matsue, M. Suzuki, M. Nishizaki, R. Hojo, Y. Hashimoto, and H. Sakurada, "Clinical implications of an implantable cardioverter-defibrillator in patients with vasospastic angina and lethal ventricular arrhythmia," *Journal of the American College of Cardiology*, vol. 60, no. 10, pp. 908–913, 2012.

[5] Y. Takagi, S. Yasuda, R. Tsunoda et al., "Clinical characteristics and long-term prognosis of vasospastic angina patients who survived out-of-hospital cardiac arrest: multicenter registry study of the Japanese Coronary Spasm Association," *Circulation: Arrhythmia and Electrophysiology*, vol. 4, no. 3, pp. 295–302, 2011.

[6] S. Stern and A. Bayes de Luna, "Coronary artery spasm: a 2009 update," *Circulation*, vol. 119, no. 18, pp. 2531–2534, 2009.

[7] M. Aoki, S. Koyanagi, K. Sakai et al., "Exercise-induced silent myocardial ischemia in patients with vasospastic angina," *American Heart Journal*, vol. 119, no. 3, pp. 551–556, 1990.

16

Ventricular Rupture due to Myocardial Infarction without Obstructive Coronary Artery Disease

Hendrik Lapp,[1] Marcel Keßler,[1] Thomas Rock,[1] Franz X. Schmid,[2] Dong-In Shin,[1] Alexander Bufe,[1,3] Heinrich G. Klues,[1] and Christian Blockhaus[1]

[1]*Department of Cardiology, Heart Centre Niederrhein, Helios Clinics Krefeld, Germany*
[2]*Department of Cardiothoracic Surgery, Heart Centre Niederrhein, Helios Clinics Krefeld, Germany*
[3]*University Witten/Herdecke, Germany*

Correspondence should be addressed to Hendrik Lapp; hendrik.lapp@ukbonn.de

Academic Editor: Antonio de Padua Mansur

An 87-year-old woman presenting with myocardial infarction and ST-segment elevation in the electrocardiogram suffered from pericardial effusion due to left ventricular rupture. After ruling out obstructive coronary artery disease and aortic dissection, she underwent cardiac surgery showing typical infarct-macerated myocardial tissue in situ. This case shows that even etiologically unclear and small-sized myocardial infarctions can cause life-threatening mechanical complications.

1. Introduction

Ischaemic heart disease is the most common cause of death worldwide. In Europe, acute myocardial infarction with ST-segment elevation (STEMI) has an incidence of 43 to 144 per 100.000 per year [1]. Compared to heart failure due to myocardial dysfunction or arrhythmic events, mechanical complications are less prevalent but nevertheless life-threatening and often associated with a lethal outcome. The rates of in-hospital mortality in patients with mechanical complications after myocardial infarction are described to be higher than 40%, highlighting ventricular septal defect, papillary muscle rupture, and complete ventricular free wall rupture as main complications [2]. In either case, rapid and efficient cardiothoracic surgery is the state-of-the-art medical treatment. Here, we describe the case of a patient with left ventricular wall rupture after acute myocardial infarction without obstructive coronary artery disease.

2. Case Report

An 87-year-old woman was transferred to our emergency department presenting with acute myocardial infarction. After syncope followed by acute chest pain in the morning during geriatric attendance in an external hospital, the immediately recorded electrocardiogram (ECG) showed significant ST-segment elevations in leads I and aVL and corresponding ST-segment depressions in all other leads, mainly II, III, and aVF (Figure 1). Upon arrival in our chest pain unit at 9:53 a.m., emergency physical examination revealed the woman to be suffering from dyspnea (oxygen saturation 96% while 10 l oxygen flow) at rest and severe cardiogenic shock with sinus tachycardia (117 bpm) and hypotension (blood pressure 82/50 mmHg). Varying doses of catecholamines (dobutamine/norepinephrine) were required to preserve a stable haemodynamic state. The patient was vigilant and fully orientated at all times. Emergency echocardiography revealed reduced left ventricular function, ventricular hypertrophy, and significant pericardial effusion. Based on the primary diagnostics and case history, aortic dissection type Stanford A was immediately excluded by computer tomography (CT). Subsequently, the patient was transferred to the cardiac catheterization laboratory. The levels of meanwhile analyzed high-sensitive Troponin T and creatine kinase were 1498 pg/ml and 92 U/l, respectively, indicating severe myocardial damage. Upon arrival in the cardiac catheterization laboratory, the pericardial effusion was instantaneously drained due to progressive haemodynamic

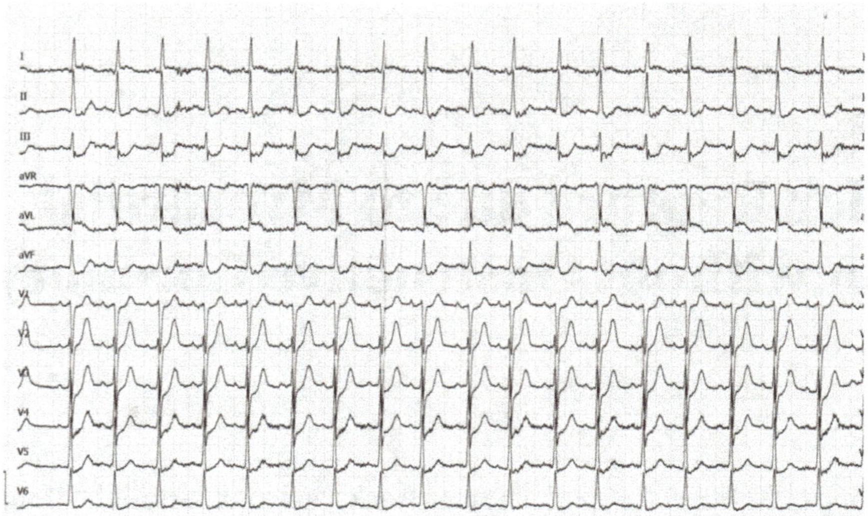

FIGURE 1: Initial ECG recording showing significant ST-segment elevations in leads I and aVL and corresponding ST-segment depressions in II, III, and aVF.

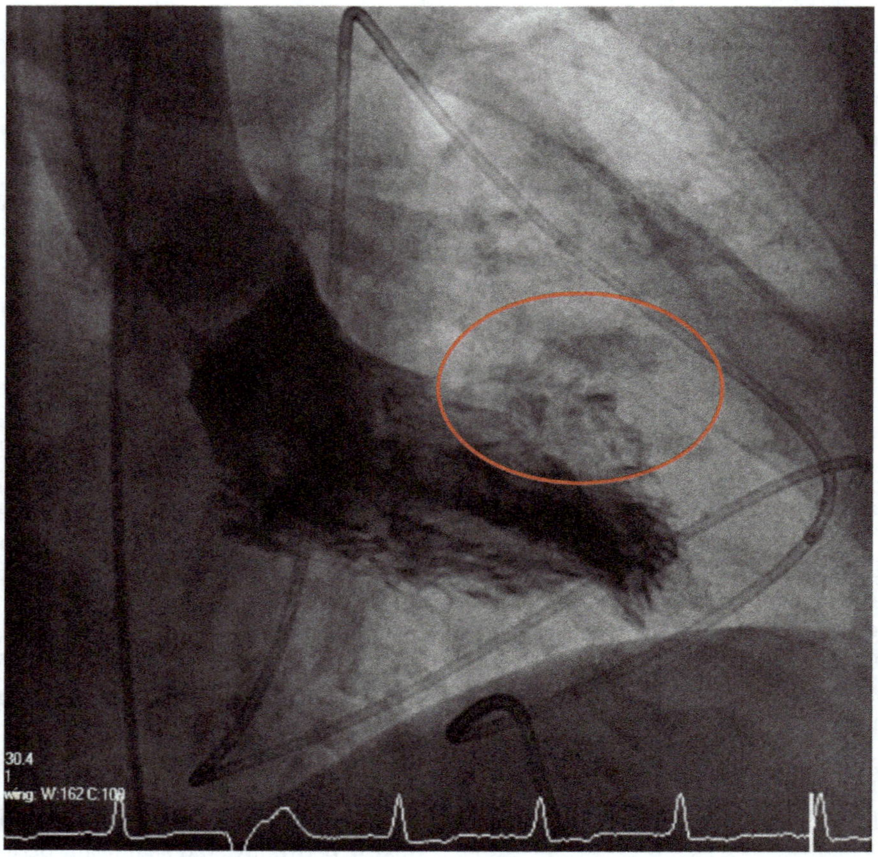

FIGURE 2: Laevocardiography showing evasion of contrast agent at the anterolateral ventricular wall.

instability. During further examination, the coronary arteries showed no signs of obstructive coronary artery disease, dissection, plaque rupture, or vasospasm. Invasive measurements demonstrated mid- to high-grade aortic stenosis. Laevocardiography revealed evasion of the contrast agent at the anterolateral ventricular wall due to ventricular rupture (Figure 2)—as already suspected in the initial computer tomography. After initial pericardiocentesis, the patient haemodynamic state showed a rapid deterioration, and increasing doses of vasopressors became necessary. Continuous pericardiocentesis with retransfusion of the blood over a 6F access in the femoral vein was necessary to obtain stable circulation followed by emergency transfer to our cardiothoracic surgery department for emergency surgery. After sternotomy and application of the heart-lung machine without complications, the left ventricular rupture in vivo showed signs of subsided myocardial infarction. The initially applied polypropylene sutures in the region of rupture were not sufficient due to macerated myocardial tissue after myocardial infarction. In a second attempt, the cardiac surgeons successfully used a bovine pericardial patch to cover the defect. After complex surgery taking several hours, active ventricular bleeding vanished and the patient was transferred to the cardiothoracic surgery intensive care unit. Subsequently, the patient demonstrated a dramatic and rapid increase of catecholaminergic substances without an adequate blood pressure response. On echocardiography, left ventricular function deteriorated finally leading to lethal cardiogenic shock within one hour after arrival at the cardiothoracic surgery intensive care unit.

3. Discussion

Ventricular rupture and overall mechanical complications after myocardial infarction are life-threatening events with high mortality. It occurs more frequently in elderly patients, females, or anterior infarctions often without previous symptoms of angina pectoris. There are three types of cardiac rupture described in literature [3]. Type I is an abrupt tear within the first 24 hours after myocardial infarction, type II is due to progressive myocardial damage, and type III is aneurysm-dependent wall thinning. Overall, the incidence declined significantly over the last decades with emerging primary coronary intervention [4]. Due to the rapid onset presenting with sudden hypotension, chest pain or cardiac murmurs after 2.6 days on average after acute myocardial infarction lethal outcomes remain still high [5]. Emergency echocardiography is the diagnostic tool of choice [1]. It is obvious that cardiothoracic surgery is the standard treatment, but powerful randomized controlled trials for best techniques and perioperative management are still missing. In smaller cohorts published by expert centers, it is suggested to cover the rupture site by autologous or synthetic pericardial patches in case of oozing bleedings, as well as the use of polypropylene sutures (direct suture techniques) in case of haemodynamically more challenging blowout bleedings [6]. Both state-of-the-art techniques were used in the presented case, but due to advanced macerated tissue, a sufficient cover of the rupture was challenging. Indeed, initial cardiac catheter examination exluded coronary artery disease and type I myocardial infarction [7] making spontaneous recanalization of plaque rupture unlikely, but there is evidence for myocardial infarction with nonobstructive coronary arteries (MINOCA) due to prolonged vasospasms, local thrombus formation, or embolization from other sites and for coronary microvascular dysfunction or obstruction potentially leading to small infarction size [8]. Only a few case reports of mechanical complications after myocardial infarction without coronary artery disease are published [9]. In the presented case, the exact underlying mechanism leading to myocardial infarction and subsequent cardiac rupture remains unclear; however, we suppose a temporary thrombotic occlusion is the most likely underlying pathology. Interestingly, in this case, emergency pericardiocentesis in the catheterization lab led to progressive haemodynamic deterioration. We suppose that an initial balance between LV hypertrophy, pericardial effusion, and tachycardia with autotamponading effect of the focal rupture in the hypertrophied myocardium may have occurred. This fragile haemodynamic stability was then abolished through the pericardiocentesis due to lowering external compression on the rupture site finally leading to progressive ventricular bleeding. In the literature, overall in-hospital survival rates between 38 and 78% are described [6], showing the current unpredictable influence of underlying pathology, patient-individual factors, comorbidities, time delay, and expertise of the center and the cardiothoracic surgeon.

4. Conclusion

At present, mechanical damages after myocardial infarction still remain a highly lethal complication. Ventricular rupture after MINOCA is a rare event but has to be kept in mind with the need for emergency, interdisciplinary and expert-based patient-focused individual treatment.

References

[1] B. Ibanez, S. James, S. Agewall et al., "2017 ESC guidelines for the management of acute myocardial infarction in patients presenting with ST-segment elevation: the task force for the management of acute myocardial infarction in patients presenting with ST-segment elevation of the European Society of Cardiology (ESC)," *European Heart Journal*, vol. 39, no. 2, pp. 119–177, 2018.

[2] A. Elbadawi, I. Y. Elgendy, K. Mahmoud et al., "Temporal trends and outcomes of mechanical complications in patients with acute myocardial infarction," *JACC. Cardiovascular Interventions*, vol. 12, no. 18, pp. 1825–1836, 2019.

[3] A. E. Becker and J. P. van Mantgem, "Cardiac tamponade. A study of 50 hearts," *European Journal of Cardiology*, vol. 3, no. 4, pp. 349–358, 1975.

[4] J. Figueras, O. Alcalde, J:. A. Barrabés et al., "Changes in hospital mortality rates in 425 patients with acute ST-elevation myocardial infarction and cardiac rupture over a 30-year period," *Circulation*, vol. 118, no. 25, pp. 2783–2789, 2008.

[5] F. Formica, S. D'Alessandro, and G. Singh, "Left ventricular free wall rupture after myocardial infarction: still a challenging complication," *The Journal of Thoracic and Cardiovascular Surgery*, vol. 158, no. 3, pp. e97–e98, 2019.

[6] F. Formica, S. Mariani, G. Singh et al., "Postinfarction left ventricular free wall rupture: a 17-year single-centre experience," *European Journal of Cardio-Thoracic Surgery*, vol. 53, no. 1, pp. 150–156, 2018.

[7] K. Thygesen, J. S. Alpert, A. S. Jaffe et al., "Fourth universal definition of myocardial infarction (2018)," *European Heart Journal*, vol. 40, no. 3, pp. 237–269, 2018.

[8] S. Pasupathy, T. Air, R. P. Dreyer, R. Tavella, and J. F. Beltrame, "Systematic review of patients presenting with suspected myocardial infarction and nonobstructive coronary arteries," *Circulation*, vol. 131, no. 10, pp. 861–870, 2015.

[9] C. P. Roth, M. Qarmali, S. H. Litovsky, and B. C. Brott, "Myocardial rupture after small acute myocardial infarction in the absence of coronary artery disease," *Cardiovascular Pathology*, vol. 37, pp. 26–29, 2018.

17

Conservative Treatment of Postinfarction Left Ventricular Free Wall Rupture

Anh Tuan Vo, Thu Trang Nguyen, Thanh Thuy Tran, and Dinh Hoang Nguyen

Department of Cardiovascular Surgery, University Medical Center, University of Medicine and Pharmacy at Ho Chi Minh City, Ho Chi Minh City, Vietnam

Correspondence should be addressed to Dinh Hoang Nguyen; nguyenhoangdinh@yahoo.com

Academic Editor: Ertugrul Ercan

Left ventricular free wall rupture is a fatal complication of acute myocardial infarction. Emergency surgical repair is usually indicated to treat this condition. However, in very high surgical risk cohort, conservative treatment can also be considered. We report a case of left ventricle pseudoaneurysm that was successfully treated conservatively in a 4-year period.

1. Introduction

Postinfarction rupture of the left ventricular free wall is a rare complication but often fatal. Emergent surgical repair is usually the treatment of choice. However, in very high-risk patient with stable hemodynamics, conservative therapy might also be an alternative therapy. We report a case of left ventricular free wall rupture that survived with medical treatment alone.

2. Case Report

An 87-year-old man was admitted to the emergency department of a local hospital due to orthopnea and severe retrosternal chest pain radiating to his jaw. The patient had a past history of myocardial infarction (10 years ago), paroxysmal atrial fibrillation, hypertension, type 2 diabetes mellitus, and stage D chronic obstructive pulmonary disease (COPD). After three days of medical treatment, the patient's condition did not improve; he was then transferred to our hospital.

On admission, the patient was conscious with a heart rate of 125 bpm, irregular rhythm, and blood pressure of 140/80 mmHg, and room air oxygen saturation was 93–95%. On physical examination, auscultation revealed irregular and distant heart sounds, radial and femoral pulses were normally detected, and breath sounds were good bilaterally. A 12-lead ECG showed an atrial fibrillation with moderate ventricular response, QS wave in V1–V4, and no ST elevation detected. Initial cardiac enzyme was found to be nearly normal with Troponin T level of 0.016 ng/mL and CKMB level of 28 U/L (normal range: <25 U/L).

Emergency transthoracic echocardiography (TTE) showed a massive pericardial effusion with maximum diameter of 38 mm without tamponade signs, mild mitral regurgitation, and severe left ventricular dysfunction with an ejection fraction of 27%. The anterolateral wall of the left ventricle near the apex was ruptured and the left ventricular chamber connected to the pericardium sac through a hole of 19 mm in diameter. The perforation was covered by a thrombus and thus created a false aneurysm with a diameter of 40 mm × 30 mm (Figure 1).

The patient and his family were informed about the critical situation. Due to the very high surgical risk, the family refused surgical treatment and accepted the risk of sudden death. The patient was discharged 3 days later, when his blood pressure and heart rate were stabilized (on July 2016). The medical treatment on discharge included low dose beta blocker and angiotensin-converting enzyme inhibitor (ACEi) to keep the systolic blood pressure around 100 mmHg. No anticoagulation/antiplatelet therapy was prescribed at this moment, and a prolonged bed rest was recommended.

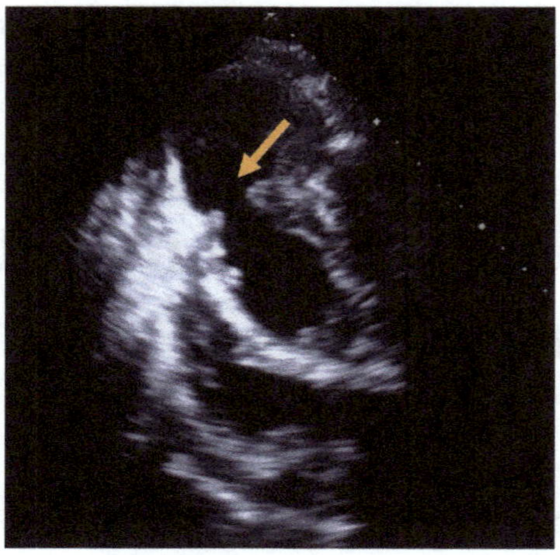

FIGURE 1: Left ventricular pseudoaneurysm formation, the perforation located at the apex with the size of 19 mm.

The patient was then followed up by a local cardiologist. Warfarin was initiated 6 months later, and the International normalized ratio (INR) was maintained around 2.0. After 45 months, the patient still survives the disease. He can now perform personal activities by himself. The last echocardiography performed on March 2020 showed that the pericardial effusion size decreased dramatically, and the old pseudoaneurysm was reinforced by a large thrombus in the pericardial sac. Color Doppler showed an active blood flow between the pseudoaneurysm and left ventricle (Figure 2).

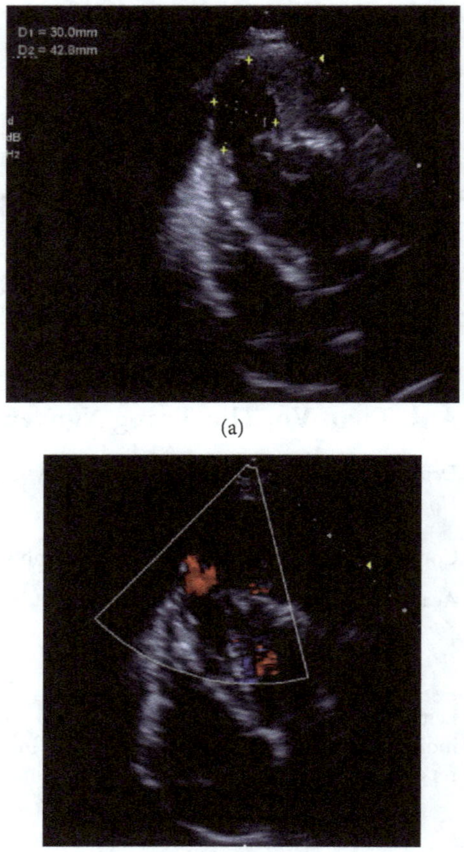

(a)

(b)

FIGURE 2: Four-chamber view TTE: the pseudoaneurysm did not change in the size (a) and active bloodstream to the pseudoaneurysm on color Doppler (b).

3. Discussion

Postinfarction rupture of the left ventricular free wall is a catastrophic complication. It consists of about 4.7% of myocardial infarction cases according to a report [1]. The incidence of ventricular rupture after myocardial infarction has reduced when percutaneous coronary intervention revascularization developed. The risk factors for postinfarction left ventricular free wall rupture include age greater than 60 years, female gender, preexisting hypertension, absence of left ventricular hypertrophy, first myocardial infarction, and midventricular or lateral wall transmural infarctions [2].

Rupture of anterolateral wall is not commonly seen. A case report of 290 patients with left ventricular pseudoaneurysms showed that the rupture located most commonly at posterior site (43%), followed by lateral (28%), apical (24%), inferior (19%), anterior (18%), and basal area (14%) [3].

Left ventricular rupture is the third cause of death in acute myocardial infarction, accounted for 4-24% among necropsy cases [4]. Nowadays, the surgical treatment is preferred to conservative treatment, but the postoperative mortality and morbidity remain high [5]. Medical treatment and less invasive modalities, such as percutaneous fibrin-glue injection, have also been reported, but the outcomes are still controversial [6]. Our patient survived the primary phase of left ventricular rupture owing to the subacute formation of a pseudoaneurysm rather than a blow-out rupture, which prevented the leakage of blood to the pericardial cavity. And medical treatment was decided based on lack of hemodynamic instability, advanced age, accompanying comorbidities, and substantially high surgical mortality. Conservative treatment included prolong bed rest, beta blockers, and strict blood pressure control to minimize the pseudoaneurysm rupture risk. However, the prognosis of this pseudoaneurysm is unpredictable, and sudden death can occur [6]. Nevertheless, he has no significant health issues after 4 years follow-up. Long-term survival was reported by Moreno et al., in a series of 10 patients, with a survival rate at 4 years as high as 74.1% [7]. On the other hand, the outcome of patients with this condition treated conservatively has been assumed to be poor, with a 2-year mortality of around 50% in one series [8].

In conclusion, postinfarction left ventricular rupture is a usually fatal condition, and surgery is the treatment of choice with a fairly high morbidity and mortality. In very high-risk patient, conservative treatment could be considered, but the long-term outcome is unpredictable.

References

[1] R. E. London and S. B. London, "Rupture of the heart," *Circulation*, vol. 31, no. 2, pp. 202–208, 1965.

[2] K. P. Batts, D. M. Ackermann, and W. D. Edwards, "Postinfarction rupture of the left ventricular free wall: clinicopathologic correlates in 100 consecutive autopsy cases," *Human Pathology*, vol. 21, no. 5, pp. 530–535, 1990.

[3] C. Frances, A. Romero, and D. Grady, "Left ventricular pseudoaneurysm," *Journal of the American College of Cardiology*, vol. 32, no. 3, pp. 557–561, 1998.

[4] S. G. Reddy and W. C. Roberts, "Frequency of rupture of the left ventricular free wall or ventricular septum among necropsy cases of fatal acute myocardial infarction since introduction of coronary care units," *American Journal of Cardiology*, vol. 63, no. 13, pp. 906–911, 1989.

[5] M. Matteucci, D. Fina, F. Jiritano et al., "Treatment strategies for post-infarction left ventricular free-wall rupture," *European Heart Journal Acute Cardiovascular Care*, vol. 8, no. 4, pp. 379–387, 2019.

[6] A. Nasir, M. Gouda, A. Khan, and A. Bose, "Is it ever possible to treat left ventricular free wall rupture conservatively?," *Interactive Cardiovascular and Thoracic Surgery*, vol. 19, no. 3, pp. 488–493, 2014.

[7] R. Moreno, E. Gordillo, J. Zamorano et al., "Long term outcome of patients with postinfarction left ventricular pseudoaneurysm," *Heart*, vol. 89, no. 10, pp. 1144–1146, 2003.

[8] K. Csapo, L. Voith, T. Szuk, I. Edes, and D. J. Kereiakes, "Postinfarction left ventricular pseudoaneurysm," *Clinical Cardiology*, vol. 20, no. 10, pp. 898–903, 1997.

18

A Steep Increase in the HeartLogic Index Predicts COVID-19 Disease in an Advanced Heart Failure Patient

Ward Heggermont,[1,2] Pham Anh Hong Nguyen,[3] Chirik-Wah Lau,[1] and Kurt Tournoy[3,4]

[1]*Cardiovascular Research Center, Department of Cardiology, OLV Ziekenhuis Aalst-Asse-Ninove, Aalst, Belgium*
[2]*Cardiovascular Research Institute Maastricht, Maastricht, Netherlands*
[3]*Department of Respiratory Medicine, OLV Ziekenhuis Aalst-Asse-Ninove, Aalst, Belgium*
[4]*Faculty of Medicine and Life Sciences, Ghent University, Ghent, Belgium*

Correspondence should be addressed to Ward Heggermont; ward.heggermont@olvz-aalst.be

Academic Editor: Takatoshi Kasai

We present a patient with severe nonischemic cardiomyopathy in whom the HeartLogic algorithm was activated on her Boston Scientific cardioverter defibrillator. She had an out-of-alert state for several months and had clinically "stable" heart failure with no hospitalizations in the last 6 months. A sudden and fast increase of the HeartLogic index preceded her presentation in the emergency ward by several days. The detailed readout of HeartLogic however had some atypical features for heart failure decompensation. The patient presented at the emergency department with an increased dyspnea and a dry cough. Clinical exam showed desaturation and was suggestive for an acute respiratory infection. Subsequent imaging with CT thorax and nasopharyngeal real-time polymerase chain reaction (RT-PCR) confirmed SARS-CoV-2 viral pneumonia (COVID-19). This case illustrates that a timely and detailed analysis of HeartLogic alerts could help in the early differentiation of disease in patients with severe heart failure.

1. Introduction

The COVID-19 pandemic, caused by SARS-Coronavirus-2 (SARS-CoV-2), is rapidly changing our daily clinical practice around the globe [1]. Due to restrictions in normal clinical practice and the reservation of crucial hospital and physician's capacity to treat critically ill COVID-19 patients, a shift from routine ambulatory follow-up consultations to focused patient contacts based on disease severity, telemedicine, and device-based monitoring is being observed [2].

Remote monitoring of patients with internal cardioverter defibrillators (ICDs) and cardiac resynchronization therapy (CRT-pacing or CRT-defibrillator) is already common these days [3]. However, these devices also increasingly allow for device-based telemonitoring of the patient's disease state, especially for heart failure. Older examples of these kinds of applications are OptiVol and CorVue [4, 5]. Recently, HeartLogic emerged as a potent predictor of impending heart failure decompensation [6–11].

HeartLogic (HL) is a multiparametric algorithm that combines different device-based features (first and third heart sounds, thoracic impedance, respiratory rate, tidal volume, tidal volume variation, heart rate, and physical activity) into a single alert number. A predefined threshold, standard set at 16, defines whether the patient is in "cardiac homeostasis"—usually referred to as an euvolemic state in heart failure (index below 16), versus whether an impending heart failure episode is about to happen (index of 16 or more). However, HL holds promise to be useful for the early detection of alternative diagnoses besides cardiac decompensation. Here, we present a case in which a sudden and steep increase of HeartLogic with atypical features of heart failure decompensation increased the suspicion for an alternative diagnosis and helped in the early detection of a severe COVID-19 pneumonia. To

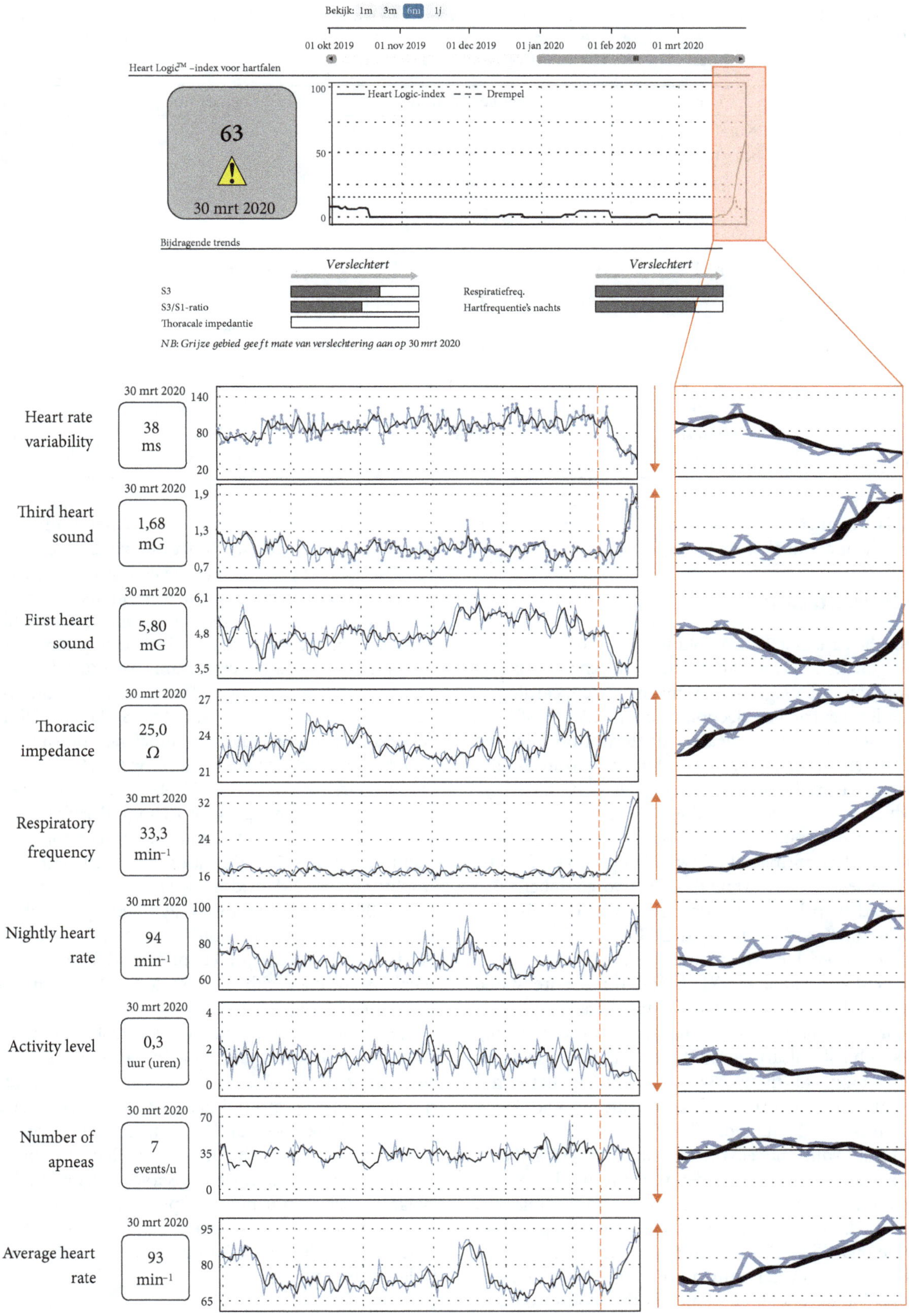

Figure 1: Overview of HeartLogic general evolution and contributing trends. Here, the general evolution of HL parameters is shown with a rapid and steep increase in the last seven days. It is observed that the third heart sound (S3), respiratory frequency, and nightly heart rate contribute to the increased HL index. Also, surprisingly, thoracic impedance rapidly increases. In contrast, heart rate variability and activity level significantly decreased. Also, due to the increased respiratory frequency, the number of apneas decreased.

TABLE 1: Overview of blood work parameters and comparison with reference blood work upon last ambulatory cardiology consultation. The last outpatient visit was six months before the admission to the emergency ward, and the patient was in NYHA class II heart failure without signs of decompensation at that time.

Parameter	Unit	Emergency ward	Last consultation	Reference value
WBC count	Number/mcL	3520	4250	4000-10000
Lymphocytes	Number/mcL	930	—	1200-3600
D-dimer	mcg/L	4607	—	<500
Hemoglobin	g/dL	11.8	10.9	12-16
INR	—	1.2	1.0	0.8-1.2
NT-pro-BNP	ng/L	2503	1757	<125
LDH	IU/L	301	—	135-250
CRP	mg/L	70.6	8.5	<5.0
Glucose	mg/dL	98	—	<100
Creatinine	mg/dL	1.06	0.75	<0.90
eGFR	mL/min	51	76	>90
Sodium	mmol/L	137.6	142.6	135-145
Potassium	mmol/L	4.4	4.24	3.5-4.9

date, this is the first case in which COVID-19 disease is revealed by the individual HeartLogic parameters.

2. Case Presentation

We present the case of a 72-year-old woman (nonsmoker) of African origin. In 2017, an idiopathic nonischemic dilated cardiomyopathy was diagnosed by means of echocardiography, with a left ventricular ejection fraction (LVEF) of 25%. Subsequent left and right heart catheterization revealed normal coronary arteries. The only known cardiovascular risk factor she had at the time of diagnosis was arterial hypertension which was treated accordingly. Magnetic resonance imaging revealed strong suspicion of left ventricular noncompaction and confirmed the low LVEF of 28%. Genetic analysis revealed no abnormalities. A two-chamber ICD was implanted in primary prevention. It was on this ICD (Boston Scientific G447 LV-plugged CRT-D) that the HeartLogic feature was enabled since June 2018.

The patient was stable in NYHA class II for more than 6 months under the following heart failure therapy: spironolactone 50 mg uid, bumetanide 1 mg bid, bisoprolol 2.5 mg bid, and sacubitril valsartan 49/51 mg bid. She also takes L-thyroxin 0.1 mg uid, thiamazol 10 mg uid (for hyperthyroidism), pantoprazole 40 mg uid, acetylsalicylic acid 80 mg uid, and simvastatin 20 mg uid.

Concordant with the euvolemic state, the HeartLogic (HL) index was consistently under the threshold level for more than 6 months (Figure 1). Seven days before admission, however, the HL index started to rise extremely fast, starting from a value of 9 till a HL index of 63 on the day of presentation at the emergency department. (Figure 1, Supplemental Figure (available here). The parameters that contributed to the out of hospital alert were a decreased heart rate variability, a strongly increased third heart sound, a rapidly changing first heart sound (i.e., a strong decrease followed by a steep increase), an increased thoracic impedance, an increased respiratory rate, an increased nightly heart rate, and a lower activity level. Concomitantly, a decreased number of apneas and an average increased heart rate were observed.

This patient presented at the emergency department with severe dyspnea. The dyspnea symptoms started 36 hours before admission. A few days prior, the patient suffered from a dry cough. She could not recall to having experienced fever; no fever was measured upon admission (36.2 degrees Celsius). She had not been visiting COVID-19-risk regions, but a close neighbor was diagnosed with SARS-CoV-2. Clinical exam revealed the known mitral insufficiency murmur as well as a normal pulmonary auscultation without wheezes or rhonchi. Respiratory rate was 25-30/min. Blood pressure was 137/80 mmHg with a pulse of 70 bpm. Peripheral oxygen saturation was 92% in ambient air. Electrocardiography showed a sinus rhythm of 70/min with signs of left ventricular hypertrophy and a QRS width of 110 ms, identical to previous ECGs. Blood analysis showed slight leucopenia, absolute lymphocyte count of 930 mcg/L, D-dimer of 4701 ng/L, LDH 301 IU/L, a C-reactive protein of 70 mg/L and an acute chronic renal insufficiency with an estimated GFR of 50 mL/min (normally 70 mL/min) (Table 1).

A chest CT scan without contrast was performed to diagnose and assess the lung involvement since the high suspicion of COVID-19. The CT scan revealed bilateral multifocal subpleural ground glass opacities, with peribronchovascular distribution and partial consolidation, and thin pleural strands in both lower lobes. No pulmonary edema and no pleural effusion were observed (Figure 2). A nasopharyngeal swab confirmed the presence of SARS-CoV-2 by means of PCR assay; the patient was subsequently hospitalized in a dedicated COVID-19 ward with the required isolation measures.

3. Discussion

This is a timely case report wherein device-based telemonitoring delivered a warning signal that was atypical for heart failure alone, holding the promise to help in the early

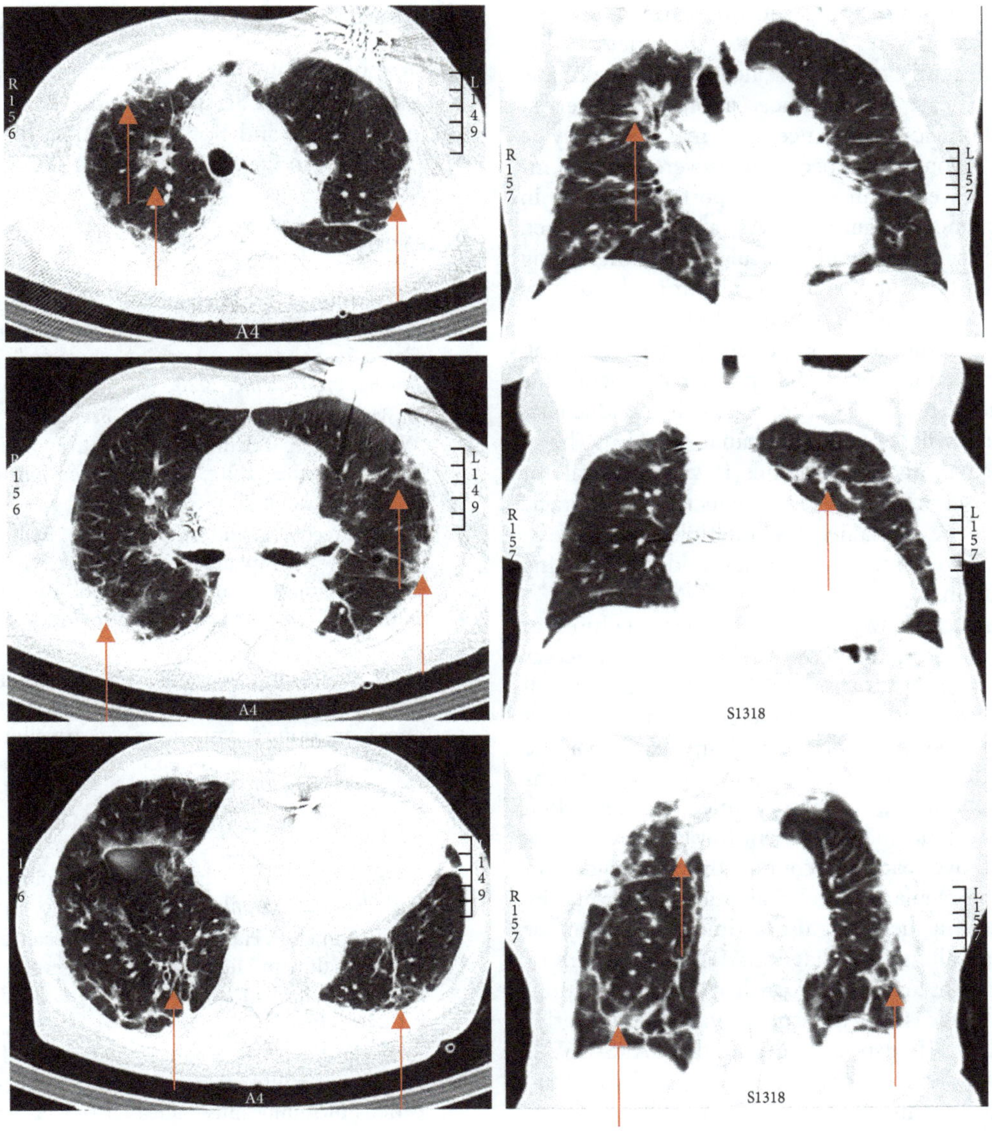

Figure 2: Overview of thoracic CT-scan revealing important COVID-19 disease. The arrows show the bilateral multifocal subpleural ground glass opacities, peribronchovascular infiltrates with partial consolidation, and thin pleural strands in both lower lobes.

diagnosis of other health problems such as a viral pneumonia, here caused by SARS-CoV-2. Device-based telemonitoring is rapidly emerging as an interesting tool for remote follow-up in heart failure patients with a pacemaker, ICD, or CRT device [3]. Also, in other branches of medicine (wireless follow-up of glycaemia in diabetic patients, follow-up of therapeutic adherence to continuous positive airway pressure therapy in obstructive sleep apnea [12, 13]), remote patient follow-up allows for faster processing of specific patient data to control larger patient cohorts. These features rapidly evolved from "gadgets" to useful tools, especially when overall health care system capacity is stretched to its maximum, as is the case with this COVID-19 pandemic.

The HeartLogic device helps in the early detection of heart failure. Based on the validation study [6], the median time between the rise-above-threshold of HL and the clinical event was more than 30 days, allowing for corrective measures in order to prevent heart failure hospitalizations. Two large studies currently investigate the broader clinical applicability of HeartLogic: the MANAGE-HF study (ClinicalTrials.gov Identifier: NCT03237858) which tests the clinical usefulness of HeartLogic to prevent heart failure and related mortality and the PREEMPT-HF study (ClinicalTrials.gov Identifier: NCT03579641) which tests the clinical usefulness of HeartLogic to detect other (non-HF-related) meaningful clinical problems.

This case report supports this idea and hints at the possibility to make a differential diagnosis of dyspnea in heart failure patients using the HL device during the current SARS-CoV-2 pandemic. The rapidly increasing respiratory frequency together with an *increasing* thoracic impedance pleads against a pure cardiac decompensation with subsequent fluid overload and hints towards an important alternative diagnosis, a hypothesis that was corroborated by the

CT scan findings and finally by showing SARS-CoV-2 in the nasopharyngeal swab. Indeed, the parameters that contributed significantly to the alert helped to differentiate COVID-19 from heart failure exacerbation. We observed an *increased* thoracic impedance, whereas normally a lower impedance would be expected for severe HF decompensation [14], as well as an out-of-proportion increase in respiratory frequency (Figure 1). As a matter of fact, thoracic impedance is generally calculated by measuring the energy needed to send a small current from the battery of a device (the "extrathoracic component") to an intracardiac lead (the "intrathoracic component"). If lung alveoli are progressively filled up with water (pulmonary edema due to decompensation), resistance decreases as the conductivity for electric current is higher for water than for air [15]. Therefore, an increased thoracic impedance is very atypical for cardiac decompensation. In this case, the increase in thoracic impedance might be explained by multiple factors, e.g., strongly increased respiratory frequency and air trapping due to hyperinflation.

Also, in many cases with established heart failure, an increased heart rate is explained by atrial fibrillation whereas here a sinus tachycardia was noted. In addition, the overall speed of changes increased the suspicion of an alternative diagnosis. It is however important to emphasize that the infection with SARS-CoV-2 will have contributed to worsening heart failure. Indeed, respiratory infections are often sufficient to flip a euvolemic HF patient towards decompensation and fluid overload. Of course, the HL algorithm cannot replace the regular clinical evaluation but should be seen as an interesting help to raise a timely suspicion for the presence of an alternative diagnosis for heart failure or at least a diagnosis that can trigger cardiac decompensation.

An important issue is how to respond timely to the "early" changes detected by HL. Especially during this SARS-CoV-2 pandemic, hospital services are being reorganized for a full focus on the control of this infection. However, the permanent vigilance for aberrant "typical" or "atypical" alert patterns on the home-monitoring devices in these patients with heart failure might hold the promise for the early detection of a diagnosis of cardiac origin and beyond. In this case, it was a potentially lethal viral infection with SARS-CoV-2.

4. Conclusion

Device-based telemonitoring of heart failure patients can help to detect noncardiac diseases that significantly alter overall homeostasis. Moreover, detailed analysis of the HeartLogic algorithm can help to shed light on the diagnosis. To the best of our knowledge, this is the first case report in which a sudden increase in HeartLogic preceded a diagnosis of COVID-19.

Consent

The patient provided written informed consent to publish this case report with related figures.

Disclosure

WH is a heart failure specialist actively implanting cardiac devices from Abbott St. Jude Medical, Biotronik, Medtronic, MicroPort CRM, and Boston Scientific; the latter company has an interest in developing the HeartLogic algorithm.

References

[1] E. J. Rubin, D. P. Harrington, J. W. Hogan, C. Gatsonis, L. R. Baden, and M. B. Hamel, "The urgency of care during the Covid-19 pandemic - learning as we go," *The New England Journal of Medicine*, 2020.

[2] R. Bashshur, C. R. Doarn, J. M. Frenk, J. C. Kvedar, and J. O. Woolliscroft, "Telemedicine and the COVID-19 pandemic, lessons for the future," *Telemedicine Journal and E-Health*, vol. 26, no. 5, pp. 571–573, 2020.

[3] N. A. Freedberg and A. Feldman, "Remote monitoring of patients with Implantable Cardioverter Defibrillators (ICD): a cute gimmick or an essential tool for clinical excellence?," *Journal of Cardiovascular Electrophysiology*, vol. 25, no. 7, pp. 771–773, 2014.

[4] V. M. Conraads, L. Tavazzi, M. Santini et al., "Sensitivity and positive predictive value of implantable intrathoracic impedance monitoring as a predictor of heart failure hospitalizations: the SENSE-HF trial," *European Heart Journal*, vol. 32, no. 18, pp. 2266–2273, 2011.

[5] J. A. Palfy, J. Benezet-Mazuecos, J. Martinez Milla et al., "CorVue algorithm efficacy to predict heart failure in real life: unnecessary and potentially misleading information?," *Pacing and Clinical Electrophysiology*, vol. 41, no. 8, pp. 948–952, 2018.

[6] J. P. Boehmer, R. Hariharan, F. G. Devecchi et al., "A multisensor algorithm predicts heart failure events in patients with implanted devices," *JACC Heart Failure*, vol. 5, no. 3, pp. 216–225, 2017.

[7] R. S. Gardner, J. P. Singh, B. Stancak et al., "Correction to: HeartLogic multisensor algorithm identifies patients during periods of significantly increased risk of heart failure events: results from the MultiSENSE Study," *Circulation: Heart Failure*, vol. 11, no. 8, p. e000029, 2018.

[8] R. S. Gardner, J. P. Singh, B. Stancak et al., "HeartLogic multisensor algorithm identifies patients during periods of significantly increased risk of heart failure events: results from the MultiSENSE study," *Circulation. Heart Failure*, vol. 11, no. 7, article e004669, 2018.

[9] L. Santini, K. Mahfouz, V. Schirripa et al., "Preliminary experience with a novel multisensor algorithm for heart failure monitoring: the HeartLogic index," *Clinical Case Reports*, vol. 6, no. 7, pp. 1317–1320, 2018.

[10] A. Capucci, L. Santini, S. Favale et al., "Preliminary experience with the multisensorHeartLogicalgorithm for heart failure monitoring: a retrospective case series report," *ESC Heart Failure*, vol. 6, no. 2, pp. 308–318, 2019.

[11] L. Santini, A. D'Onofrio, A. dello Russo et al., "Prospective evaluation of the multisensorHeartLogicalgorithm for heart failure monitoring," *Clinical Cardiology*, 2020.

[12] J. L. Pepin, R. Tamisier, D. Hwang, S. Mereddy, and S. Parthasarathy, "Does remote monitoring change OSA management and CPAP adherence?," *Respirology*, vol. 22, no. 8, pp. 1508–1517, 2017.

[13] J. L. Pépin, I. Jullian-Desayes, M. Sapène et al., "Multimodal remote monitoring of high cardiovascular risk patients with OSA initiating CPAP: a randomized trial," *Chest*, vol. 155, no. 4, pp. 730–739, 2019.

[14] Y. Aizawa, S. Takatsuki, S. Kashimura et al., "Thoracic impedance as a therapeutic marker of acute decompensated heart failure," *International Journal of Cardiology*, vol. 174, no. 3, pp. 840–842, 2014.

[15] C. M. Yu, L. Wang, E. Chau et al., "Intrathoracic impedance monitoring in patients with heart failure," *Circulation*, vol. 112, no. 6, pp. 841–848, 2005.

19

Bacillus cereus Subacute Native Valve Infective Endocarditis and its Multiple Complications

Jemimah Nallarajah and M. I. Mujahieth

Department of Medicine, Colombo South Teaching Hospital, Sri Lanka

Correspondence should be addressed to Jemimah Nallarajah; njemmy@gmail.com

Academic Editor: Assad Movahed

Bacillus cereus causing infective endocarditis (IE) in a native valve is an extremely rare event, but it is reported mostly in intravenous drug abusers and other risk factors as immunosuppression, malignancy, and valvular heart disease including prosthetic heart valves. We report a case of *B.cereus* native mitral valve infective endocarditis in a 58-year-old Sri Lankan male who is not a drug abuser who presented with painless hematuria with reduced urine output. During hospital stay, he developed frequent episodes of brief focal seizures. He had undergone multiple investigations that revealed splenic abscesses, cerebral vasculitis, and glomerular nephritis with positive rheumatoid factor, cytoplasmic antineutrophil cytoplasmic antibody (C-ANCA), and cryoglobulin. The appropriate antibiotic was the prime therapeutic intervention which carried an excellent prognosis. This case highlights an unusual organism in the blood culture that caused IE warranting thorough physical examination and investigations.

1. Introduction

Infective endocarditis (IE) is a life-threatening condition that typically affects a person with congenital heart disease or rheumatic valvular disease or prosthetic heart valves, but there are risk factors as central venous catheter, pace maker, implantable cardioverter-defibrillator (ICD), immunosuppressive state, and malignancy which also play a role in IE. The most commonly identified causative organisms are *Staphylococcus* and *Streptococcus* (1). *Bacillus cereus* is known for its association with acute gastroenteritis and is a rare causative organism of native valve IE, but that has been reported in IVDA and in the presence of other risk factors mentioned above (2). IE causes various vascular and immunological manifestations leading to life-threatening complications. Early identification and appropriate interventions save lives.

2. Case Presentation

A 58-year-old male presented with intermittent low-grade fever and painless hematuria of one-month duration. On further inquiry, he had a significant weight loss of 6 kg in the period of the same duration. He was on long-term medication for diabetes mellitus without any micro- or macrovascular complications, and his glycemic control was satisfactory with oral hypoglycemic drugs. He was a school principal and not an alcoholic or smoker and denied usage of any recreational drugs.

On 10th day of hospital admission, he developed three episodes of left-sided focal seizures without loss of consciousness, and each episode lasted for about two minutes.

On preliminary examination, he was afebrile, has thin built with body mass index (BMI) of 19.3 kg/m^2, and severely pale with finger clubbing. There were no other peripheral stigmata of infective endocarditis or lymphadenopathy identified. The pulse rate was irregularly irregular with a rate of 70 beats per minute and a pansystolic murmur best heard at the apex which radiated to the axilla; apart from that, other systemic examinations were unremarkable.

He had to undergo several (Tables 1 and 2 and Figures 1–3) investigations for his diagnostic workup.

The transthoracic echocardiography demonstrated mitral regurgitation with tiny vegetation attached to the anterior mitral leaflet which was $0.8 \times 0.4\,cm^2$ in size (Figure 1 (arrow)). Electrocardiography (ECG) showed multiple ventricular extra systoles without atrial fibrillation.

TABLE 1: Summary of basic investigations.

	Normal range	1st day	20th day	40th day	60th day
White cell ($\times 10^9$)	4-11	9.34	23.5	14.8	5.82
Neutrophils ($\times 10^9$)	1.5–8.0	6.2	21.6	9.3	2.46
Hemoglobin (g/dL)	13.5–16.5	6.9	7.8	9.8	10.1
Platelet ($\times 10^9$/L)	150-450	206	305	228	196
Sodium (mmol/L)	135-145	136	133	137	138
Potassium (mmol/L)	3.5-5.0	3.9	3.8	3.6	3.8
Creatinine (μmol/L)	50-120	457	524	362	103
CRP (mg/L)	<6	129	194	128	16
ESR (mm/1st hour)	<20	68	110	92	32
Protein (g/L)	66-83	59.2	57.2	58.8	60.3
Albumin (g/L)	35-50	22.6	24.7	25.1	31.3
Globulin (g/L)		36.6	32.5	33.7	29.0
Total bilirubin (μmol/L)	5-17	11	12.3	10	6.2
ALP (IU/L)	40-140	181	155	121	92.1
ALT (U/L)	10-40	21.9	20.3	16.7	11.8
AST (U/L)	10-40	48.5	40.1	29.8	18.6
Corrected Ca (mmol/L)	2.2–2.6	2.33	2.31	2.30	2.36
Phosphate (mg/dL)	3.4–4.5	5.3	3.3	1.0	1.2
Magnesium (mmol/L)	0.85–1.1	1.0	0.99	0.89	0.9
Urine full report		Field full red cells Protein 3+	Field full red cells Protein +	58–45 Protein-nil	Nil
Urine protein creatinine ratio (>3.5 nephrotic range)		2.61			

TABLE 2: Other investigations.

Blood culture–2 sets	*Bacillus cereus*
Urine culture	No growth
Cryoglobulin	Positive
C-ANCA	Positive
P-ANCA	Negative
IgG (mg/dL) (569-1919)	1290
IgM (mg/dL) (47-147)	152
IgA (mg/dL) (61-330)	156
C_3 (mg/dL) (55-120)	119
C_4 (mg/dL) (20-50)	26
Hepatitis B surface antigen	Negative
Hepatitis C antibody	Negative
Cytomegalovirus IgM/IgG	Negative
Epstein-Barr virus IgM/IgG	Negative
Retroviral study	Negative
VDRL	Negative
Typhus Weil-Felix	Negative
Brucella antibody	Negative
Urine Bence Jones protein	Negative
Serum protein electrophoresis	No monoclonal bands
Antinuclear antibody (ANA)	Negative
Urine dysmorphic red cells	7%
Endoscopic studies of GIT	Unremarkable

The magnetic resonance imaging (MRI) of the brain revealed multiple foci of hemorrhage in the bilateral cerebral hemispheres and cerebellum that are suggestive of cerebral vasculitis, and there were no space-occupying lesions or cerebral abscess. Eye screening was negative for vasculitis or endophthalmitis.

The contrast-enhanced computed tomography (CECT) of the chest and abdomen showed two splenic abscesses on the parenchyma and the lateral wall (Figure 3 (arrow)); apart from that, it was unremarkable.

He developed oliguria with progressively rising creatinine and had to undergo hemodialysis twice with blood transfusions. A renal biopsy was performed that demonstrated focal segmental glomerulosclerosis (FSGS) with acute and chronic tubular interstitial nephritis. No immunosuppressive therapy had been used for rapidly progressive renal failure, but the patient recovered with antibiotic therapy.

Intravenous (IV) ciprofloxacin had been administrated for 8 weeks which was sensitive for *Bacillus cereus* that has been identified by an automated identification and susceptibility testing system (BD Phoenix). He had a protracted and prolonged hospital stay for about two months. However, he made a complete recovery. There are no relapses for two years of clinic follow-up.

3. Discussion

Bacillus cereus is an aerobic spore barer and a facultative anaerobe found in the environment and certain types of food and also can be found in the gut flora which can be isolated

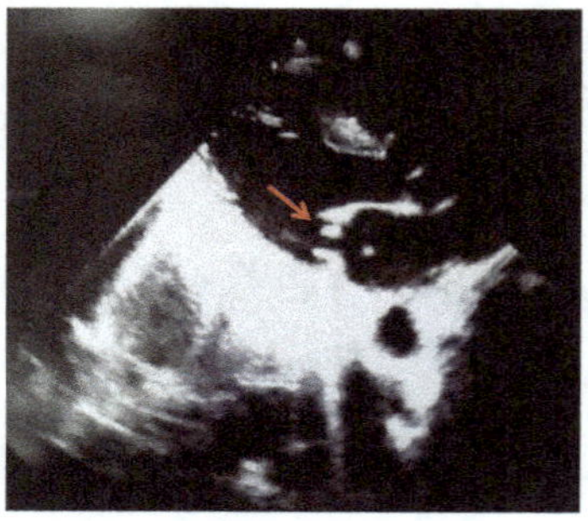

Figure 1: Transthoracic echocardiography; tiny $0.8 \times 0.4\,cm^2$ vegetation attached to the anterior mitral leaflet (arrow).

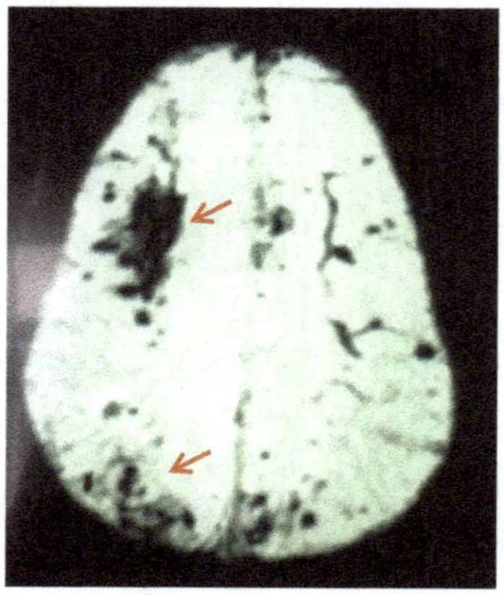

Figure 2: MRI/SWI image of the brain. There is a significant blooming with multiple peripheral and central bleeding foci in the cerebral hemispheres (arrow).

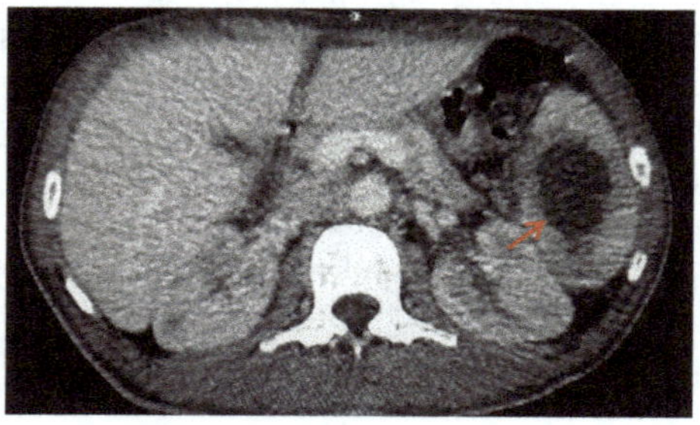

Figure 3: CECT abdomen; irregular hypodense ring-enhancing lesion in the parenchyma of the spleen (arrow).

from the human feces. When the spores overcome the immunity of the body, they become infective and can cause systemic infections such as abscess of various sites, endophthalmitis, pneumonia, and osteomyelitis (3, 4). *Bacillus cereus* causing IE commonly affects males with the age group of 41–60 years. The mitral valve is more frequently affected among the valves followed by aortic and tricuspid (common in IVDA) valves. Mortality is higher in patients with a prosthetic heart valve than native valve (5).

In our patient, the portal of entry of this organism is not clear, but we speculate that the infection was acquired from a meal that contained the organism or *Bacillus cereus* bacteremia from the gut flora. However, he had diabetes mellitus as a risk factor which is a known cause for immunosuppression by reduced phagocytosis and impaired leukocyte chemotaxis that may contribute to the pathogenesis of IE. Diabetes with poor glycemic control carries poor prognosis. Our patient has been managed with insulin and had a satisfactory control during the ward stay.

The appropriate antibiotic therapy is very vital in the management of IE, and it should be given for at least six weeks. *B.cereus* is commonly sensitive to aminoglycosides, vancomycin, ciprofloxacin, linezolid, or clindamycin and showed resistance to beta-lactamase and cephalosporin (5).

Acute kidney injury (AKI) presented as hematuria in our case as a complication of IE. He had been offered hemodialysis for the rapidly progressive nature of renal disease and also continued the antibiotics without any immunosuppressant, and the ultimate outcome was excellent. We strongly emphasize here that cardiac auscultation is very important in the cases of hematuria to avoid misdiagnosis. In our case, especially the presence of ANCA, rheumatoid factor and cryoglobulin associated with hematuria definitely direct to a diagnosis of small vessel vasculitis, and the management with immunosuppressant could further exacerbate the infection that leads to an adverse outcome. IE is a mimicker of vasculitis. Immunological phenomena of IE may result in a positivity of cryoglobulin, ANCA, and rheumatoid factor that will become negative once the infection is completely treated (6).

Most cases of glomerulonephritis associated with subacute IE are presented as hematuria with AKI. Glomerulonephritis causing hematuria is almost always painless, and rapidly progressive glomerulonephritis (RPGN) is the most common anticipated complication or a presenting manifestation of glomerulonephritis. There are several mechanisms that have been identified in IE which cause renal manifestations: immune complex deposition, septic emboli-related infarction and abscess, antibiotic-related interstitial nephritis, and thrombotic microangiopathy. FSGS is rarely found in the association of IE which has been reported in the literature that presents as proteinuria, hematuria, and hypertension. In our case, apart from hypertension, other features were found. FSGS is the result of immune complex deposition in the glomerular basement membrane that usually is associated with hypocomplimentemia. In our patient, the compliments were normal that could be due to the antibiotic therapy prior to renal biopsy (7, 8).

A splenic abscess is a rare and a fatal complication of IE (9). Our patient did not have any symptoms or signs related to the abscess apart from low-grade fever, but it has been found incidentally on the imaging. Percutaneous aspiration had been attempted however which did not yield an adequate sample for culture. The patient had been managed effectively with antibiotics, and follow-up images showed complete resolution.

The common neurological complications are mainly due to septic emboli and present as seizure, stroke, aneurysm, and cerebral abscess (10, 11). Our patient had developed cerebral vasculitis; it is an uncommon and rare manifestation and causes microbleeds that are commonly found in the brain parenchyma or in the subarachnoid space (10). Cerebral vasculitis can be primary or secondary that needs further evaluation to exclude the differential diagnoses. A brain biopsy is the gold standard investigation to make the diagnosis of cerebral vasculitis (10). However, in the presence of IE, we did not perform it, and the patient also showed a marked clinical improvement with antibiotics only without a need of any corticosteroid pulses. Neurological complications are commonly life-threatening if left untreated. *Staphylococcus aureus* causing IE is commonly identified with neurological complications (12).

The guideline of the American Association for Thoracic Surgery has mentioned several indications and timing of surgical interventions which are considered in patients who have signs of heart failure, persistent sepsis despite adequate antibiotic therapy for more than five to seven days, severe valve dysfunction, large mobile vegetation, recurrent systemic embolization, paravalvular abscess, or cardiac fistula and the presence of neurological complications (recurrent strokes, cerebral mycotic aneurysm) (13). Even though our patient developed a neurological complication (vasculitis), it was managed successfully with antibiotics.

4. Conclusion

IE must be considered in any atypical presentation of a critically ill patient, and it needs to be ruled out. *Bacillus cereus* is an uncommon organism to cause native valve IE, and it warrants thorough investigations if identified in blood cultures. Timely diagnosis matters with regard to appropriate therapeutic intervention.

Abbreviations

AKI:	Acute kidney injury
ALP:	Alkaline phosphatase
ALT:	Alanine transaminase
AST:	Aspartate transaminase
BMI:	Body mass index
C-ANCA:	Cytoplasmic antineutrophil cytoplasmic antibody
CECT:	Contrast-enhanced computed tomography
CRP:	C-reactive protein
ESR:	Erythrocyte sedimentation rate
FSGS:	Focal segmental glomerulosclerosis
GIT:	Gastrointestinal tract
IE:	Infective endocarditis
IV:	Intravenous
IVDA:	Intravenous drug abuser
MRI:	Magnetic resonance imaging
SWI:	Susceptibility weighted imaging
VDRL:	Venereal disease research laboratory.

Acknowledgments

We would like to thank the consultant cardiologist, microbiologists, nephrologist, radiologist, and histopathologist and their team in Colombo South Teaching Hospital for their assistance and generous support.

References

[1] T. J. Cahill, L. M. Baddour, G. Habib et al., "Challenges in infective endocarditis," *Journal of the American College of Cardiology*, vol. 69, no. 3, pp. 325–344, 2017.

[2] M. Shah, S. Patnaik, S. Wongrakpanich, Y. Alhamshari, and T. Alnabelsi, "Infective endocarditis due to Bacillus cereus in a pregnant female: a case report and literature review," *IDCases.*, vol. 2, no. 4, pp. 120–123, 2015.

[3] W. F. Wright, "Central venous access device-related Bacillus cereus endocarditis: a case report and review of the literature," *Clinical Medicine & Research*, vol. 14, no. 2, pp. 109–115, 2016.

[4] M. Mols and T. Abee, "Bacillus cereus responses to acid stress," *Environmental Microbiology*, vol. 13, no. 11, pp. 2835–2843, 2011.

[5] A. Gopinathan, A. Kumar, A. C. Sen et al., "A case series and review of Bacillus cereus endocarditis from India," *The Open Microbiology Journal*, vol. 12, no. 1, pp. 28–33, 2018.

[6] F. B. Kamar and T. L.-A. Hawkins, "Antineutrophil cytoplasmic antibody induction due to infection: a patient with infective endocarditis and chronic hepatitis C," *Can J Infect Dis Med Microbiol.*, vol. 2016, pp. 1–6, 2016.

[7] C. L. Boils, S. H. Nasr, P. D. Walker, W. G. Couser, and C. P. Larsen, "Update on endocarditis-associated glomerulonephritis," *Kidney International*, vol. 87, no. 6, pp. 1241–1249, 2015.

[8] J. M. Boulton-Jones, J. G. P. Sissons, D. J. Evans, and D. K. Peters, "Renal lesions of subacute infective endocarditis," *British Medical Journal*, vol. 2, no. 5909, pp. 11–14, 1974.

[9] A. Elasfar, A. AlBaradai, Z. AlHarfi, M. Alassal, A. Ghoneim, and F. AlGhofaili, "Splenic abscess associated with infective endocarditis; case series," *Journal of the Saudi Heart Association*, vol. 27, no. 3, pp. 210–215, 2015.

[10] P. Berlit and M. Kraemer, "Cerebral vasculitis in adults: what are the steps in order to establish the diagnosis? Red flags and pitfalls," *Clinical and Experimental Immunology*, vol. 175, no. 3, pp. 419–424, 2014.

[11] N. A. Morris, M. Matiello, J. L. Lyons, and M. A. Samuels, "Neurologic complications in infective endocarditis: identification, management, and impact on cardiac surgery," *The Neurohospitalist.*, vol. 4, no. 4, pp. 213–222, 2014.

[12] T. Kitazawa, M. Totsuka, Y. Yoshino, I. Koga, and Y. Ota, "Bacillus cereusNative Valve Endocarditis with Multiple Brain," *Clin Res*, vol. 2, no. 2, p. 1019, 2015.

[13] G. B. Pettersson and S. T. Hussain, "Current AATS guidelines on surgical treatment of infective endocarditis," *ASVIDE*, vol. 6, pp. 336–336, 2019.

20

Ventricular Arrhythmia Precipitated by Severe Hypocalcaemia Secondary to Primary Hypoparathyroidism

S. Ashwin Reddy

Papworth Hospital, Papworth Everard, Cambridge, UK

Correspondence should be addressed to S. Ashwin Reddy; ashwin.reddy@cantab.net
Academic Editor: Kathleen Ngu

Hypocalcaemia causes neuromuscular and myocardial symptoms, including QT interval prolongation, and cardiac arrhythmias. Prompt detection and calcium replacement may reverse the pathology, following which the underlying cause should be diagnosed and treated to prevent recurrence. I present the case of a young man presenting with collapse who was found to have sinus rhythm with significant QT interval prolongation on admission electrocardiogram (ECG) associated with profound hypocalcaemia secondary to primary hypoparathyroidism.

1. Introduction

The evaluation of blackout in the emergency setting can be challenging due to the myriad potential diagnoses ranging from the benign (such as vasovagal or postural syncope) to the potentially fatal (such as seizure or ventricular tachyarrhythmia). Ventricular arrhythmias may be precipitated by disordered ventricular repolarisation, manifested on the 12-lead electrocardiogram as prolongation of the QT interval beyond 450 ms in males and 470 ms in females when corrected for heart rate. A common but often overlooked cause of QT prolongation are electrolyte disorders, and prompt identification and treatment of these can lead to normalisation of the QT interval.

Primary hypoparathyroidism is a rare condition with a prevalence of 17-22 per 100,000 [1, 2]. Serum hypocalcaemia resulting from this condition can predispose to QT prolongation and present with potentially life-threatening ventricular arrhythmias [3, 4].

2. Case Report

A previously healthy 20-year-old Caucasian man was presented to the emergency department following two episodes of loss of consciousness occurring at rest over a fortnight. A witness described collapse followed by shaking of all four limbs but no other epileptiform activity. Spontaneous recovery occurred after a few minutes. The patient denied alcohol or drug use and had an otherwise unremarkable medical history. He had no family history of blackout, collapse, or unexplained sudden death. Physical examination was entirely normal, with specifically no evidence of cardiac failure, no audible murmurs, no tetany, and no facial dysmorphia. He was haemodynamically stable. An initial diagnosis of "seizure" was made in the emergency department pending for further investigations.

His ECG demonstrated sinus rhythm with a prolonged corrected QT interval of 588 ms (normal <450) (Figure 1). The PR interval and QRS duration were within normal limits. Admission bloods revealed a corrected calcium of <1.25 mmol/L (normal range 2.2-2.5), phosphate 2.88 mmol/L (0.8-1.4), and alkaline phosphatase (ALP) 172 μ/L (35-135). The rest of his bloods, including magnesium, potassium, and renal function, was normal. Endocrine investigations showed a parathyroid hormone (PTH) of <3 ng/mL (14-72), vitamin D 24.1 nmol/L (25-50), and normal thyroid function tests. Echocardiography showed no structural abnormality and preserved ventricular size and function. Computerised tomography (CT) head was also unremarkable.

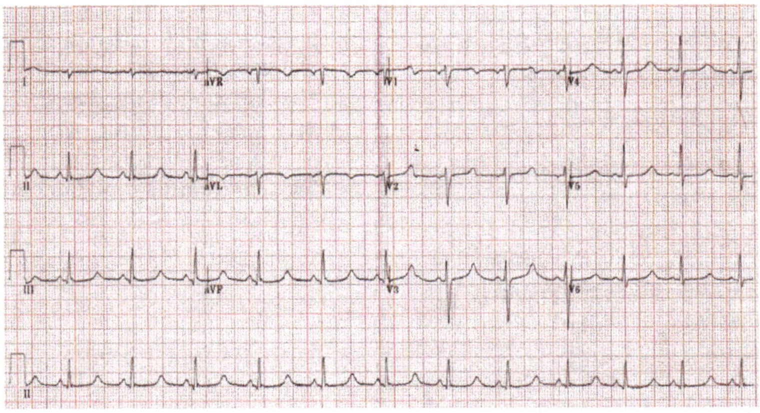

FIGURE 1: ECG demonstrating sinus rhythm, normal atrioventricular conduction, normal QRS duration, and markedly prolonged QTc.

The patient was admitted to a monitored bed and commenced on intravenous calcium replacement (10 mls 10% calcium gluconate bolus over 30 minutes, followed by infusion of 1% calcium gluconate in one litre of normal saline at a rate of 50 mls/hour). Whilst on the cardiac monitor he was observed to have short episodes of nonsustained polymorphic ventricular tachycardia (VT) which spontaneously resolved; some of these were associated with dizziness but no loss of consciousness. As his serum calcium rose, his ECG normalised and he had no further presyncopal episodes. Once the serum calcium and QTc were within normal limits, he was discharged on oral calcium and vitamin D supplement (Calcichew D3 one tablet twice daily) and 1-alphacalcidol 1 mcg once daily with early follow-up.

Screening of the patient's mother and younger brother revealed that they too had low levels of PTH and hypocalcaemia but to a less severe degree. His mother's ECG demonstrated a QTc at the upper limit of normal whilst his brother's was within normal limits. The patient was estranged from his father. The family underwent extensive genotyping to identify an underlying cause for their hypoparathyroidism but as yet no clear genetic variant has been identified.

At initial follow-up, the patient's serum calcium and ECG parameters have remained within the normal range, and he has suffered no further syncopal episodes.

3. Discussion

Hypocalcaemia predisposes to arrhythmias by affecting both depolarisation and repolarisation of cardiac myocytes. Normally, calcium blocks sodium channels and prevents depolarisation. Decreases in calcium allow increased sodium passage and lowers the depolarisation threshold, causing greater myocardial irritability [5].

Furthermore, hypocalcaemia causes the opening of L-type calcium channels during the repolarisation phase of the cardiac action potential [6], prolonging the QT interval. Late calcium influx and early after-depolarisation then occurs. If the depolarisation threshold is reached, a new action potential can be triggered. As neighbouring myocytes may be at different stages of refractoriness, this may lead to reentrant tachyarrhythmias (namely, torsades de pointes and ventricular fibrillation), thus causing loss of cardiac output and collapse or sudden death. Both the myocardial irritability and QTc prolongation can be reversed by correcting serum calcium.

Aside from QTc prolongation, severe hypocalcaemia may also present with atrioventricular (AV) block, paresthaesia, abdominal cramps, fatigue, altered mood, and tetany. Tetany can sometimes manifest clinically as Chvostek's sign (facial twitching on tapping over the facial nerve just anterior to the ipsilateral ear) or Trousseau's sign (carpal spasm induced by obstructing the brachial artery for 3 minutes with an inflated blood pressure cuff). Seizures and bronchospasm are more severe presentations and constitute an emergency [7, 8].

PTH acts to raise serum calcium by promoting calcium resorption from bone, reducing renal tubular calcium excretion and stimulating the synthesis of $1.25(OH)_2$ vitamin D in the kidney, thus increasing calcium absorption from the small intestine. Hypoparathyroidism thus causes hypocalcaemia [9]. Our patient had undetectably low levels of PTH which, given the serological abnormalities also present in his first degree relatives, is likely due to a presumed though hitherto unidentified genetic condition. PTH replacement therapy is in nascent stages of development: currently, the mainstay of treatment remains oral calcium and vitamin D replacement.

The QTc interval can be abnormally prolonged due to other factors, both acquired and inherited. Acquired causes include drugs (most commonly macrolide and quinolone antibiotics, tricyclic antidepressants and serotonin reuptake inhibitors, antipsychotics, amiodarone, and sotalol), other electrolyte abnormalities (hypokalaemia and hypomagnesaemia), and hypothyroidism. Removal or treatment of the underlying cause will often lead to correction of the QTc interval, often back to normal as in this case.

Inherited long QT syndrome can arise due to a mutation in a gene-encoding ion channels intrinsic to the cardiac action potential and is often inherited in an autosomal dominant manner. The identification of a specific genetic mutation in an index individual allows for cascade screening of relatives, enabling institution of therapy at a presymptomatic stage where appropriate. The mainstay of therapy in inherited long QT syndrome is beta blockade, with second line therapies including flecainide and surgical sympathectomy. In individuals at higher risk of sudden cardiac death, implantation of a transvenous or subcutaneous cardiac defibrillator is indicated. In those untreated who experience syncope or aborted sudden death, the mortality rate at 15 years is around 50%, but this decreases drastically with careful treatment to approximately 1%.

Prolongation of the QTc interval on the 12-lead ECG can be a subtle finding and can be easily missed. This is further complicated by the fact that approximately 2.5% of the normal population will have a prolonged QTc interval. Thus, in young patients presenting with a syncopal episode, particularly in the presence of myoclonic jerking, this can often lead to misdiagnosis of seizures if inadequate care is taken over initial clinical assessment. This not only delays diagnosis and appropriate treatment but also can sometimes lead to the administration of anticonvulsant therapy which has the potential to cause further harm. In this instance, the initial differential diagnosis of seizures was quickly downgraded once the ECG had been performed, and no anticonvulsant treatment was given.

4. Conclusion

This case reiterates the importance of considering cardiac arrhythmias as a cause of unexplained syncope with myoclonus and to have a low index of suspicion for considering specifically long QT-associated ventricular tachyarrhythmia. It also strongly demonstrates the importance of accounting for metabolic causes of cardiac rhythm disturbances as these are potentially easily treatable and reversible.

References

[1] T. Vadiveloo, P. T. Donnan, and G. P. Leese, "A population-based study of the epidemiology of chronic hypoparathyroidism," *Journal of Bone and Mineral Research*, vol. 33, no. 3, pp. 478–485, 2018.

[2] B. L. Clarke, E. M. Brown, M. T. Collins et al., "Epidemiology and diagnosis of hypoparathyroidism," *The Journal of Clinical Endocrinology & Metabolism*, vol. 101, no. 6, pp. 2284–2299, 2016.

[3] A. B. Rometo, L. Beerman, and G. Arora, "Electrolyte screening in the evaluation of prolonged QTc interval," *Cardiology in the Young*, vol. 25, no. 2, pp. 398-399, 2015.

[4] J. S. Mangat, J. Till, and N. Bridges, "Hypocalcaemia mimicking long QT syndrome: case report," *European Journal of Pediatrics*, vol. 167, no. 2, pp. 233–235, 2008.

[5] C. M. Armstrong and G. Cota, "Calcium block of Na^+ channels and its effect on closing rate," *Proceedings of the National Academy of Sciences of the United States of America*, vol. 96, no. 7, pp. 4154–4157, 1999.

[6] D. Bronsky, A. Dubin, S. S. Waldstein, and D. S. Kushner, "Calcium and the electrocardiogram. I. The electrocardiographic manifestations of hypoparathyroidism," *The American Journal of Cardiology*, vol. 7, no. 6, pp. 823–832, 1961.

[7] J. P. Bilezikian, A. Khan, J. T. Potts et al., "Hypoparathyroidism in the adult: epidemiology, diagnosis, pathophysiology, target-organ involvement, treatment, and challenges for future research," *Journal of Bone and Mineral Research*, vol. 26, no. 10, pp. 2317–2337, 2011.

[8] J. T. Potts Jr., "Diseases of the parathyroid gland and other hyper- and hypocalcemic disorders," in *Harrison's Principles of Internal Medicine*, vol. 16, pp. 2249–2268, McGraw-Hill, New York, NY, USA, 2005.

[9] M. L. Brandi, M. P. Bilezikian, D. Shoback et al., "Management of hypoparathyroidism: summary statement and guidelines," *The Journal of Clinical Endocrinology & Metabolism*, vol. 101, no. 6, pp. 2273–2283, 2016.

21

Endocarditis Complicated by Severe Aortic Insufficiency in a Patient with COVID-19: Diagnostic and Management Implications

David J. Sanders[1] **Joanne S. Sutter,**[1] **Antone Tatooles,**[2] **Tisha M. Suboc,**[1] **and Anupama K. Rao**[1]

[1]*Department of Internal Medicine, Section of Cardiology, Rush University Medical Center, Chicago, IL, USA*
[2]*Department of Cardiovascular and Thoracic Surgery, Rush University Medical Center, Chicago, IL, USA*

Correspondence should be addressed to David J. Sanders; david_j_sanders@rush.edu

Academic Editor: Luigi Sciarra

A 38-year-old man presented with cough, shortness of breath, and fatigue. He was diagnosed with Coronavirus Disease-2019 (COVID-19) as well as *Enterococcus faecalis* bacteremia. Imaging revealed a subaortic membrane with aortic valve endocarditis and severe aortic insufficiency. He had successful aortic valve replacement with a mechanical prosthesis and subaortic membrane resection. This case highlights some of the diagnostic and therapeutic challenges presented by COVID-19 pandemic.

1. Introduction

The Coronavirus Disease-2019 (COVID-19) pandemic is an unparalleled global crisis that has commanded health resources and public attention. Although there is an overwhelming focus on this new disease, the emergence of SARS-CoV-2, COVID-19's causative organism, has not eliminated other maladies. Patients continue to have common etiologies for their presentation, and multiple illnesses can complicate and coexist with COVID-19. Additionally, concerns about the infectivity and potential aerosolization of SARS-CoV-2 impose barriers to performing invasive procedures on such patients.

Here, we present a case of aortic valve infective endocarditis (IE) complicated by severe aortic insufficiency (AI) in a patient simultaneously diagnosed with COVID-19. We illustrate how COVID-19 can have similar clinical characteristics to IE, among other cardiovascular diseases. We also highlight our thought process on the risks and benefits of transesophageal echocardiogram (TEE) and aortic valve replacement surgery in this patient and discuss the importance of individualized decision-making.

2. Case

A 38-year-old man with end-stage renal disease from hypertensive nephropathy requiring hemodialysis through a tunneled dialysis catheter presented with two weeks of nonproductive cough, shortness of breath, and fatigue. The patient's initial vital signs were notable for a blood pressure of 84/46, pulse of 83, respirations of 20, and oxygen saturation of 97% on room air. Though initially afebrile, he mounted a temperature of 101.5°F several hours after presentation. On admission, his physical exam was notable for a II/VI systolic ejection murmur, not previously documented.

A chest X-ray revealed pulmonary vascular congestion and a right retrocardiac opacity. ECG showed sinus rhythm, borderline 1st degree AV block, and left anterior fascicular block. Laboratory evaluation demonstrated white blood cell count of 14.5 K/μL, troponin of 0.1 ng/mL, BNP of 148 pg/mL, C-reactive protein of 108 mg/L, and ferritin of 1685 ng/mL. A nasopharyngeal swab detected SARS-CoV-2 RNA, confirming the diagnosis of COVID-19. Blood cultures were also obtained on admission, which grew *Enterococcus faecalis* from consecutive specimens.

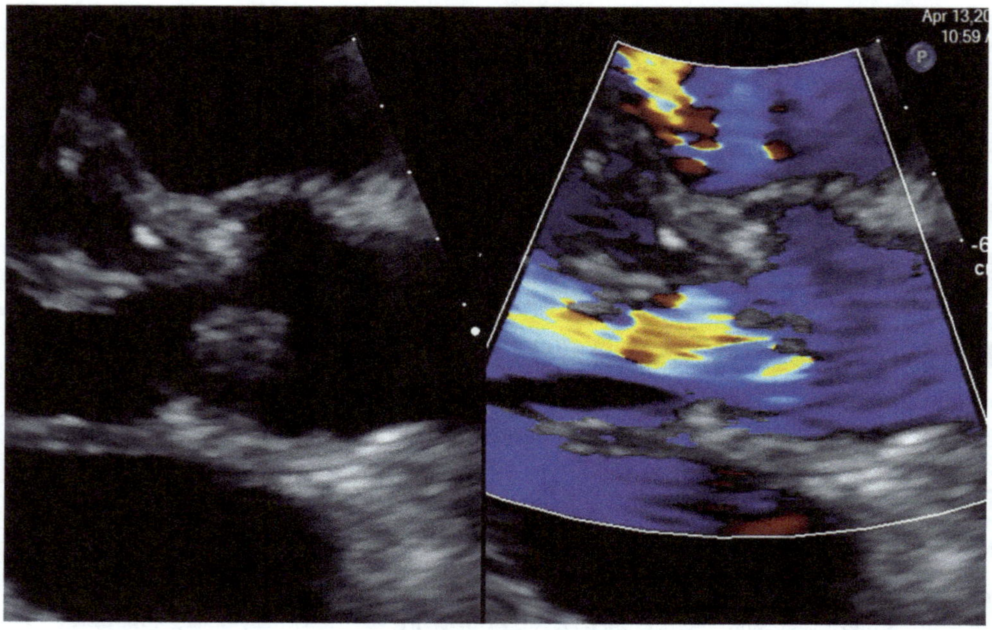

FIGURE 1: TTE from parasternal long axis view showing large echodensity on the right coronary cusp. Color Doppler demonstrates AI.

The patient was initiated on an IV antibiotic regimen of vancomycin and gentamicin. However, persistent bacteremia was noted despite several days of antibiotic therapy. His dialysis catheter was exchanged in case it was the infectious source. Given the murmur on exam and ongoing bacteremia, the patient underwent a transthoracic echocardiogram (TTE) for further evaluation. This revealed a 10 × 11 mm mobile echodensity on the right coronary cusp as well as a possible smaller vegetation on the left coronary cusp of the aortic valve. Additionally, there was eccentric aortic insufficiency (AI) graded as moderate in severity by qualitative assessment (Figure 1).

To further characterize the aortic valve and assess for paravalvular abscess, a transesophageal echocardiogram (TEE) was then performed. All personnel donned appropriate personal protective equipment (PPE) including controlled air purifying respirators (CAPR). The TEE confirmed two aortic valve vegetations: (1) 8 × 14 mm on the right coronary cusp and (2) 3 × 4 mm on the left coronary cusp. There was nonspecific thickening of the posterior aortic root, raising concern for a paravalvular abscess. Multiple parameters suggested his AI was severe: jet width ratio > 65%, jet area ratio > 60%, vena contracta of 0.6, and premature closure of the mitral valve. Interestingly, a linear structure in the left ventricular outflow tract (LVOT) was visualized, suggestive of a subaortic membrane (Figure 2).

A multispecialty team including cardiology, cardiovascular surgery, and infectious disease determined that despite his COVID-19, the patient required urgent aortic valve surgery given the severity of his AI, persistent bacteremia, vegetation size > 10 mm, and concerns for paravalvular abscess. The day following his TEE, the patient was taken to the operating room. He was found to have extensive phlegmon on the right coronary cusp and a perforation of the left coronary cusp of the aortic valve (Figure 3). Additionally, inspection of the LVOT confirmed a fibrotic subaortic membrane extending from the interventricular septum to the anterior annular region of the mitral valve (Figure 4). The native aortic valve was resected and replaced with a 25 mm St Jude mechanical prosthesis. The subaortic membrane was resected.

The patient tolerated the procedure well and did not have any postoperative complications. He was extubated a few hours following the surgery. His aortic valve culture grew *Enterococcus faecalis*. His SARS-CoV-2 PCR was also repeated and remained positive. The patient's antibiotics for IE were switched to ampicillin and ceftriaxone based on sensitivity data, and he was discharged home to complete a six-week course.

3. Discussion

As our case illustrates, the COVID-19 pandemic has presented new challenges for the diagnosis and treatment of cardiovascular disease. Patients with COVID-19 most commonly present with fever and cough and can have an array of nonspecific complaints [1]. There is a symptom overlap with other cardiovascular conditions such as acute coronary syndrome, decompensated heart failure, non-COVID-19 myocarditis, and IE. Clinicians have to remain vigilant to the possibility of these other illnesses, or they may be overlooked. Relying on heuristics, or mental shortcuts, in making a diagnosis could lead to delays and adverse outcomes [2]. In particular, the dominant focus on COVID-19 brings this diagnosis to mind more easily than others (availability bias) [2]. Attributing all of the given patient's symptoms to COVID-19 after a positive test (premature closure) may lead to other common prepandemic diagnoses, such as IE, being missed [2].

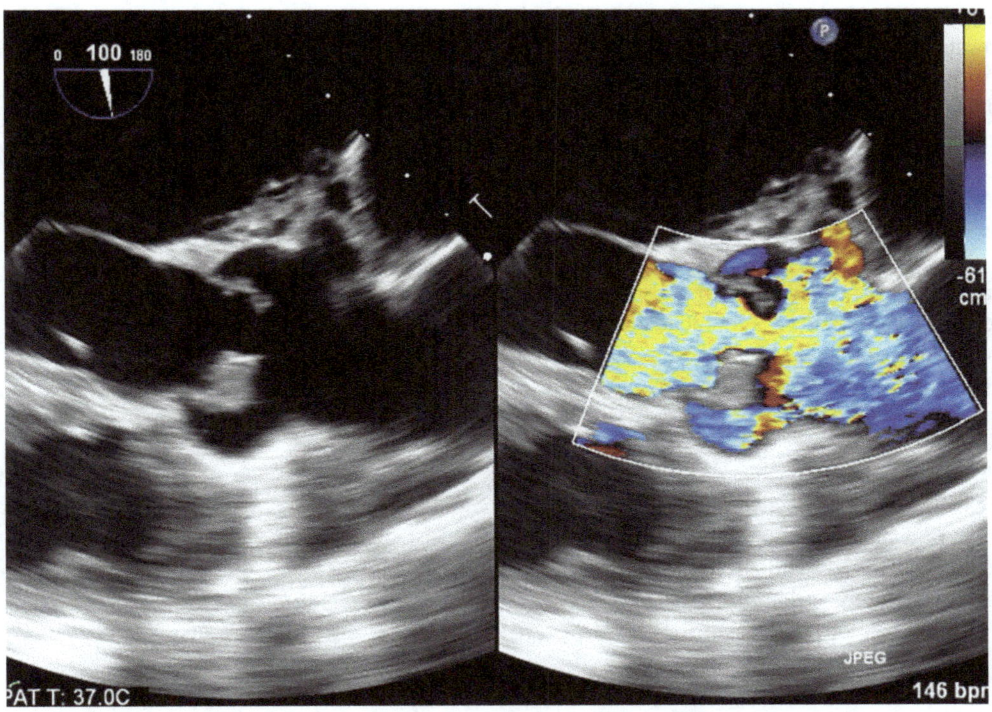

Figure 2: TEE from transgastric long axis view with beam path at 120 degrees showing aortic valve echodensity. Color Doppler demonstrates severe AI. Yellow arrow points to subaortic membrane.

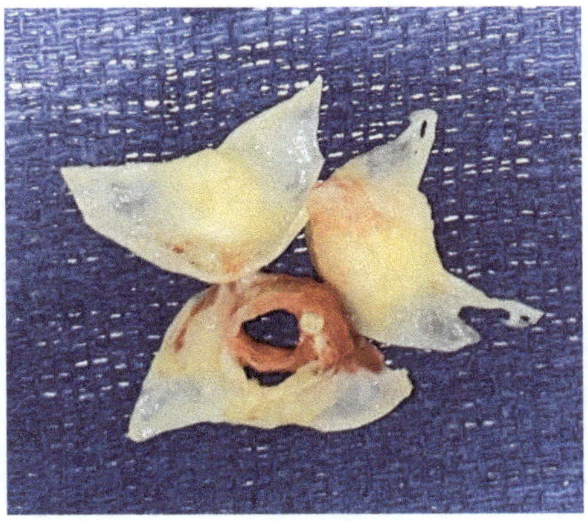

Figure 3: Resected aortic valve with vegetation on the left coronary cusp and perforation of the right coronary cusp.

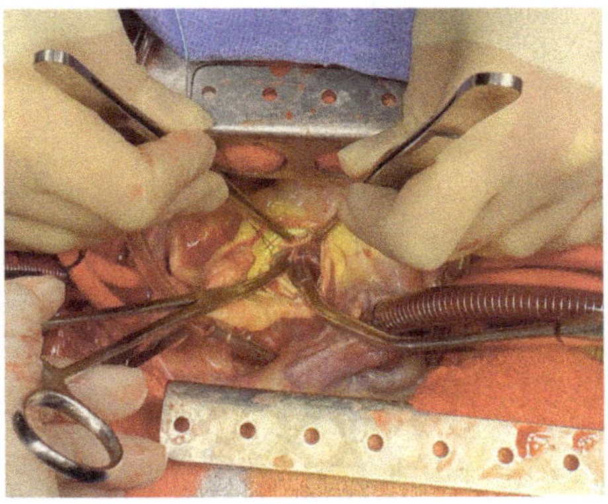

Figure 4: Intraoperative images showing the thin fibrotic subaortic membrane visible above the suction cannula.

For our patient, it was not clear which disease process caused his symptoms: COVID-19 respiratory infection, bacterial IE with pulmonary congestion from AI, or some combination of the two conditions. Testing for multiple diagnoses from the beginning was critical for timely diagnosis.

The original source for the patient's bacteremia was suspected to be his tunneled dialysis catheter. Additionally, his previously undiagnosed subaortic membrane likely created an ideal substrate for aortic valve seeding. The patient's TTE identified a vegetation > 10 mm and associated AI, high-risk features that suggested a greater chance of a complicated course or need for surgery [3]. This earned a class I indication for urgent TEE to further assess for complications [3].

In this patient with COVID-19, it was especially necessary to carefully consider the risks and benefits of a TEE. TEEs are aerosol-generating procedures that could increase the risk of transmitting SARS-CoV-2 to those involved [4, 5]. To minimize staff exposure, computed tomography (CT) or magnetic resonance imaging (MRI) can serve as an alternative for some indications [6]. While multimodality imaging might be a useful adjunct for IE, CT and MRI may not have comparable spatial and temporal resolution to a TEE for the diagnosis of endocarditis [6]. Postponing this procedure would have delayed characterizing the intracardiac complications and determining the need for surgical intervention. Thus, in our case, TEE was deemed essential and performed utilizing proper personal protective equipment (PPE).

The TEE results produced a similar dilemma for surgical planning. The study confirmed large vegetation size, severe AI, and possible early aortic root abscess, all indications for early surgery, which is associated with reduced embolic events and mortality [3, 7, 8]. Additionally, the patient had persistent bacteremia despite being on appropriate antibiotic therapy. And, given the unpredictable course of acute severe AI and potential for abrupt clinical deterioration, the multi-specialty team determined that delaying surgery would be too unsafe. Lastly, postponing surgery risked further valve destruction and, given the vegetation's location, progression to aortic root abscess formation and subsequent heart block.

Proceeding with surgery before the patient had cleared the COVID-19 infection did pose hazards to the surgical staff and required special precautions. This included minimizing the number of operating room personnel, using N95 masks and other PPE throughout surgery, and coordinated handling of equipment and specimens.

As the pandemic continues, we will have to continue to carefully weigh the risks of delaying care to the potential hazards of exposing clinical staff to the virus. Cases that are elective or time sensitive now have the potential to become urgent or emergent. As with this case, individualized decision-making may be key to providing timely and appropriate care.

Consent

Informed oral consent was given by the patient.

References

[1] W. Guan, Z. Ni, Y. Hu et al., "Clinical characteristics of coronavirus disease 2019 in China," *The New England Journal of Medicine*, vol. 382, no. 18, pp. 1708–1720, 2020.

[2] P. Croskerry, "The importance of cognitive errors in diagnosis and strategies to minimize them," *Academic Medicine*, vol. 78, no. 8, pp. 775–780, 2003.

[3] L. M. Baddour, W. R. Wilson, A. S. Bayer et al., "Infective endocarditis in adults: diagnosis, antimicrobial therapy, and management of complications. A scientific statement for healthcare professionals from the American Heart Association," *Circulation*, vol. 132, no. 15, pp. 1435–1486, 2015.

[4] N. van Doremalen, T. Bushmaker, D. H. Morris et al., "Aerosol and surface stability of SARS-CoV-2 as compared with SARS-CoV-1," *The New England Journal of Medicine*, vol. 382, no. 16, pp. 1564–1567, 2020.

[5] J. N. Kirkpatrick, C. Mitchell, C. Taub, S. Kort, J. Hung, and M. Swaminathan, "ASE statement on protection of patients and echocardiography service providers during the 2019 novel coronavirus outbreak," *Journal of the American College of Cardiology*, vol. 75, no. 24, pp. 3078–3084, 2020.

[6] P. A. Erba, M. N. Pizzi, A. Roque et al., "Multimodality imaging in infective endocarditis," *Circulation*, vol. 140, no. 21, pp. 1753–1765, 2019.

[7] T. Lalani, C. H. Cabell, D. K. Benjamin et al., "Analysis of the impact of early surgery on in-hospital mortality of native valve endocarditis," *Circulation*, vol. 121, no. 8, pp. 1005–1013, 2010.

[8] D. H. Kang, Y. J. Kim, S. H. Kim et al., "Early surgery versus conventional treatment for infective endocarditis," *The New England Journal of Medicine*, vol. 366, no. 26, pp. 2466–2473, 2012.

22

New Horizon of Intervention in Congenital Heart Disease: AFR in a Complex Cyanotic Patient

Zahra Khajali,[1] Homa Ghaderian,[1] Ata Firoozi,[1] Zahra Hosseini,[1] and Maryam Aliramezany[2]

[1]*Rajaie Cardiovascular Medical and Research Center, Iran University of Medical Sciences, Tehran, Iran*
[2]*Cardiovascular Research Center, Institute of Basic and Clinical Physiology Sciences, Kerman University of Medical Sciences Kerman, Iran*

Correspondence should be addressed to Maryam Aliramezany; maliramezany@yahoo.com
Academic Editor: Christopher S. Snyder

Double-inlet left ventricle (DILV) is the commonest form of the anatomic univentricular heart which has different ventriculoarterial connection; generally, the most prevalent type is DILV with the hypoplastic right ventricle on the left side. The disease is associated with several heart defects, and the treatment method is different based on the anatomy of the heart, but treatment methods are almost always palliative. In this paper, we described one adult patient with DILV and severe left AV (atrioventricular valve) stenosis who is managed with a novel palliative intervention; it means AFR (atrial flow regulator) device implantation for the first time.

1. Introduction

DILV is the most common form of single ventricle which both AV (atrioventricular) valves communicate into a common chamber; the prevalence of this rare anatomical anomaly is reported about 1.5-5%. There are three primary subtypes of DILV based on the relationship of the great arteries:

Type I: DILV has normally related great arteries

Type II: has a rightward and anterior aorta and rightward outlet chamber

Type III: has a leftward anterior aorta

DILV with a hypoplastic subpulmonary, rightward RV and normally related great arteries (type I) is classically referred to as the "Holmes heart" and is relatively rare. In type II, the outlet chamber is anterior and rightward, consistent with D-looped ventricles, and there is D-transposition of the great arteries (SDD). This type is associated with the obstruction of the bulboventricular foramen and, therefore, subaortic stenosis, because the aorta arises from the small chamber. Arch anomalies are reported in approximately 50% of cases.

Type III is the most common form of DILV, which consists of DILV with a left-sided, subaortic, hypoplastic right ventricle (L-loop ventricles) and L-transposition of the great arteries (SLL). Subaortic stenosis is present in approximately 67% of patients with this morphology due to a small bulboventricular foramen or obstruction by the left AV valve tissue [1–3].

Associated cardiac anomalies are commonly seen in this complex anatomical disease, such as aortic coarctation or interruption in which the systemic outflow traverses from the bulboventricular foramen, which has a tendency to narrow over time, double-outlet arterial connections, pulmonary atresia, valvular and subvalvular pulmonary stenosis, subaortic obstruction in V-A discordant type, left or right A-V valve stenosis, and conduction abnormalities [4].

Herein, we aimed to report a patient with a functional univentricle who was diagnosed with DILV type III association with severe left A-V valve stenosis who is the first Iranian experience of AFR implantation for congenital heart disease patients which led to improve in congestion symptoms and oxygenation.

2. Case Report

A 38-year-old man who was the known case of DILV and Eisenmenger syndrome and was managed with optimal medical therapy referred with progressive dyspnea (NYHA functional class IV) and cyanosis to our clinic for better evaluation. In physical exam, his hemodynamic was stable with So2: 70%. Obviously, he had severe clubbing and central cyanosis; in cardiac exam, left lateral deviation of the LV apex with loud P2 at the base of the heart and diastolic murmur grade II was heard in the left sternal border and apex.

Transthoracic echocardiography demonstrated abdominal and atrial situs solitus, levocardia, L-looped, A-V, and V-A discordance. Morphologic LV (main ventricle) was the right side of the rudimentary right ventricle with a ejection fraction of ~35%. A large inlet type ventricular septal defect (24 mm) and very small secundum type atrial septal defect (3 mm) with left-to-right shunt was illustrated. Aorta was anterior and the left side of the pulmonary artery and originated from rudimentary RV. PA derived from the main ventricle with confluent pulmonary artery branches with mild pulmonary insufficiency and severe pulmonary hypertension (mPAP:70 mmHg). The thick and hypoplastic left A-V valve was remarkable with severe stenosis (MG:15 mmHg, PG:21 mmHg, Figures 1(a)–1(d)).

Based on the TTE, DILV with CCTGA (congenitally corrected transposition of great arteries) physiology and severe left A-V valve stenosis (DILV type AIII) was confirmed for better evaluation, and cardiac catheterization was performed.

Cardiac catheterization showed RV injection which demonstrated rudimentary RV at the left side; severe systemic ventricle (LV) enlargement with moderate dysfunction which filled via a large inlet type VSD. PA originated from LV (Figure 2). Both A-V valves were connected to LV with severe left A-V valve stenosis (MG: 15 mmHg).

Regarding to his refractory symptoms and significant left A-V valve stenosis and small ASD, he was scheduled for AFR implantation to reduce LA and pulmonary capillary wedge pressure.

2.1. Procedural Technique. The procedure was performed under local anesthesia and intensive hemodynamic monitoring. Through the right femoral vein, after heparin injection to achieve ACT > 250 s, under TEE guidance, the ASD was crossed with multipurpose catheter which its tip was positioned in the LUPV and a floppy tip Amplatzer super stiff guide wire placed in the LUPV; then, sequential balloon dilatation of the atrial septum was done with peripheral balloons 10-30 mm and 12-30 mm (OTW). After that, the delivery sheath (Occlutech 14F) was crossed through the wire to mid LA, and the dilator was removed to allow back bleed. After loading the device (AFR 10 mm) and connecting to the delivery cable, the device was passed over the sheath to reach the tip of the sheath. By retracting the sheath, the distal disk was deployed in LA; then, the whole system was pulled backed toward the septum; after checking the orientation of the device by TEE, the proximal disk deployed. Eventually, after complete assessment of the device position, its stability, and the degree of left to right shunt, the device was released (Figure 3). Immediately after device implantation, hemodynamic study showed reduction of wedge pressure to 18 mmHg. Hemodynamic study before and after intervention is shown in Table 1.

The patient's daily visit after the procedure until discharge (one week) indicated that his shortness of breath had decreased. Lower extremity edema decreased, and blood oxygen saturation reached 79%.

Furthermore, at 2 months follow-up, the patient's clinical status (dyspnea and edema) improved significantly; cyanosis was decreased, and So2 increased to 79%.

Follow-up echocardiography showed the AFR device in the proper position with left-to-right shunt, and the left A-V valve mean pressure gradient was decreased to 7 mmHg, and mPAP decreased from 80 to 50 mmHg (Figure 4).

3. Discussion

In this article, we review different anatomical and hemodynamic conditions in patients with DILV and review different treatment methods in these patients. In addition, we are reviewing a new palliative treatment that has been performed for the first time in Iran in our patient.

As will be discussed below, the mentioned patient was still symptomatic with full drug treatment, and due to his condition and progression of disease to the Eisenmenger, it was not possible to perform corrective surgery for him, and we had to undergo palliative treatment.

As mentioned in studies, the most prevalent form of the univentricular heart is double-inlet ventricle in which a large ventricle, mostly with left ventricle morphology, receives both atrioventricular valves and connects to a hypoplastic ventricle through a ventricular septal defect which is called bulboventricular foramen [5]. Based on study, we have some anatomic heterogeneity in this disease [6], and therefore, the clinical presentations are variable and for this reason, there are divergent methods for palliative therapy of these patients including modified Blalock-Taussig shunt (for those with restrictive pulmonary blood flow), pulmonary artery banding (for patients with unrestrictive pulmonary blood flow), modified Norwood operation, palliative arterial switch, or arch repair plus concomitant pulmonary artery banding (for patients with systemic outflow tract obstruction or arch obstruction) [7]. Based on mentioned points, however, recent advances in the treatment of this disease have led to a major breakthrough in early and late prognosis of these patients and for some, we may not be able to do so for a variety of reasons [8].

Furthermore, in patients with left A-V valve stenosis, there is pressure gradient between LA and LV which in long-term leads to pulmonary venous congestion, pulmonary artery hypertension, and finally, irreversible elevated pulmonary vascular resistance [9].

In our patient who did not undergo any palliative strategies in a timely manner, due to the severity of his symptoms and the outstanding elevation of capillary wedge pressure and no convenient surgical options, we decided to perform percutaneous therapeutic interventions.

We had two options: dilating the interatrial septum defect or commissurotomy of the left AV valve; because of

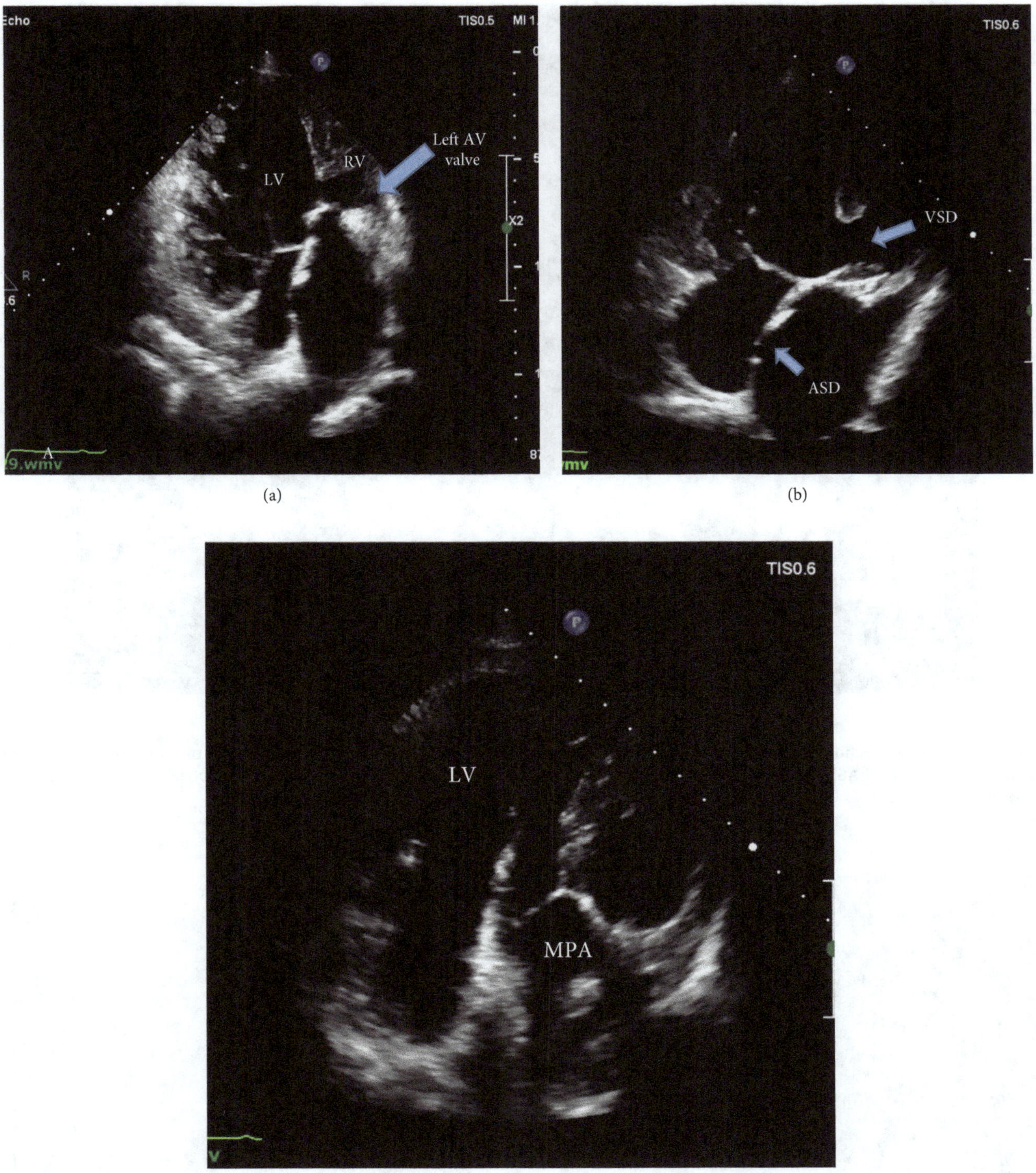

(a) (b) (c)

Figure 1: Continued.

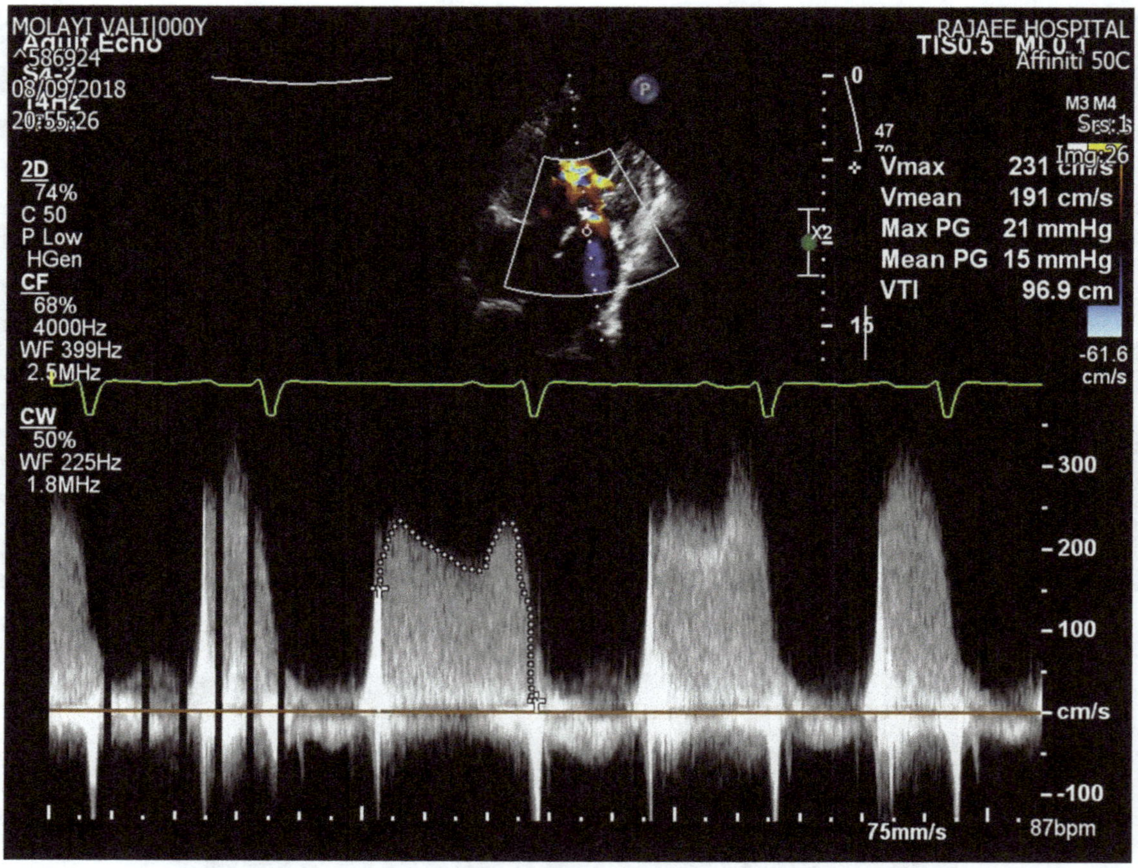

(d)

FIGURE 1: Transthoracic echocardiography in 4-chamber view shows (a) morphologic LV which is the right side of rudimentary RV, (b) large inlet type VSD, very small ASD, (C) PA originate from the main ventricle with confluent PABs, (d) Thick and hypo plastic left AV valve severe stenosis (MG:15, PG:21).

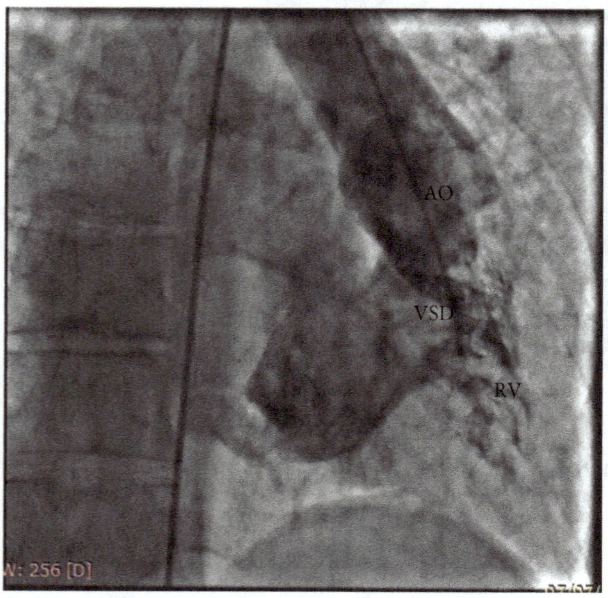

FIGURE 2: RV injection shows rudimentary systemic RV at the left side and large VSD.

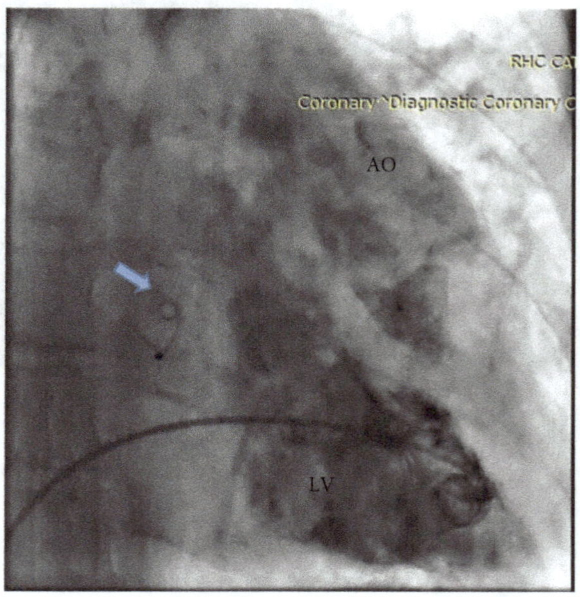

FIGURE 3: AFR is seen in the proper position.

Table 1: Hemodynamic parameters (mmHg) before and after AFR device implantation.

	LV	RV	PAP	Wedge	RA
Before	110/0-10	100/0-8	110/65	25	8
After	110/0-10	90/0-6	105/45	18	6

AFR: atrial flow regulator; LV: left ventricle; RV: right ventricle; PAP: pulmonary arterial pressure; RA: right atrium.

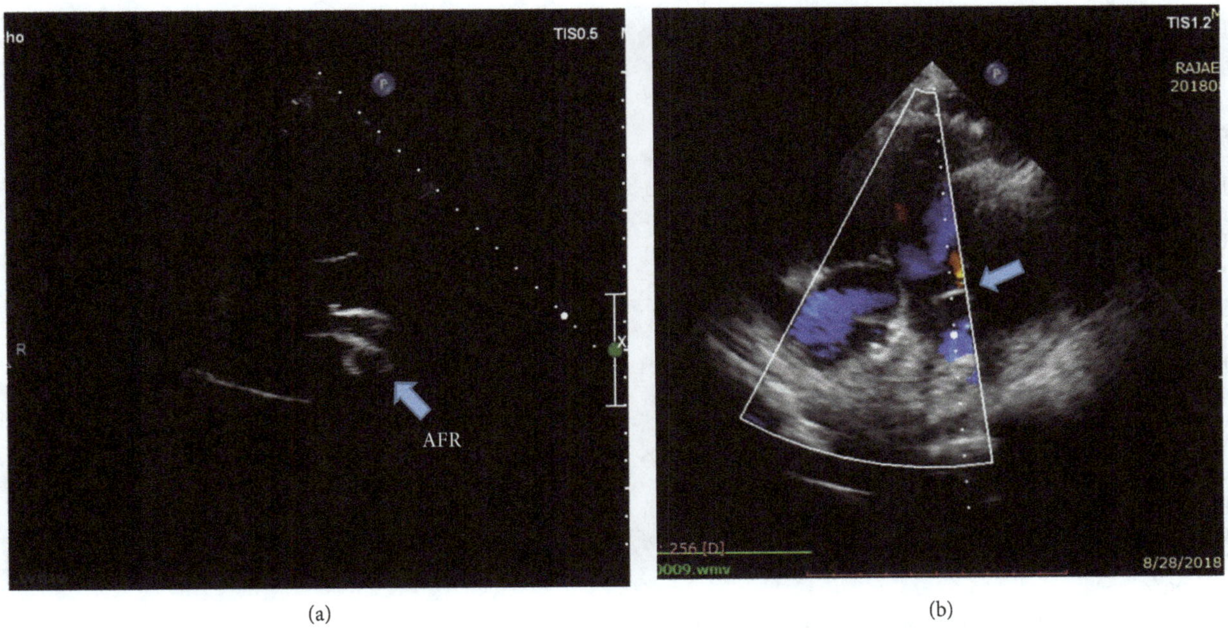

Figure 4: Follow-up echocardiography indicating the proper position of the AFR device with left-to-right shunt.

unsuitable anatomy of the AV valve for balloon dilation, we chose the first option. Isolated balloon atrial septostomy (BAS) might lead to unintentional tearing of the IAS and potential death. Also, it might occlude within the short-term due to overgrowth of intimal cells. So, we arbitrated to deploy the AFR device at the IAS to ensure that the hole remained open permanently.

The AFR device is a self-expandable double-disc nitinol wire mesh production which creates a communication between the atriums and allows blood to flow across the interatrial septum [10]. Initially, it was designed for those with severe pulmonary hypertension and RV failure with refractory symptoms for decompressing the right heart chambers via permanent right-to-left shunt which leads to elevation of the cardiac output, blood pressure, and organ perfusion despite of inducing mild systemic desaturation. Following the more experience about the role of this device, nowadays, it could be used whenever the either atrial pressure increases; so, the device would decompress the dedicated atrium. Those with elevated left atrium pressure would create a persistent left-to-right shunt which cause the reduction of LAP, PCWP, PAP, and pulmonary congestion symptoms and increase arterial blood saturation, cardiac output, blood pressure, and organ perfusion [11].

The diameter of disc varied from 16 to 23, the fenestration diameter ranges between 4 and 10 mm. and disc connective waist depending on the thickness of atrial septum varied between 2 and 0 mm.

The device is very flexible and adaptable with distinctive braiding and is currently used in patients with severe right ventricular (RV) failure due to pulmonary hypertension or left heart failure [9], left atrial congestion, and failing Fontan [12].

4. Conclusion

Transcatheter AFR device implantation could be regarded as a relatively novel palliative approach that is utilized in selective high-risk patients with pulmonary hypertension (PH).

Although it was used to be implanted in pH patients with RV overload for decompressing the right side of the heart, in this case, we implanted that to decompress the left side chambers due to severe left A-V valve stenosis in DILV patient.

To our knowledge, this case is one of the first experiences with the Occlutech AFR device implementation in adult patient with cyanotic congenital heart disease, with severe AV valve stenosis and restricted atrial septal defect.

Consent

We obtained written consent of our patient to report his case.

Authors' Contributions

ZK, MA, and AF managed the patients and drafted the paper. HG and ZH drafted the paper. All authors have read and approved the manuscript.

Acknowledgments

We thank our kind patient and our respectful colleagues who made this report possible.

References

[1] J. K. Perloff and A. Marelli, *Perloff's Clinical Recognition of Congenital Heart Disease: Expert Consult-Online and Print*, Elsevier Health Sciences, 2012.

[2] M. L. Jacobs and R. H. Anderson, "Nomenclature of the functionally univentricular heart," *Cardiology in the Young*, vol. 16, Supplement 1, pp. 3–8, 2006.

[3] B. Alsoufi, T. Slesnick, C. McCracken et al., "Current outcomes of the Norwood operation in patients with single-ventricle malformations other than hypoplastic left heart syndrome," *World Journal for Pediatric and Congenital Heart Surgery*, vol. 6, no. 1, pp. 46–52, 2015.

[4] P. Ayyıldız, "The evaluation of cases with double-inlet left ventricle-ventriculoarterial discordance," *Turkish Journal of Thoracic and Cardiovascular Surgery*, vol. 24, no. 2, pp. 213–219, 2016.

[5] J. L. Wilkinson and R. H. Anderson, "Anatomy of functionally single ventricle," *World Journal for Pediatric and Congenital Heart Surgery*, vol. 3, no. 2, pp. 159–164, 2012.

[6] C. Frescura and G. Thiene, "The new concept of univentricular heart," *Frontiers in Pediatrics*, vol. 2, p. 62, 2014.

[7] B. Alsoufi, S. Gillespie, B. Kogon et al., "Results of palliation with an initial modified Blalock-Taussig shunt in neonates with single ventricle anomalies associated with restrictive pulmonary blood flow," *The Annals of Thoracic Surgery*, vol. 99, no. 5, pp. 1639–1647, 2015.

[8] S. Tabbutt, N. Ghanayem, C. Ravishankar et al., "Risk factors for hospital morbidity and mortality after the Norwood procedure: a report from the Pediatric heart network single ventricle reconstruction trial," *The Journal of Thoracic and Cardiovascular Surgery*, vol. 144, no. 4, pp. 882–895, 2012.

[9] B. A. Carabello, "Modern management of mitral stenosis," *Circulation*, vol. 112, no. 3, pp. 432–437, 2005.

[10] A. Dąbrowska-Kugacka, D. Ciećwierz, G. Żuk et al., "Atrial flow regulator for severe drug resistant pulmonary arterial hypertension after congenital heart defect correction," *Cardiology Journal*, vol. 26, no. 1, pp. 102–104, 2019.

[11] R. Baglini, "Atrial septostomy in patients with end-stage pulmonary hypertension. No more needles but wires, energy and close anatomical definition," *Journal of Interventional Cardiology*, vol. 26, no. 1, pp. 62–68, 2013.

[12] L. Manuri, R. E. Calaciura, A. De Zorzi et al., "Atrial flow regulator for failing Fontan circulation: an initial European experience," *Interactive CardioVascular and Thoracic Surgery*, vol. 27, no. 5, pp. 761–764, 2018.

23

Early Left Ventricular Thrombus Formation in a COVID-19 Patient with ST Elevation Myocardial Infarction

Harish Sharma[1,2] **and Sudhakar George**[2]

[1]*Institute of Cardiovascular Sciences, University of Birmingham, Birmingham, UK*
[2]*University Hospitals Birmingham NHS Foundation Trust, Mindelsohn Way, Birmingham B15 2TH, UK*

Correspondence should be addressed to Sudhakar George; sudhakar.george@uhb.nhs.uk

Academic Editor: Kuan-Rau Chiou

Background. Left ventricular thrombus (LVT) is a complication of acute myocardial infarction (AMI) due to localised haemostasis. LVT is typically seen 3-12 days following AMI and is seldom seen within the first 24 hours. LVT increases the risk of mortality due to systemic thromboembolism. Patients with Coronavirus Disease-19 (COVID-19) are potentially hypercoagulable and this may promote early development of LVT. *Case.* A 50-year-old man with no past medical history was admitted with a severe diabetic ketoacidosis following a 4-day history of cough and fever. The patient tested positive for COVID-19 and required intensive care treatment for ventilation and haemofiltration. After returning to ward-based care, the patient developed chest pain and electrocadiographic changes consistent with an acute anterior ST-elevation myocardial infarction. Emergency percutaneous coronary intervention was performed to the left anterior descending artery. However, the patient developed diuretic-resistant pulmonary oedema and a bedside echocardiogram revealed significant LVT despite only 4 hours of chest pain. The thrombus was associated with the anteroseptal wall of the left ventricle which was hypokinetic but not aneurysmal. An intra-aortic balloon pump (IABP) was inserted, but the patient developed ipsilateral lower limb ischaemia due to the formation of thrombus in the femoral artery and irreversible cardiogenic shock from which he ultimately succumbed. *Conclusion.* COVID-19-positive patients are potentially hypercoagulable, and MI in this population may precipitate LVT earlier than expected. Consideration should be made for routine early screening of post-MI COVID-19 patients for LVT. If detected, anticoagulation may reduce the risk of cardiovascular mortality in this high-risk group.

1. Introduction

Left ventricular thrombus (LVT) complicates up to 15% of all acute myocardial infarction (AMI) cases [1] and 25% of patients with anterior myocardial infarction [2]. A postinfarction triad of hypercoagulability, left ventricular (LV) hypokinesia or aneurysm, and local myocardial inflammation creates an area of relatively static blood which is prone to thrombus formation.

Traditionally, LVT has been detected by transthoracic echocardiography (TTE) with the use of contrast enhancement if the LV endocardium is not clearly visualised. A serial study using TTE found that LVT is typically detected 3-4 days following myocardial infarction (MI), with very few cases detectable within the first 24 hours [3]. In another serial TTE study of 105 patients, no cases of LVT were observed within the first 11.3 ± 8 hours and the median time to the first discovery of LVT following anterior MI was 6 days. Cardiovascular magnetic resonance (CMR) imaging has superseded echocardiography as the most accurate modality for the detection of LVT [4]. Recent evidence has shown that CMR performed 9-12 days post-MI gives the highest detection rate [5].

The incidence of LVT has fallen significantly since widespread early percutaneous coronary intervention (PCI) has been widely adopted for the management of AMI. In clinical practice, LVT is most commonly seen in late-presenting MI patients. In patients who present early and undergo prompt

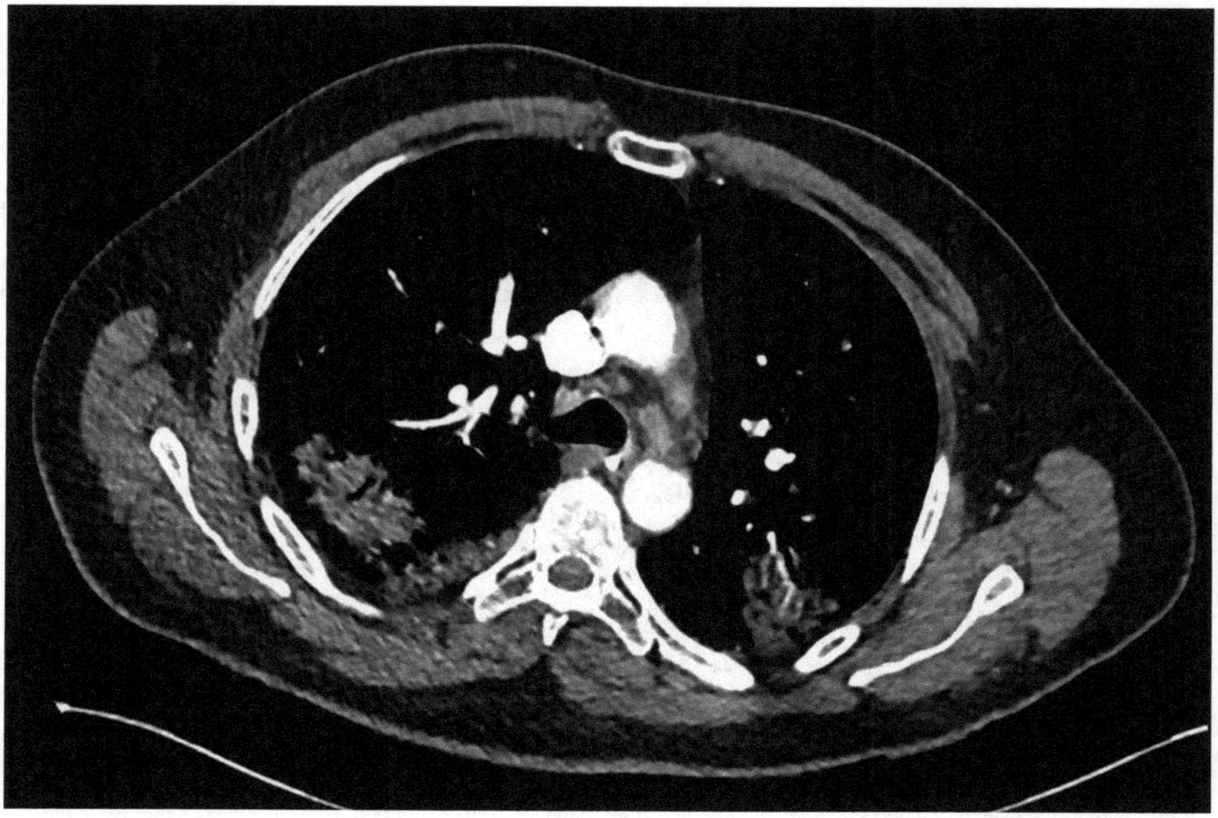

Figure 1: CTPA: bilateral patchy consolidation in keeping with COVID-19 with superadded aspergillosis infection causing cavitating lesions.

revascularisation, LVT is rarely observed, particularly within the first 24 hours of AMI.

The emergence of the novel zoonotic Severe Acute Respiratory Syndrome Coronavirus-2 (SARS-CoV-2) has resulted in Coronavirus Disease 2019 (COVID-19) becoming a major global pandemic. Although the predominant symptoms are respiratory, cardiovascular complications have also been described. Studies have reported that COVID-19 patients are subject to a significant derangement of haemostasis, resulting in hypercoagulability as seen on whole blood thromboelastography [6].

In this case, we describe a COVID-19 patient who suffered an acute anterior myocardial infarction and had readily detectable, established LVT on transthoracic echocardiography, within 4 hours of presentation.

2. History of Presentation

A 50-year old man with no past medical history was admitted to hospital by ambulance after his wife found him unresponsive. On admission, the patient was confused and agitated with a Glasgow Coma Scale (GCS) score of 11.

3. Examination

On examination, the patient had mottled legs, dry mucous membranes, and peripheral circulatory collapse. Blood pressure (BP) and peripheral oxygen saturations were unrecordable.

4. Investigations

Arterial blood gas measurements revealed a blood glucose beyond the upper limit of recordable value (despite no history of diabetes) and ketones of 3.6 mmol/L with a lactic acidosis.

Notable abnormal blood tests included an acute kidney injury (urea 41.3 mmol/L, creatinine 277 μmol/L, estimated glomerular filtration rate of 21 mL/min), hypernatraemia (Na 172 mmol/L), and hypercholersterolaemia (total cholesterol 9.0 mmol/L). The white cell count was normal (9.3×10^9), but the C-reactive protein level was raised at 53 mg/L and over the following 5 days increased to 374 mg/L.

5. Differential Diagnosis

The patient was thought to have a new diagnosis of diabetes mellitus presenting as either a diabetic ketoacidosis or hyperosmolar hyperlycaemic state provoked by COVID-19 infection.

6. Course of Disease and Management

The patient was initially treated with intravenous (IV) fluids, antibiotics, and an insulin infusion until the blood glucose reduced to acceptable levels, following which he was treated with subcutaneous insulin. A collateral history revealed that the patient had a 4-day history of cough and pyrexia. One week prior to admission, two members of his household had been unwell with COVID-19 symptoms. The patient

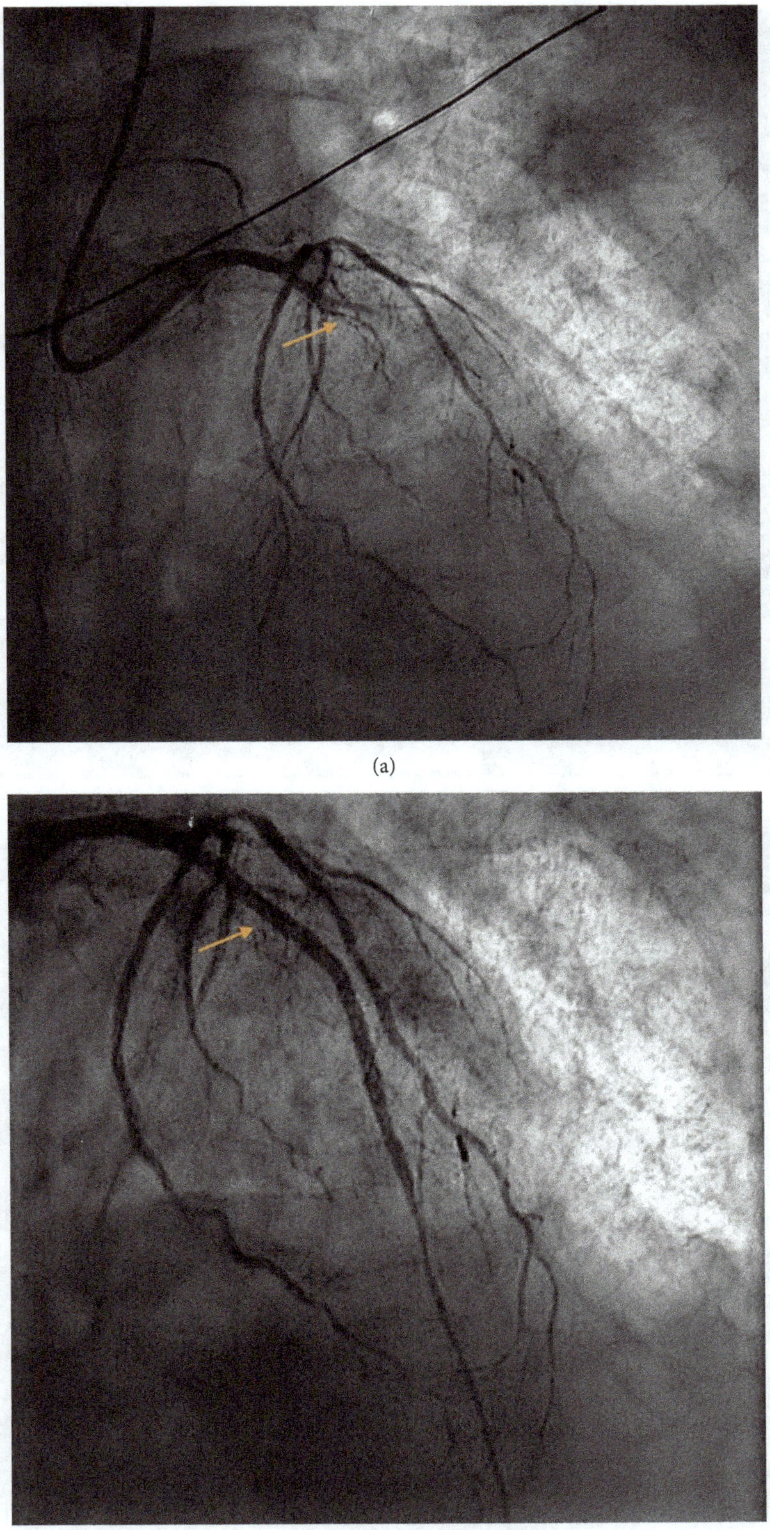

(a)

(b)

FIGURE 2: Coronary angiogram in the PA cranial view demonstrating (a) LAD occlusion before intervention and (b) reperfusion following implantation of a drug-eluting stent.

tested positive for COVID-19, and despite 3 days of ward-based treatment, his condition continued to deteriorate. Worsening respiratory failure necessitated transfer to the intensive care unit (ICU) for intubation and ventilation. The circulation was supported by vasopressors and continuous veno-venous haemofiltration was commenced.

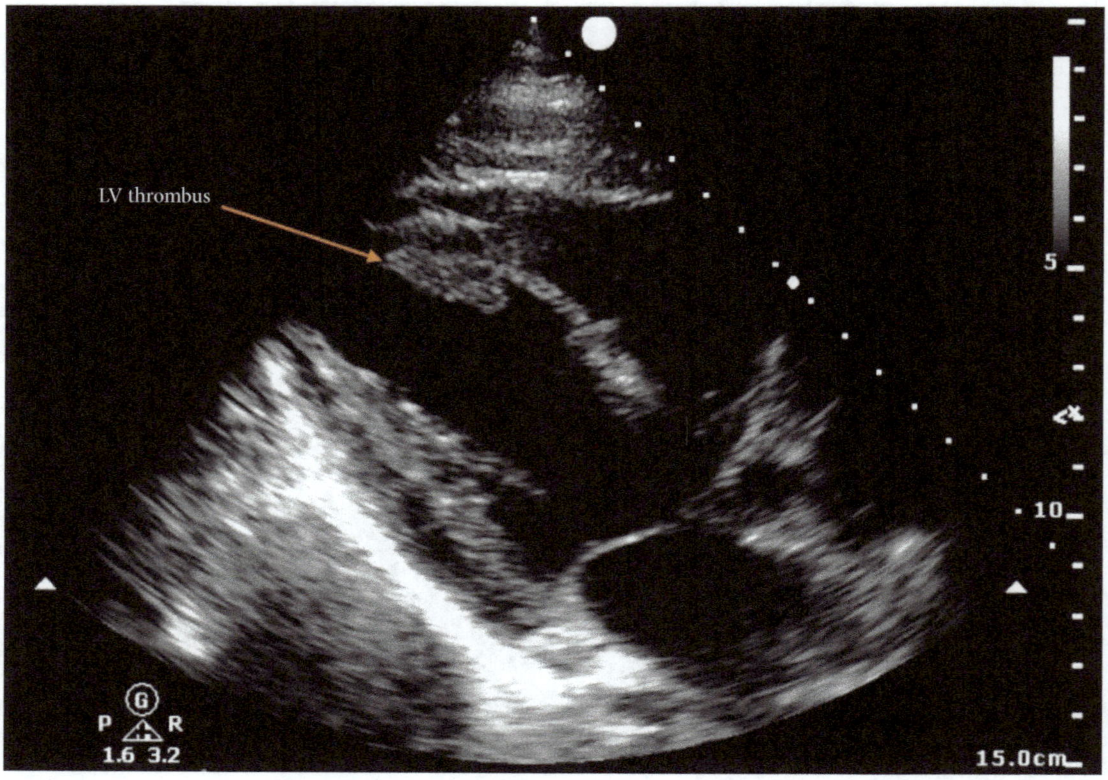

(a)

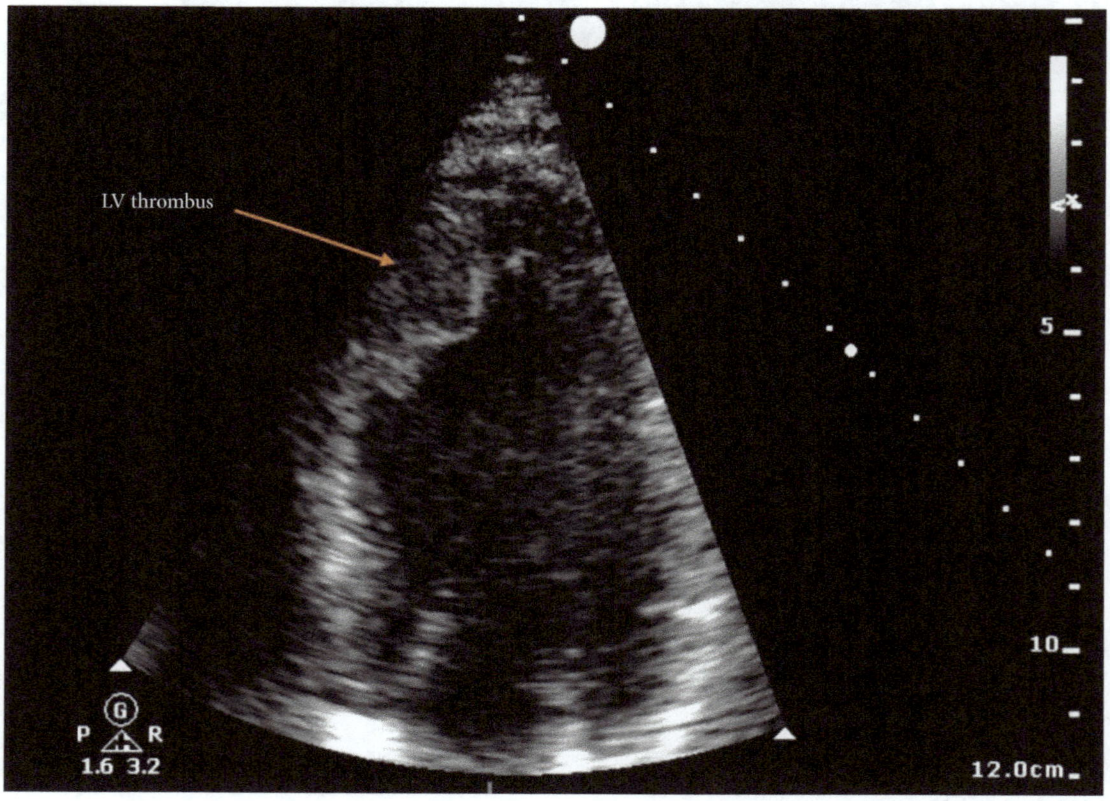

(b)

FIGURE 3: Transthoracic echocardiogram demonstrating thrombus on the mid-to-apical anteroseptal left ventricular wall in the (a) parasternal long axis view and (b) apical 4-chamber view.

Twelve days after admission, the patient was transferred back to the ward. Once again, his respiratory status declined and a computed tomography pulmonary angiogram (CTPA) revealed patchy consolidation and cavitation (Figure 1). Two sputum samples tested positive for aspergillus, and the patient was treated with voriconazole.

One month after admission, the patient suddenly developed acute chest pain. An electrocardiogram (ECG) demonstrated anterior ST-segment elevation. The patient was taken to the cardiac catheterisation suite for an emergency coronary angiogram. This demonstrated acute occlusion of the left anterior descending (LAD) artery (Figure 2(a)) and moderate bystander atheroma in the other coronary vessels. The patient was treated with primary percutaneous coronary intervention (PCI) to the LAD with implantation of a single drug-eluting stent, restoring TIMI 3 flow in the vessel. However, during the procedure, the patient developed acute pulmonary oedema with poor response to IV furosemide. Bedside transthoracic echocardiography revealed moderately impaired left ventricular (LV) function with the greatest function in the basal segments. Surprisingly, LV thrombus was noted attached to the anteroseptal LV wall, which was hypokinetic but not aneurysmal (Figure 3).

The patient was reintubated and readmitted to the intensive care unit. High-sensitive troponin I was measured at >50,000 ng/L one day postinfarction, having been only 2540 ng/L one day earlier, indicating an acute large territory myocardial infarction had occurred. The total plasma cholesterol level was rechecked and was within the normal range. The patient developed cardiogenic shock resistant to inotropes, and despite insertion of an intra-aortic balloon pump (IABP), cardiac output did not improve. Ipsilateral lower limb ischaemia developed as a result of a hypercoagulable state and IABP. Ultrasound of the right femoral artery confirmed the presence of thrombus in the vessel. Vascular surgeons did not feel that the patient would survive emergency vascular surgery, and after discussions with the family, treatment was withdrawn and the patient succumbed to cardiogenic shock.

7. Discussion

This case report describes an unusual case whereby established LVT was detected only 4 hours after the onset of acute anterior ST-elevation MI in a patient recovering from severe COVID-19 infection.

Studies have demonstrated that COVID-19 infection is associated with several cardiovascular complications including myocarditis, arrhythmias, and vascular inflammation. Localised inflammation at the plaque level may disrupt stable coronary atheroma and predispose to acute coronary syndromes [7].

Although the patient in this case did not have a history of angina, moderate multivessel coronary atheroma was found on coronary angiography, indicating preexisting asymptomatic coronary artery disease. The presence of COVID-19 infection may have not only promoted plaque instability in the LAD but also the development of early LVT.

Although the prevalence of LVT has fallen in the modern era of early revascularisation, frequency of detection is likely to increase during the COVID-19 pandemic. Firstly, patients with MI symptoms are more likely to avoid early hospital admission due to a fear of contracting COVID-19. Secondly, COVID-19 infection has been associated with markedly hypercoagulable thromboelastography profiles, increasing the risk of early LVT formation.

Detection of LVT in COVID-19 post-MI patients is paramount due to the risk of systemic thromboembolism, further increasing the risk of morbidity and mortality in this high-risk group. International guidelines recommend anticoagulation if LVT is detected [8]. This case highlights that COVID-19 patients presenting with MI are at risk of early LVT formation and should be evaluated with early inpatient echocardiography, with a low threshold for contrast echocardiography or CMR if necessary.

Additional Points

Learning Objectives. Case: a patient with COVID-19 who developed early LV thrombus. (i) Patients with COVID-19 are potentially hypercoagulable and may form LV thrombus far earlier than expected. (ii) Consider early inpatient imaging following acute MI in COVID-19 patients with echocardiography or CMR if necessary.

References

[1] S. Solheim, I. Seljeflot, K. Lunde et al., "Frequency of left ventricular thrombus in patients with anterior wall acute myocardial infarction treated with percutaneous coronary intervention and dual antiplatelet therapy," *The American Journal of Cardiology*, vol. 106, no. 9, pp. 1197–1200, 2010.

[2] R. Delewi, R. Nijveldt, A. Hirsch et al., "Left ventricular thrombus formation after acute myocardial infarction as assessed by cardiovascular magnetic resonance imaging," *European Journal of Radiology*, vol. 81, no. 12, pp. 3900–3904, 2012.

[3] C. A. Visser, G. Kan, K. I. Lie, and D. Durrer, "Left ventricular thrombus following acute myocardial infarction: a prospective serial echocardiographic study of 96 patients," *European Heart Journal*, vol. 4, no. 5, pp. 333–337, 1983.

[4] I. Roifman, K. A. Connelly, G. A. Wright, and H. C. Wijeysundera, "Echocardiography vs cardiac magnetic resonance imaging for the diagnosis of left ventricular thrombus: a systematic review," *Canadian Journal of Cardiology*, vol. 31, no. 6, pp. 785–791, 2015, 31.

[5] B. Gellen, L. Biere, D. Logeart et al., "Timing of cardiac magnetic resonance imaging impacts on the detection rate of left ventricular thrombus after myocardial infarction," *JACC: Cardiovascular Imaging*, vol. 10, no. 11, pp. 1404-1405, 2017.

[6] M. Panigada, N. Bottino, P. Tagliabue et al., "Hypercoagulability of COVID-19 patients in intensive care unit: A report of thromboelastography findings and other parameters of hemostasis," *Journal of Thrombosis and Haemostasis*, vol. 18, no. 7, pp. 1738–1742, 2020.

[7] M. Madjid, P. Safavi-Naeini, S. D. Solomon, and O. Vardeny, "Potential effects of coronaviruses on the cardiovascular System," *JAMA Cardiology*, 2020.

[8] B. Ibanez, S. James, S. Agewall et al., "2017 ESC guidelines for the management of acute myocardial infarction in patients presenting with ST-segment elevation," *European Heart Journal*, vol. 39, no. 2, pp. 119–177, 2018.

24

Rare Case of Cavernous Haemangioma of the Right Atrium with Probable Hepatic Haemangioma

Sally Harrison

Dunedin Public Hospital, Dunedin, New Zealand

Correspondence should be addressed to Sally Harrison; sally_harrison@hotmail.com

Academic Editor: Aiden Abidov

Cardiac haemangiomas are rare causes of atrial masses. This case report is of a 44-year-old male who presented with a right atrial mass that was found incidentally on a CT performed for renal colic. The mass was further investigated with a transthoracic echocardiogram that showed that it was echodense and arising from the Eustachian valve in the right atrium. Coronary angiogram revealed large well-developed atrial branches that crossed superiorly over the left atrium and entered the mass in the right atrium. Surgical resection was undertaken, and this confirmed that the mass had a fleshy, encapsulated appearance with a sessile stalk. Histology demonstrated a cavernous haemangioma. The patient had a residual small defect in the interatrial septum postoperatively but otherwise made a good recovery.

1. Introduction

Cardiac tumours are uncommon medical entities. 75% of primary cardiac tumours are benign in nature, with atrial myxomas being the most common of these, making up 75% [1].

The following case report is of a 44-year-old patient with a right atrial mass. This is an example of a mass which was suspicious for myxoma but with atypical features.

2. Case Presentation

A 44-year-old gentleman presented with an episode of right-sided renal colic and was referred for an US abdomen. On this imaging, an echogenic mass was incidentally seen within the right atrium. Due to the patient's ongoing abdominal discomfort, a CT abdomen with arterial and venous contrast was also performed.

The CT abdomen report detailed that the right atrial mass measured 38 by 35 mm with a tail extending down into the supradiaphragmatic inferior vena cava (Figure 1). Additionally, there was a round low density segment two liver lesion with minimal peripheral enhancement with contrast, possibly a haemangioma.

At this stage, the patient was referred for cardiology assessment. Further questioning revealed symptoms of intermittent chest pain. He did not exhibit any symptoms or signs of heart failure. He had no history of malignancy and no B symptoms. There was no personal or familial history of cardiac disorders. Physical exam and ECG were unremarkable.

Firstly, a transthoracic echocardiogram was performed. This depicted a large echodense mass measuring 4.5 by 3 cm in the right atrium that appeared to arise from the Eustachian valve (Figure 2). It did not seem to originate from the inferior vena cava and was not obstructing the tricuspid valve. The patient had an otherwise normal echocardiograph with left ventricular ejection fraction 55-60%, normal right ventricular function, and no valvular pathology.

Transoesophageal echocardiogram confirmed the above findings and clearly demonstrated the mass, which appeared to have morphological features consistent with myxoma (Figure 3).

Routine preoperative coronary angiogram was conducted and interestingly revealed large well-developed atrial

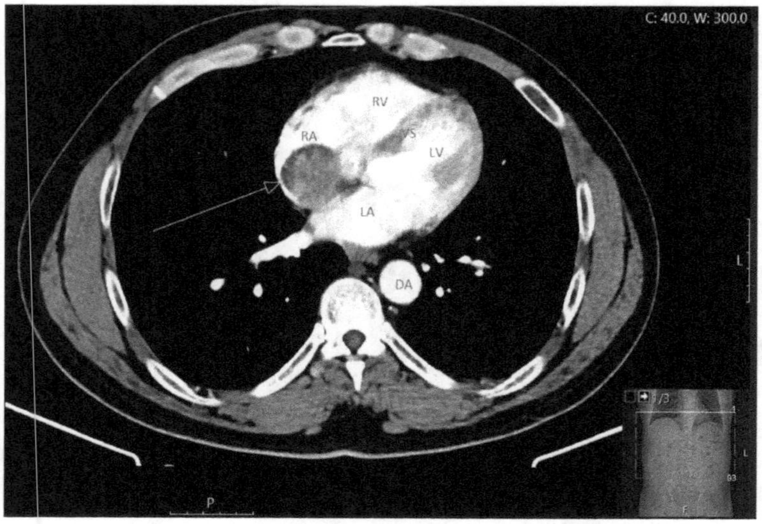

Figure 1: CT abdomen axial view with arterial contrast. Arrow pointing to the right atrial mass. RA = right atrium; RV = right ventricle; VS = interventricular septum; LV = left ventricle; LA = left atrium; DA = descending aorta.

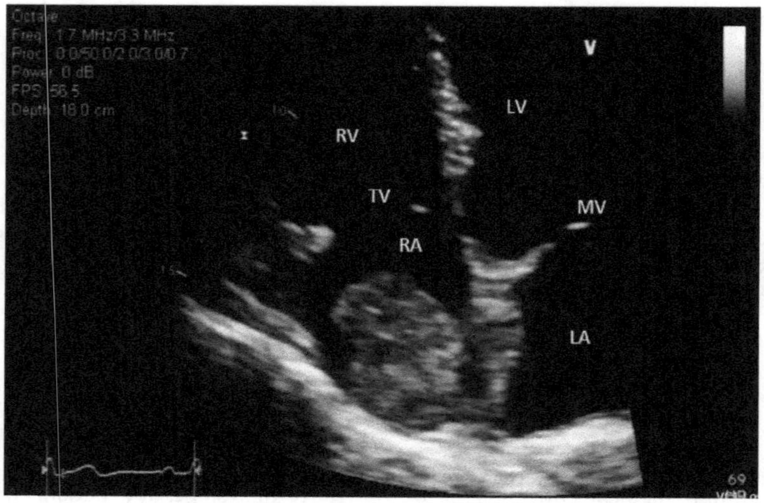

Figure 2: Transthoracic echocardiogram, four chamber view. Mass depicted in the right atrium, not obstructing the tricuspid valve. RV = right ventricle; LV = left ventricle; RA = right atrium; LA = left atrium; MV = mitral valve; TV = tricuspid valve.

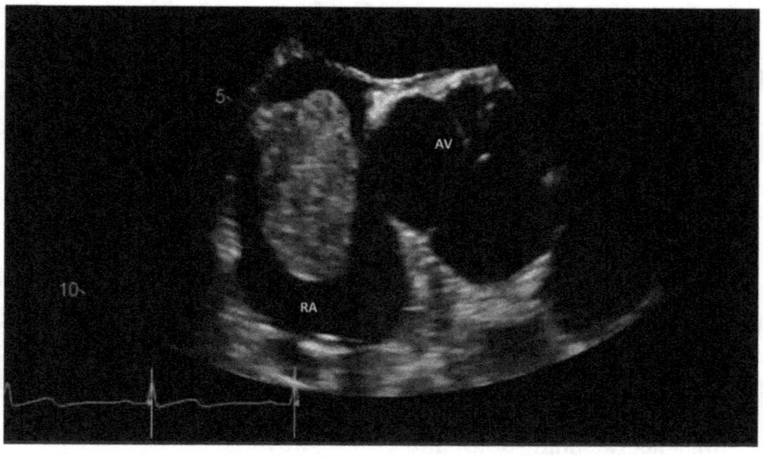

Figure 3: Transoesophageal echocardiogram mid oesophageal aortic valve short axis view demonstrating an echogenic mass in the right atrium (RA) and aortic valve (AV).

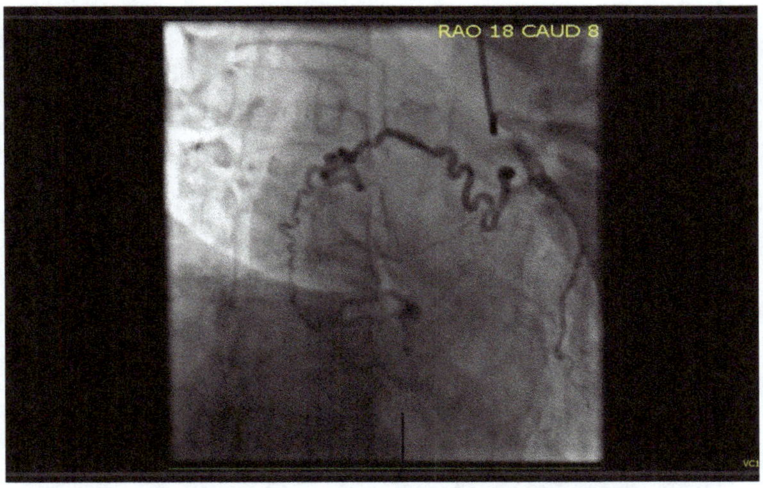

Figure 4: Coronary angiogram RAO caudal view defining the vascular nature of the right atrial mass.

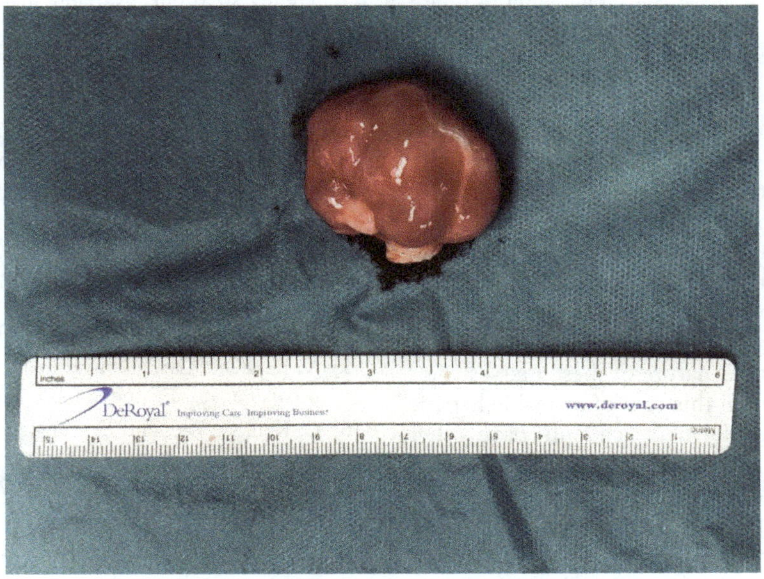

Figure 5: Operative specimen: right atrial mass.

branches that crossed superiorly over the left atrium and entered the mass in the right atrium. The vessel carried contrast, enhancing the outer layers of the mass (Figure 4).

The patient was referred for surgical removal of the right atrial mass. Intraoperative epicardial ultrasound was initially used to interrogate the inferior vena cava to ensure that bicaval cannulation was feasible. It was confirmed that the mass did not encroach into the inferior vena cava and therefore aortic and bicaval cannulation was used to place the patient on cardiopulmonary bypass. The mass was located at the inferolateral aspect of the right atrium and had a fleshy, encapsulated appearance with a sessile stalk. The mass was completely excised (Figure 5). The resulting atrial defect was closed in two layers with 4-0 Prolene.

The patient had an uneventful postoperative period and was discharged five days after his surgery.

Histology of the mass demonstrated a cavernous haemangioma composed of dilated vascular spaces lined by endothelial cells (Figure 6). There was no evidence of atypia or malignancy.

Echocardiogram performed four months after his operation depicted a small atrial shunt seen on colour Doppler. There was no residual mass in the right atrium.

3. Discussion

Cardiac cavernous haemangiomas are exceedingly rare benign tumours, representing 5% of this group [1, 2]. They are most frequently found in the right side of the heart [2]. These haemangiomas are often asymptomatic and found incidentally during investigation of other diseases [3].

Cardiac haemangiomas are most commonly seen in young adults, with a median presenting age of 43 years, similar to this case [2]. Presentation is likely to occur earlier if the haemangioma causes arrhythmia or heart failure through intracardiac obstruction or valvular involvement

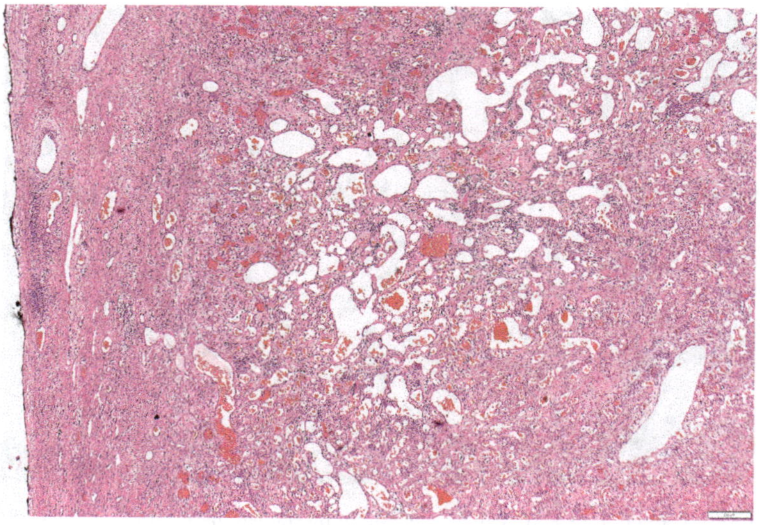

FIGURE 6: Histological photograph 40x (haemotoxylin and eosin stain). Free surface of the lesion (not attached to the wall of the atrium) to the left; occupying most of the image is a proliferation of thin-walled, differently sized but invariably dilated, capillaries lined by banal endothelial cells.

due to their size [1]. Echocardiogram is the gold standard imaging for this condition [4].

Whilst preoperative investigations suggested a myxoma, some features of this presentation were atypical. Firstly, right atrial myxomas only account for 23% of all myxomas [5]. Secondly, in this case, the rich vascularity seen on angiogram may have indicated that this was not a myxoma but a haemangioma. Cardiac MRIs and coronary angiogram are useful in determining the vascular nature of these masses prior to resection [4]. The finding in this case of probable hepatic haemangioma is not unusual—many patients have other haemangiomas including skin, pulmonary, pleural, and hepatic [3, 6]. The presence of this hepatic haemangioma may have also given a clue to the true diagnosis of this mass.

Although atrial myxomas make up the vast majority of cardiac tumours, it is prudent to remember that not all cardiac masses are myxomas, as evidenced by this case. In particular, when atypical features are present, the presumptive preoperative diagnosis of myxoma should be avoided.

Consent

The patient has provided written consent for publication of this case report.

References

[1] T. J. Vander Salm, "Unusual primary tumors of the heart," *Seminars in Thoracic and Cardiovascular Surgery*, vol. 12, no. 2, pp. 89–100, 2000.

[2] J. E. Thomas, A. T. Eror, M. Kenney, and J. Carvalho, "Asymptomatic right atrial cavernous hemangioma: a case report and review of the literature," *Cardiovascular Pathology*, vol. 13, no. 6, pp. 341–344, 2004.

[3] H. Miao, W. Yang, M. Zhou, Q. Zhu, and Z. Jiang, "Atrial hemangioma: a case report and review of the literature," *Annals of Thoracic and Cardiovascular Surgery*, vol. 25, no. 2, pp. 71–81, 2019.

[4] M. L. Grebenc, M. L. Rosado de Christenson, A. P. Burke, C. E. Green, and J. R. Galvin, "Primary cardiac and pericardial neoplasms: radiologic-pathologic correlation," *Radiographics*, vol. 20, no. 4, pp. 1073–1103, 2000.

[5] K. Reynen, "Cardiac myxomas," *The New England Journal of Medicine*, vol. 333, no. 24, pp. 1610–1617, 1995.

[6] C. Kan, C. Yae, and Y. Yang, "Left ventricular haemangioma with papillary endothelial hyperplasia and liver involvement," *Heart*, vol. 90, no. 8, article e49, 2004.

25

Cardiac and Systemic Thrombus Caused by Drug Abuse

John Eliveha, Shravani Vindhyal, and Mohinder Vindhyal

Department of Internal Medicine, University of Kansas, 1001 N Minneapolis St., Wichita, KS 67214, USA

Correspondence should be addressed to John Eliveha; jbeliveha@gmail.com

Academic Editor: Antonio de Padua Mansur

Drug abuse is an increasing concern all over the world especially in the United States. Methamphetamine have been well established to cause elevated body temperature, irregular heartbeat, seizures, and heart disease. We present a case of ventricular thrombus with systemic emboli in a patient with dilated cardiomyopathy after methamphetamine use.

1. Introduction

Methamphetamine is a sympathomimetic amine that increases synaptic concentration of serotonin, noradrenaline, and dopamine, creating hallucinogenic, euphoric, and stimulant effects [1]. Cardiovascular complications are the second leading cause of death in methamphetamine users [2]. The cardiac complications of methamphetamines are hypothesized from a variety of mechanisms such as hypertension, tachycardia, and myocardial toxicity with cellular death, fibrosis, and contraction band necrosis [3, 4].

2. Case Presentation

A 24-year-old female with a history of HIV/AIDS, nonischemic cardiomyopathy, and methamphetamine and marijuana abuse presented with acute onset lower extremity pain. The patient reported to have snorted methamphetamine overnight and woke up with severe lower extremity pain as well as inability to move. Surgical history was significant for excision of sublingual glands. Family history: mother was HIV positive; both mother and father had significant history of substance abuse. She drank one to two alcoholic drinks per week and was an everyday smoker, between 1/4 pack and 1/2 pack per day. Her vital signs were significant for tachycardia, tachypnea, and hypotension. Lower extremity examination was positive for tender lower extremities with no palpable dorsalis pedis, posterior tibial, and popliteal pulses bilaterally. Initial lab tests were significant for lactic acidosis, acute kidney injury, EKG with nonspecific ST-T wave changes (Figure 1), elevated troponin, 1.08 ng/ml, peaked at 3.5 ng/ml and urine drug screen was positive for methamphetamine and marijuana. Hemoglobin 11.9 gm/dl, white blood cells 10.4, platelets 178, sodium 139 mmol/liter, potassium 4.1 mmol/liter, chloride 104 mmol/liter, bicarbonate 20 mmol/liter, BUN 11 mg/dl, creatinine 1.3 mg/liter, blood glucose 141 mg/dl, AST 68 units/liter, ALT 41 units/liter, total bilirubin 0.9 grams/dl, alkaline phosphatase 107 IU/liter, and INR 1.8. Arterial and venous duplex of the lower extremities revealed no blood flow. CT angiogram showed large segment aortic occlusion (4 cm) just beyond the renal arteries and partial occlusive thrombus in the superior mesenteric artery with early ischemia (Figures 2 and 3). There were also multiple areas of bilateral renal infarcts left greater than right with the main renal arteries patent bilaterally. Transthoracic echocardiogram showed an echo dense mass, 2.4 cm × 2.8 cm, 1.2 cm × 2.0 cm in size, in the left ventricle with defined margins that are distinct from the endocardium seen throughout systole and diastole, consistent with left ventricular thrombus (Figures 4–6). Ejection fraction was estimated to be 15 %, with increased wall thickness and grade 3 diastolic dysfunction. There was mild to moderate mitral and tricuspid regurgitation with normal valve structure. CT head was obtained due to an altered mental status which was negative for acute bleeding. The patient became profoundly hypotensive which was likely due to cardiogenic shock despite being on maximum vasopressors. She developed limb ischemia due to compartment syndrome requiring fasciotomy. Interventional radiology and vascular surgery were consulted, surgical thrombectomy was done.

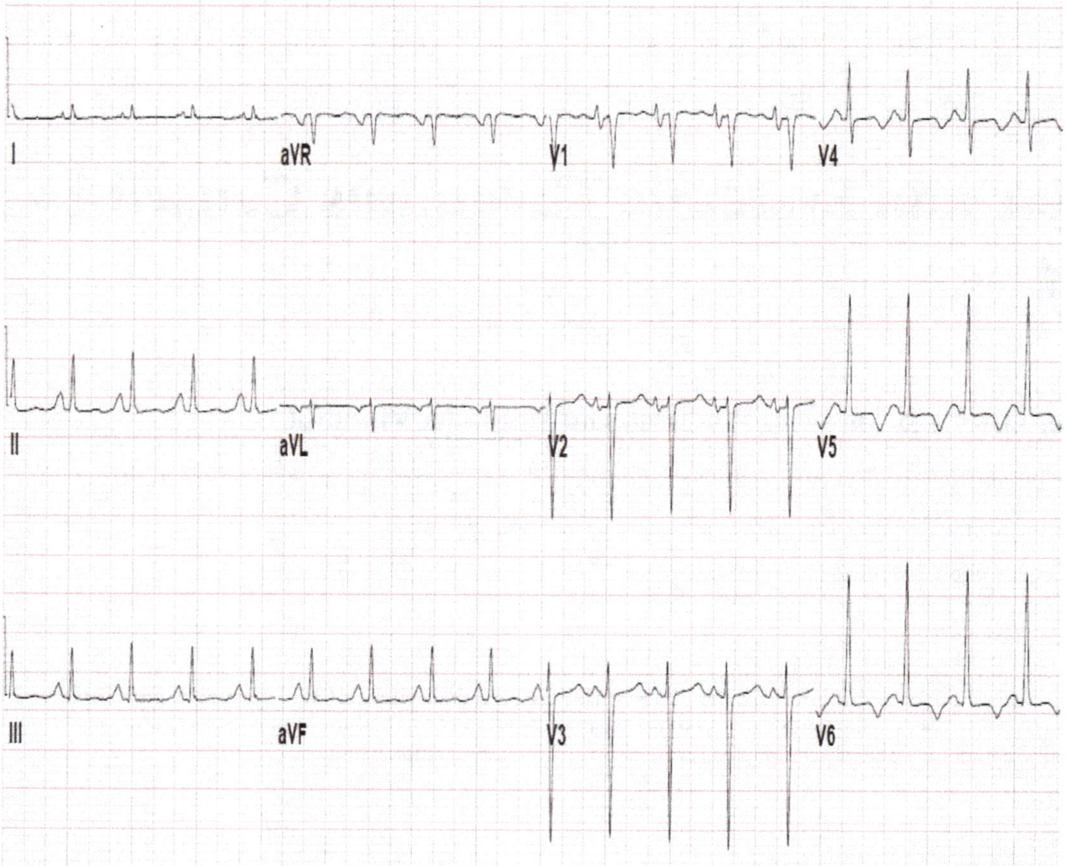

FIGURE 1: EKG showing nonspecific ST-T wave changes.

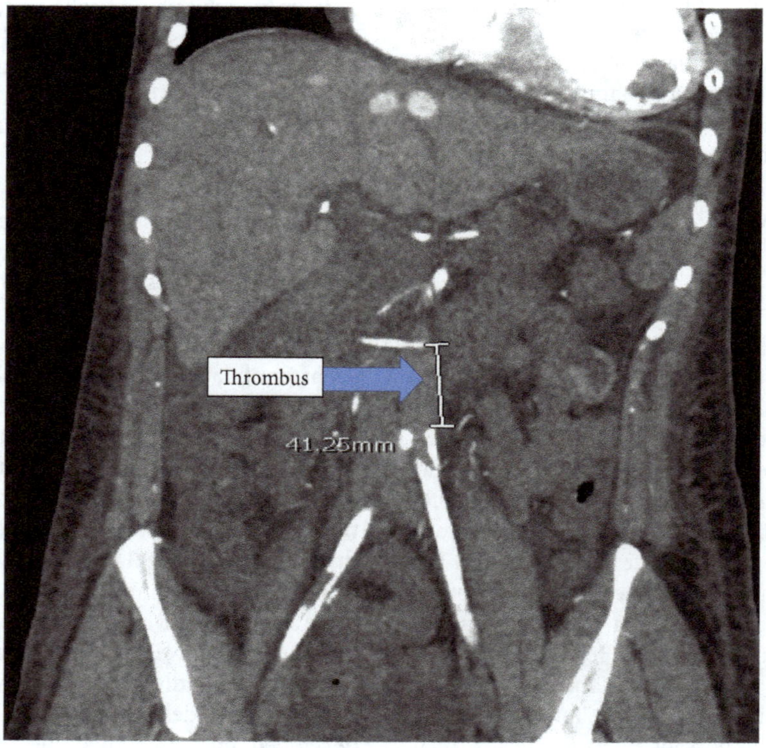

FIGURE 2: CT angiogram showing a massive AAA thrombus beyond the renal arteries.

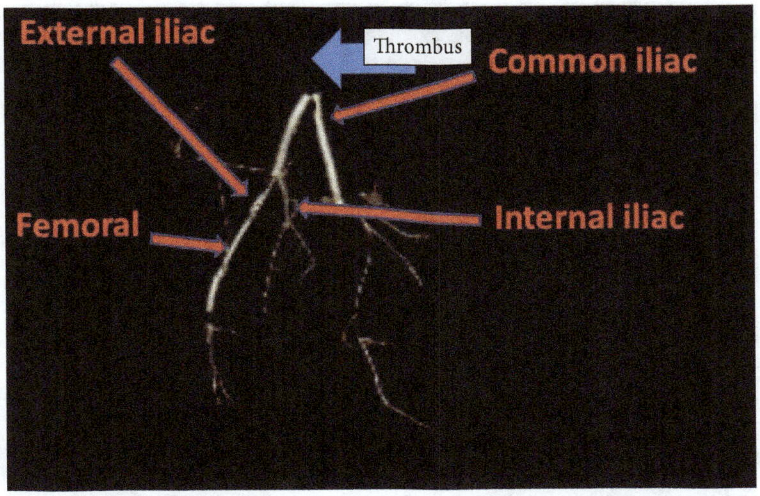

FIGURE 3: CT angiogram reconstruct showing large segmental aortic occlusions.

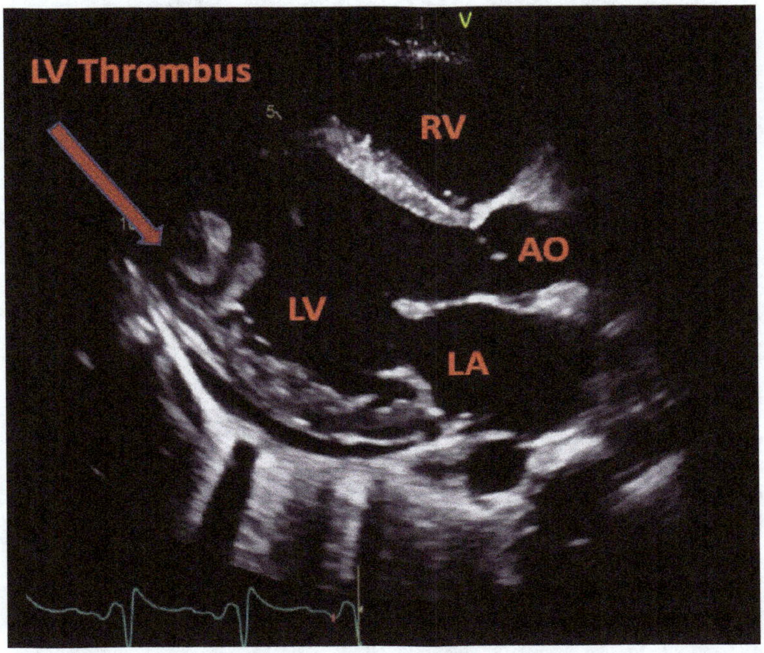

FIGURE 4: Parasternal long axis view showing LV thrombus. LA: left atrium; AO: aorta; RV: right ventricle; LV: left ventricle.

The patient's status worsened developing rhabdomyolysis, shock liver, and acute kidney injury with severe metabolic acidosis. She could not tolerate continuous renal replacement therapy. The patient had an episode of ventricular fibrillation and expired after three days of being hospitalized.

3. Discussion

Methamphetamine cause myocardial damage via multifactorial mechanisms. Excessive catecholamine activity is thought to be the primary mode underlying the cardiotoxic effects of methamphetamines, leading to excessive vasoconstriction, vasospasm, rapid heart rate, and high blood pressure [5]. Tachycardia leads to myocardial necrosis; increased blood pressure leads to fibrosis; vasospasm leads to hypertrophy of cells. Direct cardiac toxicity including hypertrophy and other damage in the heart has been well established, but the understanding of the pathophysiology is unknown [5].

A major complication of acute myocardial infarction is left ventricular thrombus formation. Risk factors for thrombus formation include large infarct size (EF < 30%), severe apical akinesia or dyskinesia, formation of ventricular aneurysms, and anterior myocardial infarction [6]. Virchow's triad is a prerequisite for in vivo thrombus formation. LV wall regional akinesia and dyskinesia result in stasis. Prolonged ischemia leads to subendocardial tissue injury with inflammatory changes. Acute MI patients have increased concentrations of prothrombin, fibrinopeptide A, and von Willebrand factor and decreased concentrations of

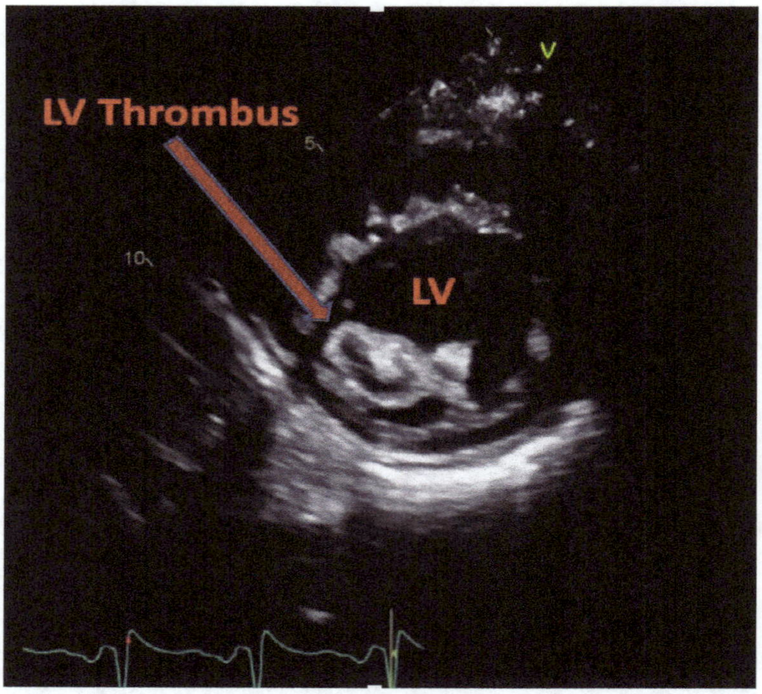

FIGURE 5: Parasternal short axis view. Mid to apical segment showing LV thrombus. LV: left ventricle.

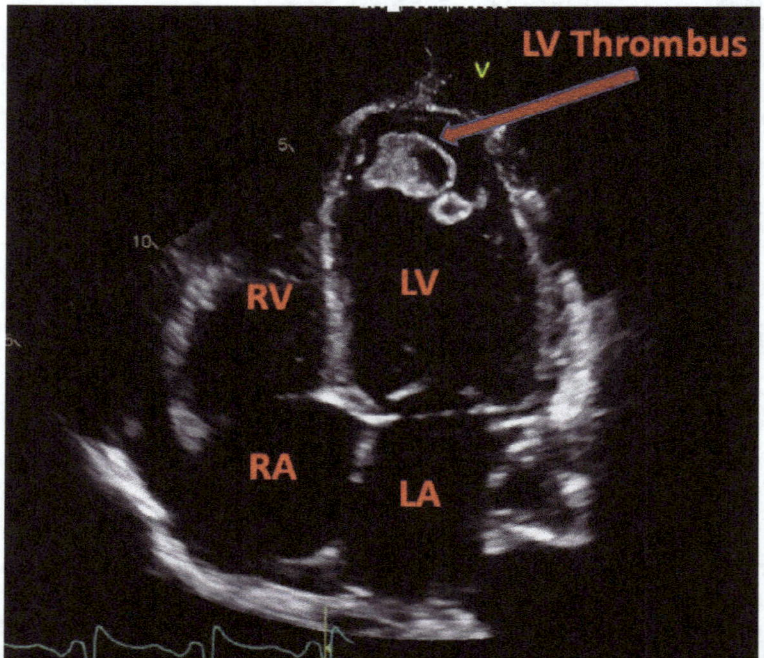

FIGURE 6: Apical four-chamber view showing LV thrombus. LA: left atrium; RA: right atrium; RV: right ventricle; LV: left ventricle.

ADAMTS 13 [7]. Left ventricular thrombus can occur within 24 hours of MI [8]. Patients can present with left ventricular thrombus after unrecognized myocardial infarction. Conditions that increase the risk for systemic embolization include severe congestive heart failure, diffuse left ventricular dilation, systolic dysfunction, previous embolization, advanced age, and the presence of left ventricular protruding or mobile thrombus [7].

Our patient had a prolonged history of methamphetamine abuse. She had chronic heart failure with reduced ejection fraction, 10-15% with severe dilated cardiomyopathy and diffuse hypokinesis. We hypothesized that catecholamine storm due to acute methamphetamine intoxication caused acute myocardial infarction. This was unrecognized mainly because of atypical presentation. Severe dyskinesia along with diffuse wall motion abnormalities led to stasis of blood and eventual thrombus formation. The patient had significant risk factors for systemic embolization including severe congestive heart failure and systolic dysfunction, leading to systemic embolization.

A high index of suspicion is paramount to making a diagnosis. Presence of risk factors, especially presence of severely reduced ejection fraction without anticoagulation, should prompt physicians to look out for left ventricular thrombus. Diagnosis can be made using two-dimensional transthoracic echocardiogram which is cheap, is readily available, and has excellent specificity, 85-90%, and sensitivity of 95% in detecting left ventricular thrombus [9]. Cardiac magnetic resonance imaging (CMR) with contrast delayed enhancement (DE) has significantly better accuracy than TTE for the diagnosis of LV thrombus, 99% specificity, and 88% sensitivity [9, 10]. DE-CMR is nowadays considered the gold standard for diagnosis. Vitamin K antagonist is the standard of treatment. The European guidelines recommend antivitamin K treatment for 3-6 months while the American guidelines recommend indefinite treatment for patients with low risk of bleeding [7].

4. Conclusion

Physicians should be aware of the cardiac complications of methamphetamine. Left ventricular thrombus with systemic emboli is a potential complication of chronic methamphetamine use.

Usually, patients with decreased ejection fraction are at a higher risk.

References

[1] S. Won, R. A. Hong, R. V. Shohet, T. B. Seto, and N. I. Parikh, "Methamphetamine-associated cardiomyopathy," *Clinical Cardiology*, vol. 36, no. 12, pp. 737–742, 2013.

[2] S. Schürer, K. Klingel, M. Sandri et al., "Clinical characteristics, histopathological features, and clinical outcome of methamphetamine-associated cardiomyopathy," *JACC: Heart Failure*, vol. 5, no. 6, pp. 435–445, 2017.

[3] M. N. Islam, H. Kuroki, B. Hongcheng et al., "Cardiac lesions and their reversibility after long term administration of methamphetamine," *Forensic Science International*, vol. 75, no. 1, pp. 29–43, 1995.

[4] N. Nishida, N. Ikeda, K. Kudo, and R. Esaki, "Sudden unexpected death of a methamphetamine abuser with cardiopulmonary abnormalities," *Medicine, Science and the Law*, vol. 43, no. 3, pp. 267–271, 2003.

[5] S. Kaye and R. McKetin, *National Drug and Alcohol Research Centre (Australia) Cardiotoxicity associated with methamphetamine use and signs of cardiovascular pathology among methamphetamine users*, NDARC, Sydney, 2005.

[6] J. W. Weinsaft, H. W. Kim, A. L. Crowley et al., "LV thrombus detection by routine echocardiography: insights into performance characteristics using delayed enhancement CMR," *JACC: Cardiovascular Imaging*, vol. 4, no. 7, pp. 702–712, 2011.

[7] R. Delewi, F. Zijlstra, and J. J. Piek, "Left ventricular thrombus formation after acute myocardial infarction," *Heart*, vol. 98, no. 23, pp. 1743–1749, 2012.

[8] H. M. M. T. B. Herath, S. P. Pahalagamage, L. C. Lindsay et al., "Takotsubo cardiomyopathy complicated with apical thrombus formation on first day of the illness: a case report and literature review," *BMC Cardiovascular Disorders*, vol. 17, no. 1, p. 176, 2017.

[9] M. B. Srichai, C. Junor, L. L. Rodriguez et al., "Clinical, imaging, and pathological characteristics of left ventricular thrombus: a comparison of contrast-enhanced magnetic resonance imaging, transthoracic echocardiography, and transesophageal echocardiography with surgical or pathological validation," *American Heart Journal*, vol. 152, no. 1, pp. 75–84, 2006.

[10] N. R. Mollet, S. Dymarkowski, W. Volders et al., "Visualization of ventricular thrombi with contrast-enhanced magnetic resonance imaging in patients with ischemic heart disease," *Circulation*, vol. 106, no. 23, pp. 2873–2876, 2002.

26

Treatment and Imaging Modalities of Giant Coronary Aneurysms Resulting from Kawasaki Disease and Presenting as Acute Inferior Wall Myocardial Infarction

Mahmood Abu Akel,[1] Yaron M. Hellman,[1] Shtiwi Sawaed,[2] Erez Sharoni,[2] Amnon Eitan,[1] and Moshe Y. Flugelman[1]

[1]*Department of Cardiovascular Medicine, Lady Davis Carmel Medical Center and Rappaport Faculty of Medicine, Technion Israel Institute of Technology, Haifa, Israel*
[2]*Department of Cardiothoracic Surgery, Lady Davis Carmel Medical Center and Rappaport Faculty of Medicine, Technion Israel Institute of Technology, Haifa, Israel*

Correspondence should be addressed to Moshe Y. Flugelman; myf@technion.ac.il

Academic Editor: Assad Movahed

Giant coronary aneurysms are late sequelae of Kawasaki disease (KD). We describe a 53-year-old patient who presented with acute myocardial infarction and proximal aneurysms of all three coronary arteries. Coronary angiography demonstrated the aneurysms, but CT angiography allowed accurate assessment of the real dimensions of the aneurysms and making the decision on the preferred method of revascularization. The patient underwent coronary bypass surgery and is asymptomatic at follow-up.

1. Introduction

Kawasaki disease (KD) is an acute multisystem vasculitis of unknown etiology, which predominantly affects infants and young children. Fifteen to twenty-five percent of untreated patients with acute KD have coronary aneurysms or ectasia [1, 2]. Symptomatic coronary heart disease (CAD) develops in 5% of patients during long-term follow-up [3, 4]. Symptomatic CAD is due to narrowing or thrombosis of the coronary arteries secondary to the coronary aneurysms [5–7].

We present a 53-year-old man who presented with myocardial infarction and was found to have giant coronary aneurysms, probably due to KD. We discuss clinical management and review the relevant imaging modalities and potential therapies.

2. Case Presentation

A 53-year-old man presented to the emergency department with chest pain that started on the day of admission. He was a smoker, with dyslipidemia treated by atorvastatin 20 mg, with no family history of cardiac disease or significant pediatric history. He was in good general condition and had no signs of heart failure. His ECG showed sinus rhythm and ST segment elevation in the inferior leads (Figure 1(a)).

The patient underwent emergency coronary angiography. The right coronary artery (RCA) was totally occluded with an aneurysm involving the ostium (Figure 1(b)). Filling of the distal RCA from the left coronary system was observed. Giant aneurysms in the proximal portions of the left anterior descending (LAD) and left circumflex coronaries (Figure 1(c)) were demonstrated. A second marginal branch was demonstrated with slow flow and filling defects.

An attempt to pass a guide wire to the proximal RCA through the ostial aneurysm failed, and the patient was transferred to the coronary care unit and treated with aspirin, clopidogrel, fractionated heparin, and morphine.

Echocardiography showed good left ventricular contraction with an estimated ejection fraction of 55% and wall motion abnormalities in the inferior and posterior walls. Peak troponin T was 1027 ng/l on the second day of hospitalization

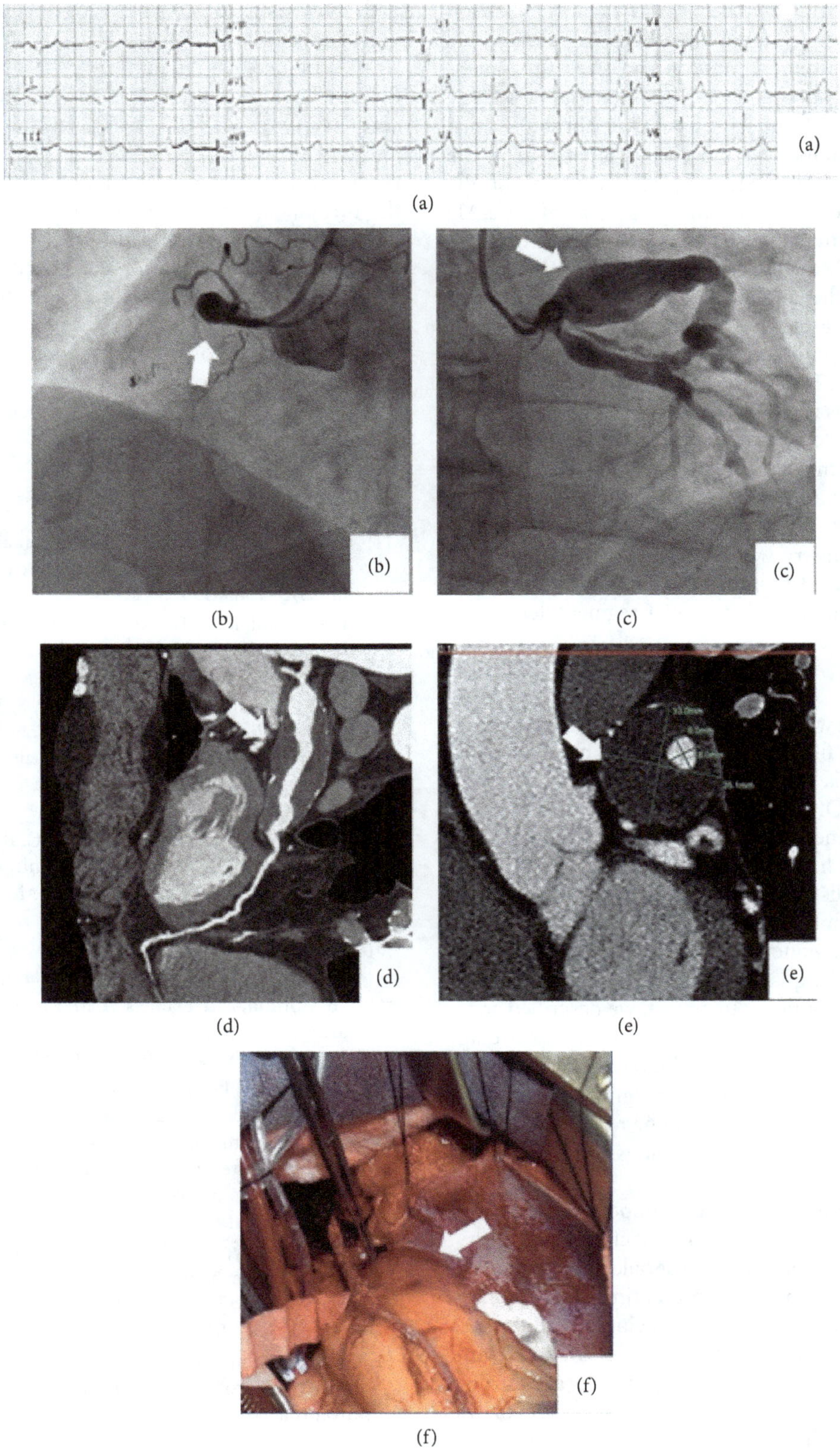

FIGURE 1: (a) Twelve-lead ECG on admission. ST segment elevation in leads II, III, and AVF is evident. Acute ST elevation inferior wall infarction was confirmed by troponin T dynamics over the following week. (b) Coronary angiography showing a large coronary aneurysm involving the proximal right coronary artery (white arrow) with complete occlusion of the artery. (c) Coronary angiography showing large coronary aneurysms involving the left anterior descending (black arrow) and circumflex (white arrow) coronary arteries. (d) CT angiography showing the gigantic proximal left anterior descending coronary artery aneurysm (white arrow). (e) Actual measurements of the left anterior descending coronary artery (LAD) aneurysm (white arrow): the maximal outer size of the LAD aneurysm is 35×33 mm, and the size of the lumen of the LAD is 9×11 mm. (f) A view from the operation showing the large aneurysm involving the left anterior descending artery (forceps tip and white arrow).

and decreased to 226 ng/l on the 7th day of hospitalization (normal < 13 ng/l). The angiographic findings were attributed to KD based on the proximal location and size of the aneurysms and the lack of another explanation for these findings.

A cardiac computed tomography was performed, which revealed a giant thrombotic nonocclusive aneurysm in the proximal LAD with calcifications of the margins of the aneurysm (Figure 1(d)); the maximal outer size of the LAD aneurysm is 35 × 33 mm, and the size of the lumen of the LAD is 9 × 11 mm. Moderate aneurysmal dilatation of the proximal left circumflex and an ostial thrombotic aneurysm of the right coronary artery were observed.

One week after admission, the patient underwent coronary bypass surgery. The giant aneurysm of the proximal LAD (Figure 1(e)) was identified by the surgeons, and the left internal mammary artery was connected to the distal LAD. The right internal mammary artery was connected to the first marginal branch, and a saphenous vein graft was connected to the distal RCA.

Recovery from surgery was unremarkable, and a graded exercise test performed 3 months after surgery showed good aerobic capacity with no complaints or ST segment deviations.

3. Discussion

We describe a patient with an unusual cause of acute myocardial infarction at the fifth decade of life. The most probable etiology is thrombosis of coronary aneurysms, which are a late sequel of KD. Only a few reports have documented patients with giant aneurysms presenting for the first time in the fifth decade of life [7, 8]. Although diagnostic criteria have not been established for KD at the chronic phase of the disease, our probable diagnosis is based on the proximity and size of the coronary aneurysms and lack of signs of other syndromes that could explain coronary aneurysms, such as Behcet's disease [9]. In a previous report, we described acute coronary syndrome in a patient with KD, which was diagnosed retrospectively based on childhood medical records [10]. Since KD in childhood can be misdiagnosed or ignored, diagnosis during late phases of KD can be reached only with high probability based on anatomic findings and lack of signs of other relevant syndromes.

Our case report highlights several important issues. (a) KD can present late in life with no relevant childhood history. Although this is a rare presentation, it should be kept in mind in both young and older patients presenting with coronary aneurysms. (b) Combining different imaging modalities was important for better understanding of the anatomy and pathophysiology. We used coronary angiography and cardiac computed tomography and showed the exact size of the aneurysms and the healthier parts of the coronary tree that were suitable for bypass grafting. The use of multiple modalities shed light on the pathology of aneurysms in Kawasaki disease [11]. As shown in Figure 1(d), the lumen of the LAD is filled with contrast medium, while the area between the patent LAD lumen and the outer borders of the aneurysm is filled by "greyish" material that can be either organized thrombus or myofibroblastic proliferation and the resulting extracellular matrix [11]. Calcifications are also part of the pathophysiology of chronic Kawasaki disease affecting the vasculature [11].

Percutaneous interventions, bypass surgery, and medical therapy have been prescribed for KD presenting with acute coronary syndrome [6, 12–14]. In our patient, we decided jointly with our surgeons that the best therapeutic modality is coronary bypass surgery, based on the assumption that the thrombosed proximal coronary aneurysms can further limit coronary flow and cause additional myocardial injury and infarction. The size of the infarct was limited in our patient due to filling of the distal RCA from collaterals from the left system.

The relevance of our case report is highlighted by the potential increase of patients with Kawasaki disease-like syndrome during the COVID-19 pandemic [15–17].

References

[1] H. Kato, T. Sugimura, T. Akagi et al., "Long-term consequences of Kawasaki Disease," *Circulation*, vol. 94, no. 6, pp. 1379–1385, 1996.

[2] A. S. Dajani, K. A. Taubert, M. A. Gerber et al., "Diagnosis and therapy of Kawasaki disease in children," *Circulation*, vol. 87, no. 5, pp. 1776–1780, 1993.

[3] J. W. Newburger, M. Takahashi, A. S. Beiser et al., "A single intravenous infusion of gamma globulin as compared with four infusions in the treatment of acute Kawasaki syndrome," *The New England Journal of Medicine*, vol. 324, no. 23, pp. 1633–1639, 1991.

[4] J. W. Newburger, M. Takahashi, J. C. Burns et al., "The treatment of Kawasaki syndrome with intravenous gamma globulin," *The New England Journal of Medicine*, vol. 315, no. 6, pp. 341–347, 1986.

[5] J. C. Burns and M. P. Glodé, "Kawasaki syndrome," *Lancet*, vol. 364, no. 9433, pp. 533–544, 2004.

[6] J. B. Gordon, L. B. Daniels, A. M. Kahn et al., "The spectrum of cardiovascular lesions requiring intervention in adults after Kawasaki disease," *JACC. Cardiovascular Interventions*, vol. 9, no. 7, pp. 687–696, 2016.

[7] B. W. McCrindle, C. Manlhiot, J. W. Newburger et al., "Medium-term complications associated with coronary artery aneurysms after Kawasaki disease: a study from the International Kawasaki Disease Registry," *Journal of the American Heart Association*, vol. 9, no. 15, p. e016440, 2020.

[8] P. D. Crawley, W. J. Mahlow, D. R. Huntsinger, S. Afiniwala, and D. C. Wortham, "Giant coronary artery aneurysms: review and update," *Texas Heart Institute Journal*, vol. 41, no. 6, pp. 603–608, 2014.

[9] P. T. Kariyanna, P. Shah, A. Jayarangaiah, Y. S. Chowdhury, and D. Lazaro, "Acute coronary syndrome in Behcet's syndrome: a systematic review," *European Journal of Rheumatology*, 2020.

[10] M. Y. Flugelman, Y. Hasin, M. M. Bassan, R. Leor, and M. S. Gotsman, "Acute myocardial infarction 14 years after an acute episode of Kawasaki's disease," *The American Journal of Cardiology*, vol. 52, no. 3, pp. 427-428, 1983.

[11] J. M. Orenstein, S. T. Shulman, L. M. Fox et al., "Three linked vasculopathic processes characterize Kawasaki disease: a light and transmission electron microscopic study," *PLoS One*, vol. 7, no. 6, article e38998, 2012.

[12] E. Tsuda, H. Fujita, T. Yagihara, O. Yamada, S. Echigo, and S. Kitamura, "Competition between native flow and graft flow after coronary artery bypass grafting. Impact on indications for coronary artery bypass grafting for localized stenosis with giant aneurysms due to Kawasaki disease," *Pediatric Cardiology*, vol. 29, no. 2, pp. 266–270, 2008.

[13] T. Ino, K. Akimoto, M. Ohkubo et al., "Application of percutaneous transluminal coronary angioplasty to coronary arterial stenosis in Kawasaki disease," *Circulation*, vol. 93, no. 9, pp. 1709–1715, 1996.

[14] M. Ariyoshi, J. Shiraishi, M. Kimura et al., "Primary percutaneous coronary intervention for acute myocardial infarction due to possible sequelae of Kawasaki disease in young adults: a case series," *Heart and Vessels*, vol. 26, no. 1, pp. 117–124, 2011.

[15] E. M. Dufort, E. H. Koumans, E. J. Chow et al., "Multisystem inflammatory syndrome in children in New York state," *The New England Journal of Medicine*, vol. 383, no. 4, pp. 347–358, 2020.

[16] L. R. Feldstein, E. B. Rose, S. M. Horwitz et al., "Multisystem inflammatory syndrome in U.S. children and adolescents," *The New England Journal of Medicine*, vol. 383, no. 4, pp. 334–346, 2020.

[17] S. Sokolovsky, P. Soni, T. Hoffman, P. Kahn, and J. Scheers-Masters, "COVID-19 associated Kawasaki-like multisystem inflammatory disease in an adult," *The American Journal of Emergency Medicine*, vol. S0735-6757, no. 20, pp. 30542–30548, 2020.

27

Acute Stent Thrombosis Associated with Eptifibatide-Induced Profound Thrombocytopenia

Amer Aljundi,[1] Alaa Rahhal ,[1] and Wafer Dabdoob[2]

[1]*Pharmacy Department, Heart Hospital, Hamad Medical Corporation, Doha, Qatar*
[2]*Cardiology and Cardiovascular Surgery Department, Heart Hospital, Hamad Medical Corporation, Doha, Qatar*

Correspondence should be addressed to Alaa Rahhal; arahhal1@hamad.qa
Academic Editor: Domingo A. Pascual Figal

Background. Eptifibatide is an inhibitor of the platelet glycoprotein (GP) IIb/IIIa receptor that is commonly used in patients undergoing percutaneous coronary intervention (PCI). *Case.* We describe a case of a 62-year-old female patient admitted with acute ST-elevation myocardial infarction (STEMI) treated by primary coronary intervention (primary PCI) with a drug-eluting stent placement. She developed profound thrombocytopenia within 8 hours of first administration of eptifibatide and subsequent acute stent thrombosis next day. Other causes of thrombocytopenia were excluded and intravascular ultrasound (IVUS) showed good stent expansion and opposition to the coronary wall. Platelet count gradually returned to normal after discontinuation of eptifibatide. *Conclusion.* Although Eptifibatide has been associated with the development of thrombocytopenia, to the best of our knowledge, this is the first case report in the medical literature that associates acute stent thrombosis and eptifibatide-induced thrombocytopenia.

1. Introduction

There are several agents that are used in the treatment of acute coronary syndromes (ACS) that were reported to cause drug-induced thrombocytopenia [1, 2]. Eptifibatide is a synthetic cyclic heptapeptide and a selective inhibitor of the platelet glycoprotein (GP) IIb/IIIa receptor that blocks the final common pathway of platelet aggregation. It is commonly used in patients with acute coronary syndromes and in those undergoing PCI to reduce the risk of acute cardiac ischemic events [3–6].

Recent literature has suggested an association between eptifibatide exposure and the development of thrombocytopenia. However, to the best of our knowledge, this is the first case report in the medical literature that associates acute stent thrombosis and eptifibatide-induced thrombocytopenia.

2. Case Presentation

A 62-year-old female with a history of diabetes mellitus and hypertension presented to the emergency department with a two-hour history of retrosternal chest pain radiating to both shoulders and associated with profuse sweating and vomiting. She denied any previous history of blood dyscrasia or thrombocytopenia. She had no history of drug abuse and denied any history of a previous hospitalization where she may have received heparin or eptifibatide. She does not have any known allergies. Her past medication history included the use of amlodipine 5 mg daily, atorvastatin 20 mg daily, metformin 500 mg daily, aspirin 100 mg daily, carvedilol 25 mg twice daily, and lisinopril 20 mg/hydrochlorothiazide 12.5 mg daily.

Vital signs at presentation included a temperature of 36.8°C, regular pulse of 98 bpm, brachial blood pressure of 140/70 mmHg, respirations of 20 per minute, and oxygen saturation of 98% on room air. The physical exam demonstrated an alert and oriented patient in moderate distress from chest pain. There were no signs of peripheral edema or cyanosis. The patient had bilateral basilar crackles at the bases. The heart was regular, with no murmurs, rubs, and gallops. The abdomen was soft with no organomegaly.

Her electrocardiogram (ECG) showed ST-segment elevation in lead II, III, aVF, Q wave in III, and reciprocal ST-segment depression in I and aVL (Figure 1). Transthoracic echocardiography showed inferior left ventricular (LV) wall motion akinesia with normal LV systolic function (as demonstrated by an LV ejection fraction of 55-60%) and mild concentric LV hypertrophy. Other findings included a mild mitral regurgitation with normal other valves and chambers. At baseline, the patient had a white blood cell count of 12.000/mm3, a hemoglobin level of 13.9 g/dL, and a platelet count of 378,000/mm3. Cardiac markers were creatine kinase myoglobin (CK MB) level of 87.40 ng/ml and troponin T level of 4040 ng/mL. The values of prothrombin time (PT) and activated partial thromboplastin time (aPTT) were within normal limits. Similarly, liver function tests and kidney function tests were within normal limits. Due to the patient's ischemic symptoms and ECG changes consistent with an acute inferior STEMI, she was taken for urgent cardiac catheterization. Coronary angiography revealed a dominant RCA with a 99% stenosis with a thrombolysis in myocardial infarction (TIMI) grade 0 flow and a 40% stenosis of the left circumflex artery (LCx). Angiography also showed normal left main coronary artery (LMCA) and left anterior descending (LAD) coronary artery.

Following our local protocol, before catheterization, the patient received aspirin 300 mg; clopidogrel 600 mg; one dose of intravenous unfractionated heparin 7000 units; and eptifibatide 180 μg/kg as a bolus dose then 2-μg/kg/min infusion. A 3.0×24 mm XIENCE™ Everolimus Eluting Coronary stent was deployed in the distal RCA with a very satisfying angiographic result (TIMI grade 3 flow) with no complications. Once flow was restored in the RCA, the patient became pain-free with the resolution of her ST-segment elevation (Figure 2). She was then transferred in a stable condition to the coronary intensive care unit (CICU). Postpercutaneous coronary intervention (PCI) medications included dual antiplatelet therapy (DAPT) with aspirin 100 mg daily and clopidogrel 75 mg daily, ramipril 5 mg daily, metoprolol tartrate 25 mg twice daily, rosuvastatin 20 mg daily, and the eptifibatide intravenous infusion was to be continued for 18 hours.

Approximately eight hours post-PCI and eptifibatide initiation, the patient developed a profound thrombocytopenia, with her platelet count dropping by over 90% from baseline to 17,000/mm3. The rest of her complete blood count at this time included hemoglobin 13.2 g/dL, hematocrit 39.6%, and white blood cell count 18.8×109/L. The platelet count trend through hospitalization is summarized in Figure 3.

After the acute platelet drop, eptifibatide was discontinued. Intravenous lepirudin 14.5 mg/h was initiated due to a high clinical suspicion for heparin-induced thrombocytopenia (HIT).

On the next day (approximately 18 hours after primary PCI), our patient developed chest pain with nausea and vomiting. Her electrocardiogram (ECG) showed diffuse STEMI of the II, III, aVF, and reciprocal ST-segment depression in I and aVL (Figure 4). Urgent angiography revealed thrombosed mid and distal RCA with intravascular ultrasound (IVUS) study conforming thrombus formation (Figures 5 and 6). Export catheter™ was utilized to extract clot fragments with satisfying results (TIMI grade 2 flow). The subsequent IVUS study confirmed excellent stent expansion and apposition to the vessel indicating the optimal stent deployment (Figure 7).

3. Discussion

Eptifibatide is a potent adjunct medication that significantly improves outcomes in patients undergoing PCI among those presenting with ACS [3–6]. Eptifibatide works by preventing the binding of fibrinogen, von Willebrand factor, and other ligands to the GP IIb/IIIa receptor, thereby reversibly inhibiting platelet aggregation and subsequent thrombosis [1, 2]. Drug-induced acute profound thrombocytopenia can be defined as a decrease in platelet count to below 20,000/mm3 within 24 hours of exposure to the drug, which was the case in our patient having reached a low as 17,000/mm3 [7].

Our patient was exposed to several agents other than eptifibatide that are well known to be associated independently with profound thrombocytopenia, including heparin and clopidogrel [8]. These agents are usually coadministered before PCI which can make it difficult to discern causation in the setting of drug-induced thrombocytopenia.

Treatment with GP IIb/IIIa antagonists has been reported to be associated with pseudothrombocytopenia [9]. Pseudothrombocytopenia is an artificial laboratory process resulting from the adherence of platelets to leukocytes. This process typically occurs when blood samples are collected in EDTA tubes. Pseudothrombocytopenia in our scenario was ruled out by confirmation of thrombocytopenia in an EDTA-free tube and by direct review of the peripheral blood smear which showed no signs of platelet clumping. Moreover, there was no evidence of microangiopathic hemolytic anemia consistent with thrombotic thrombocytopenic purpura–hemolytic uremic syndrome (TTP-HUS) due to the administration of clopidogrel [10]. Additionally, other than thrombocytopenia, our patient did not manifest any other hallmarks of the disease which include fever, neurologic manifestations, and renal insufficiency. Moreover, our patient received only one loading dose of clopidogrel 600 mg six hours before the drop in her platelet count making it unlikely that clopidogrel was the culprit for the observed thrombocytopenia.

Use of the Naranjo scale to assess the probability of drug adverse events also indicated a probable relationship between the administration of eptifibatide and the development of profound thrombocytopenia (score of 5), while the relation was possible with heparin and clopidogrel (score 1) [11].

Heparin is well known to be associated with thrombocytopenia; however, the timing of thrombocytopenia in this patient was consistent with eptifibatide-induced thrombocytopenia as it occurred within less than 24 hours of stating eptifibatide. Heparin-induced thrombocytopenia (HIT) type I usually develops early within the first two days of starting heparin and is usually mild and transient (rarely <100,000 platelet/mm3). Heparin-induced thrombocytopenia type II, on the other hand, is an immune-mediated reaction with a typical onset of 5-10 days after the administration of heparin without previous heparin exposure and can be as early as hours due to circulating heparin/platelet factor 4 from a previous exposure [12]. Our patient had a severe form of thrombocytopenia ruling out HIT type I, while the time

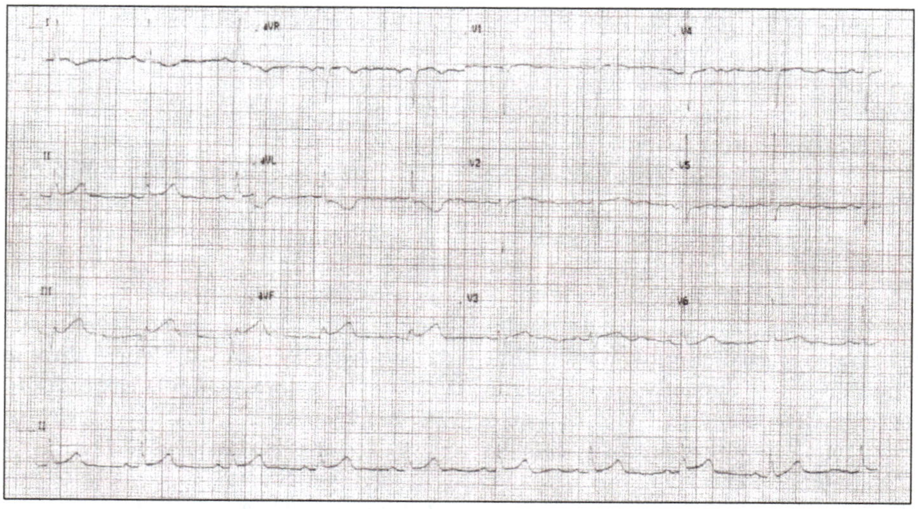

Figure 1: Electrocardiogram (ECG) showing ST-segment elevation in lead II, III, aVF, Q wave in III, and reciprocal ST-segment depression in I and aVL at presentation.

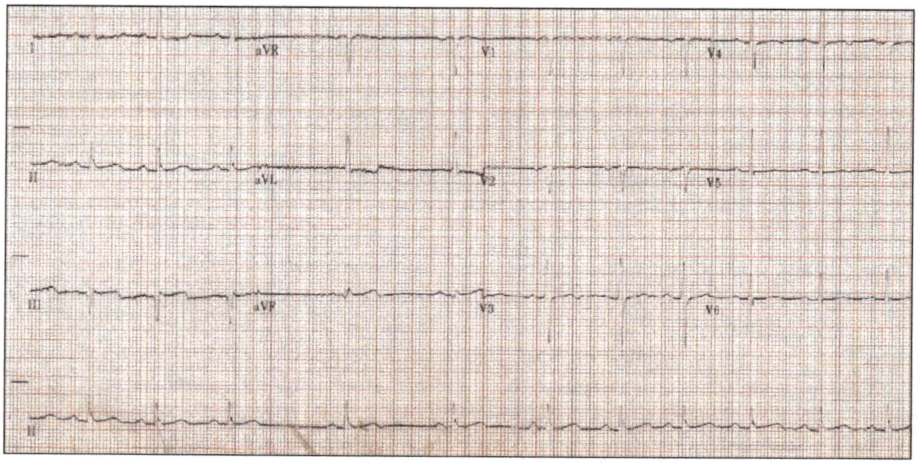

Figure 2: ECG showing resolution of ST-segment elevation after PCI to RCA.

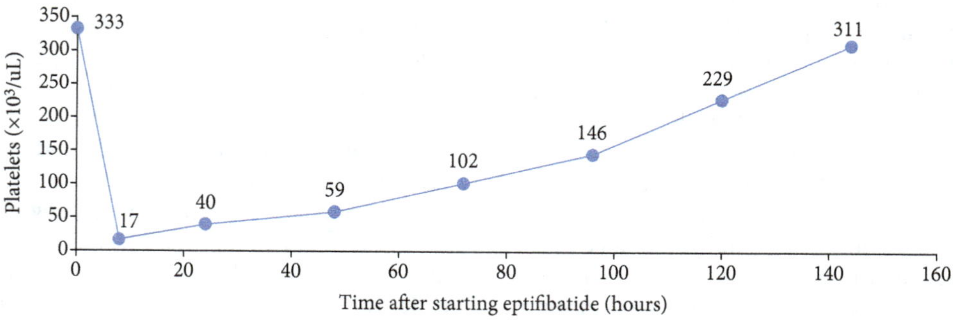

Figure 3: Platelet count during hospital stay.

frame for developing thrombocytopenia was not consistent with HIT type II as our patient had no previous exposure to heparin. Additionally, ELISA immunoassay was performed and was negative for heparin-platelet factor 4 antibodies. The patient's platelet count started to improve after discontinuing eptifibatide. These factors suggested that eptifibatide was the most likely cause of thrombocytopenia associated with acute stent thrombosis.

The mechanisms by which GP IIb-IIIa inhibitors cause thrombocytopenia are poorly understood. One possible mechanism is the formation of antibodies to a group of epitopes, called ligand-induced binding sites (LIBSs), which are normally hidden on the surface of the platelet. Binding of the GP IIb-IIIa inhibitor to the receptor induces a conformational change exposing LIBSs in the platelet. This permits the binding of the anti-LIBS antibodies and can eventually

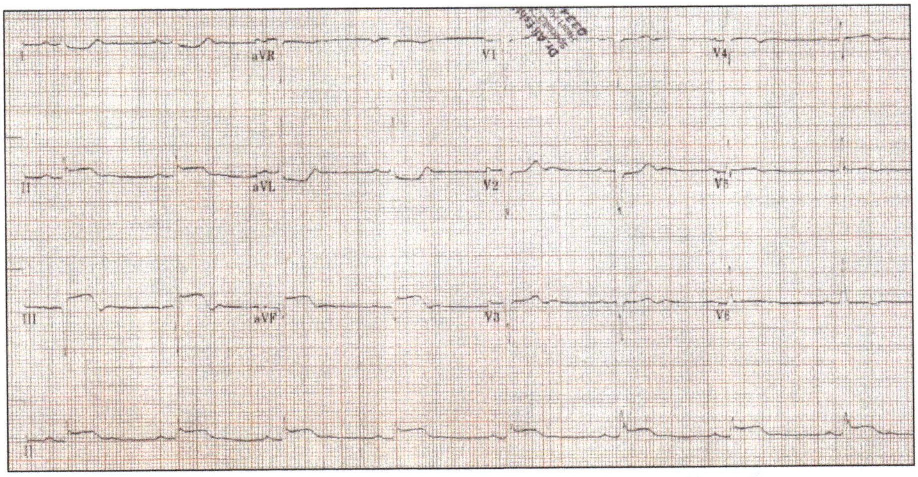

Figure 4: ECG showing diffuse ST elevation in lead II, III, aVF, and reciprocal ST-segment depression in I and aVL.

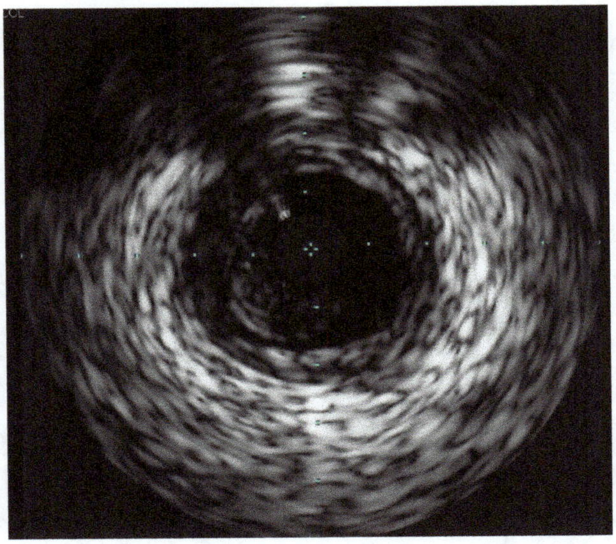

Figure 5: IVUS showing thrombus in mid RCA at 5 to 11 o'clock.

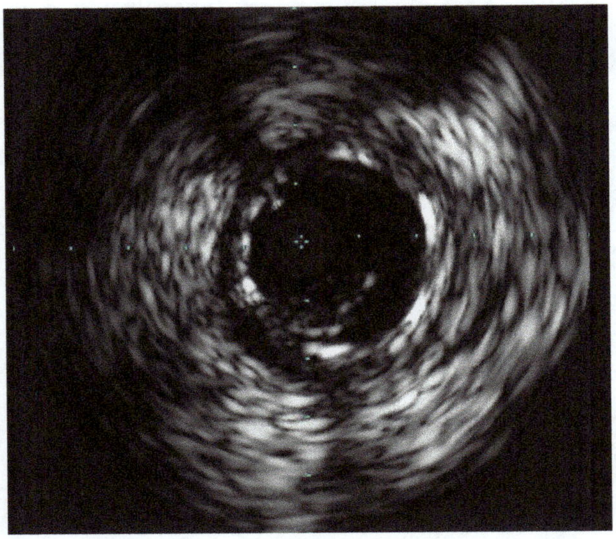

Figure 6: IVUS showing thrombus at 3 to 8 o'clock within the stent.

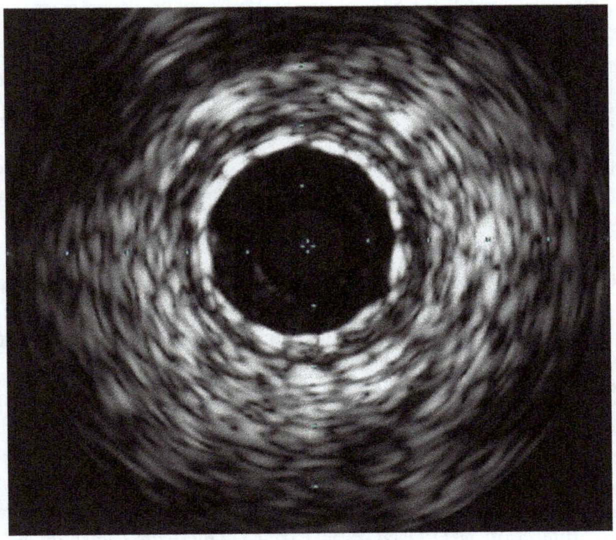

Figure 7: IVUS showing well-expanded and opposed stent.

lead to subsequent clearance of platelets by the reticuloendothelial system [13].

A proposed mechanism for thrombosis, however, is that LIBS antibodies can activate platelets by stabilizing the open, or active, conformation of the GP IIb/IIIa receptor, enabling the binding of multivalent ligands such as fibrinogen. Antibody-mediated fibrinogen binding can lead to bridging of adjacent platelets and platelet activation responses with subsequent generation of cell-surface procoagulant activity [14].

4. Conclusion

Eptifibatide is known to cause severe thrombocytopenia; however, this the first report of this being associated with subsequent acute stent thrombosis. Despite being uncommon, it is a clinically important complication of eptifibatide. This report highlights the importance of close monitoring platelet counts, before and after starting eptifibatide. A high index of suspicion of acute stent thrombosis should be raised if a patient develops new onset chest pain following successful PCI in the setting of eptifibatide-induced thrombocytopenia.

Consent

A written informed consent for publishing patient's information and images were obtained from the patient.

References

[1] M. A. Rizvi, K. Kojouri, and J. N. George, "Drug-induced thrombocytopenia: an updated systematic review," *Annals of Internal Medicine*, vol. 134, no. 4, 2001.

[2] R. H. Aster, "Drug-induced immune thrombocytopenia: an overview of pathogenesis," *Seminars in Hematology*, vol. 36, 1 Suppl 1, pp. 2–6, 1999.

[3] J. E. Tcheng, "Impact of eptifibatide on early ischemic events in acute ischemic coronary syndromes: a review of the IMPACT II trial. Integrilin to Minimize Platelet Aggregation and Coronary Thrombosis," *The American Journal of Cardiology*, vol. 80, no. 4, pp. 21B–28B, 1997.

[4] The PURSUIT Trial Investigators, "Inhibition of platelet glycoprotein IIb/IIIa with Eptifibatide in patients with acute coronary syndromes," *New England Journal of Medicine*, vol. 339, no. 7, pp. 436–443, 1998.

[5] The ESPRIT investigators, "Novel dosing regimen of eptifibatide in planned coronary stent implantation (ESPRIT): a randomised, placebo-controlled trial," *The Lancet*, vol. 356, no. 9247, pp. 2037–2044, 2000.

[6] ADVANCE MI Investigators, "Facilitated percutaneous coronary intervention for acute ST-segment elevation myocardial infarction: Results from the prematurely terminated ADdressing the Value of facilitated ANgioplasty after Combination therapy or Eptifibatide monotherapy in acute Myocardial Infarction (ADVANCE MI) trial," *American Heart Journal*, vol. 150, no. 1, pp. 116–122, 2005.

[7] S. D. Berkowitz, R. A. Harrington, M. M. Rund, and J. E. Tcheng, "Acute Profound Thrombocytopenia After c7E3 Fab (Abciximab) Therapy," *Circulation*, vol. 95, no. 4, pp. 809–813, 1997.

[8] I. E. Fahdi, J. F. Saucedo, T. Hennebry, M. Ghani, S. Sadanandan, and L. Garza-Arreola, "Incidence and time course of thrombocytopenia with *abciximab* and *eptifibatide* in patients undergoing percutaneous coronary intervention," *The American Journal of Cardiology*, vol. 93, no. 4, pp. 453–455, 2004.

[9] D. C. Sane, L. V. Damaraju, E. J. Topol et al., "Occurrence and clinical significance of pseudothrombocytopenia during abciximab therapy," *Journal of the American College of Cardiology*, vol. 36, no. 1, pp. 75–83, 2000.

[10] C. L. Bennett, B. Kim, A. Zakarija et al., "Two mechanistic pathways for thienopyridine- associated thrombotic thrombocytopenic purpura: a report from the SERF-TTP Research Group and the RADAR Project," *Journal of the American College of Cardiology*, vol. 50, no. 12, pp. 1138–1143, 2007.

[11] C. A. Naranjo, U. Busto, E. M. Sellers et al., "A method for estimating the probability of adverse drug reactions," *Clinical Pharmacology and Therapeutics*, vol. 30, no. 2, pp. 239–245, 1981.

[12] T. E. Warkentin, A. Greinacher, A. Koster, and A. M. Lincoff, "Treatment and Prevention of Heparin-Induced Thrombocytopenia," *Chest*, vol. 133, no. 6, pp. 340S–380S, 2008.

[13] M. Madan and S. D. Berkowitz, "Understanding thrombocytopenia and antigenicity with glycoprotein IIb-IIIa inhibitors," *American Heart Journal*, vol. 138, no. 4, pp. S317–S326, 1999.

[14] C. Gao, B. Boylan, D. Bougie et al., "Eptifibatide-induced thrombocytopenia and thrombosis in humans require FcgammaRIIa and the integrin beta3 cytoplasmic domain," *The Journal of Clinical Investigation*, vol. 119, no. 3, pp. 504–511, 2009.

Life-Threatening Coronary Vasospasm Treated by Implantable Cardioverter Defibrillator: The Warning Signs

Deborah Adepoju, Jamie A. L. Smith, and Stephen J. Leslie

Cardiac Unit, Raigmore Hospital, Inverness IV2 3UJ, UK

Correspondence should be addressed to Deborah Adepoju; deborah.adepoju@nhs.scot

Academic Editor: Gopal Chandra Ghosh

Coronary artery vasospasm is the sudden narrowing of an artery caused by rapid prolonged contraction. It reduces blood supply to the heart and can present with typical cardiac chest pain symptoms. Vasospasm can lead to fatal arrhythmic complications such as ventricular fibrillation. Our case report describes an example of this occurring in a 53-year-old female, and the management plan that ensued. We look at the importance of accurate and prompt diagnosis of vasospasm and how this can have implications for treatment options. One of the available treatments for vasospasm is placement of an implantable cardioverter defibrillator (ICD). This delivers a shock in the event of future life-threatening arrhythmia, with the aim of preventing cardiac arrest. ICD placement, however, is not always a suitable option. This case report discusses the various challenges that arose while making the decision for ICD placement and gives insight into the best available treatment options for coronary artery vasospasm. We also highlight early warning signs that predict life-threatening vasospastic events and how this can be diagnosed and treated appropriately.

1. Learning Objectives

Coronary vasospasm causing chest pain is relatively common. Life-threatening arrhythmias are an important complication of vasospasm. Recurrent episodes of chest pain in the absence of coronary artery disease could be indicative of severe vasospasm. Coronary angiogram and medical therapy should be considered to prevent the onset of vasospasm-induced arrhythmic events. Current literature suggests the best means of preventing death in vasospasm is by combining medical therapy with an implantable cardioverter defibrillator. This decision, however, is not always straight forward and requires careful evaluation, considering all aspects of the clinical case including patient's wishes.

2. Introduction

Coronary vasospasm was first described in 1959 as an important cause of myocardial ischaemia [1]. It can manifest in different ways, from asymptomatic ischaemia to sudden cardiac death. Vasospasm is an important cause of life-threatening cardiac arrhythmias in patients without any hemodynamically significant coronary artery disease [1].

Many different factors such as can coronary artery inflammation, oxidative stress, endothelial dysfunction, and lifestyle choices can all increase the likelihood of developing vasospasm. [2]

Although the two often occur together, the diagnosis of vasospasm can often be mislabelled purely as atherosclerotic disease. [3] Accurate diagnosis of vasospasm relies on the use of coronary angiography. When vasospasm leads to a life-threatening arrhythmic event, lifestyle modification is often combined with medical therapy and placement of an implantable cardioverter defibrillator (ICD) to prevent recurrence. The decision to opt for ICD placement is not always simple. Patient factors must be considered, and the benefit-risk assessment must be carefully weighed. An article by Ishihara et al. discussed the pathophysiology behind vasospasm in detail. They further discussed the use of ICD treatment in vasospasm patients postventricular fibrillation-

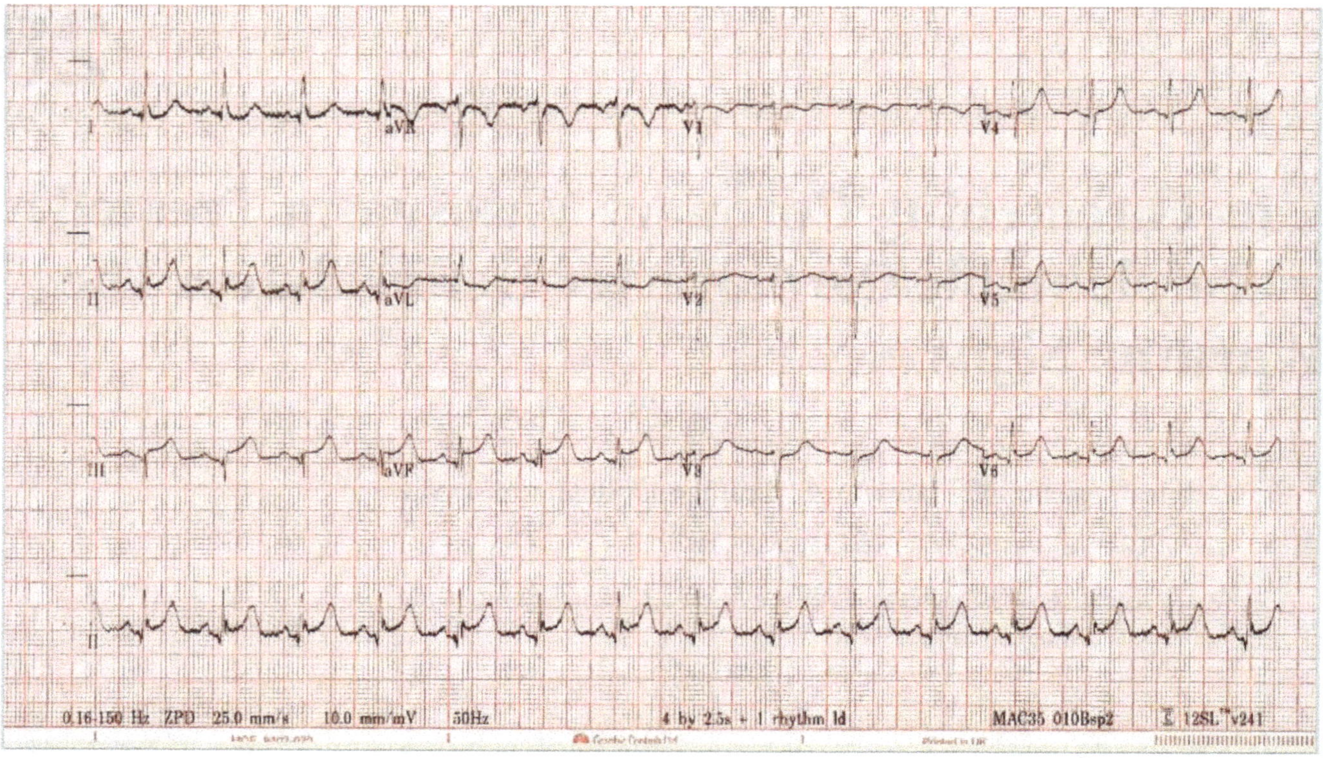

FIGURE 1: 'Abnormal ECG.' This figure is a 12-lead ECG which was taken after resuscitation from cardiac arrest. It shows ST elevation at the J point in leads II, III, and aVF.

(VF-) induced cardiac arrest and the importance of carefully weighing up the potential benefit of ICD implantation with a reasonable risk stratification beforehand [4].

This report is an example of a classic presentation of spasm-induced cardiac arrest. We discuss some of the difficulties that arose while deciding about ICD placement and how these difficulties were overcome, along with some warning signs that preceded cardiac arrest.

3. Case Report

A 53-year-old female chef with a previous history of non ST-elevated myocardial infarction (NSTEMI) and recurrent episodes of chest pain, presented to the Emergency Department after a collapse and confirmed VF arrest. The patient required 2 direct current shocks before return of spontaneous circulation.

Her past medical history includes hypertension, chronic obstructive pulmonary disease (COPD), asthma, and a transient ischemic attack (TIA). She also had a 30 pack-year smoking history and body mass index of 30.3 kg/m^2. Medications included atorvastatin 40 mg, aspirin 75 mg, and lansoprazole 30 mg.

On physical exam, she was sweaty with cool peripheries. Pulse was 113 beats per minute, respiratory rate was 24 breaths per minute, and blood pressure was 86/61 mmHg. A 12-lead ECG revealed ST elevation at the J point in leads II, III, and aVF (Figure 1). Plasma high-sensitivity troponin increased from 27 ng/L to 50 ng/L over four hours. Urea and electrolytes were all within normal limits, and the lipid profile showed cholesterol of 7 mmol/L and triglycerides of 5.7 mmol/L. The clinical diagnosis, supported by ECG, was acute occlusive myocardial infarction, and she was transferred for emergency coronary angiography. ECG had normalized on arrival in the catheterization laboratory; however, coronary angiography showed considerable restriction of the right coronary artery (RCA) lumen (Figure 2(a)), accompanied by recurrent gross ST elevation on the ECG monitor. The patient was given 400 micrograms of intracoronary nitrate. This resulted in a dramatic resolution of the RCA stenosis and ST segments on ECG (Figure 2(b)). Severe vasospasm in the RCA was diagnosed as the primary problem due to the quick resolution of the dynamic ECG changes and near-normal coronary angiogram findings following nitrate administration.

Following angiography, the patient was started on vasodilator therapy with diltiazem (240 mg) and a long acting nitrate (Elantan 50 mg). There were no recurrences of arrhythmia, and all subsequent resting ECGs showed a return to normal sinus rhythm (Figure 3). An echocardiogram demonstrated preserved LV function. Due to the presentation with a VF arrest, ICD placement was discussed with the patient. This was successfully performed and, coupled with lifestyle modification and medical therapy, she has shown no recurrences of chest pain, ECG changes, or arrhythmias at follow-up.

4. Discussion

This patient had multiple risk factors for coronary vasospasm. She was middle aged, a chronic smoker with obesity,

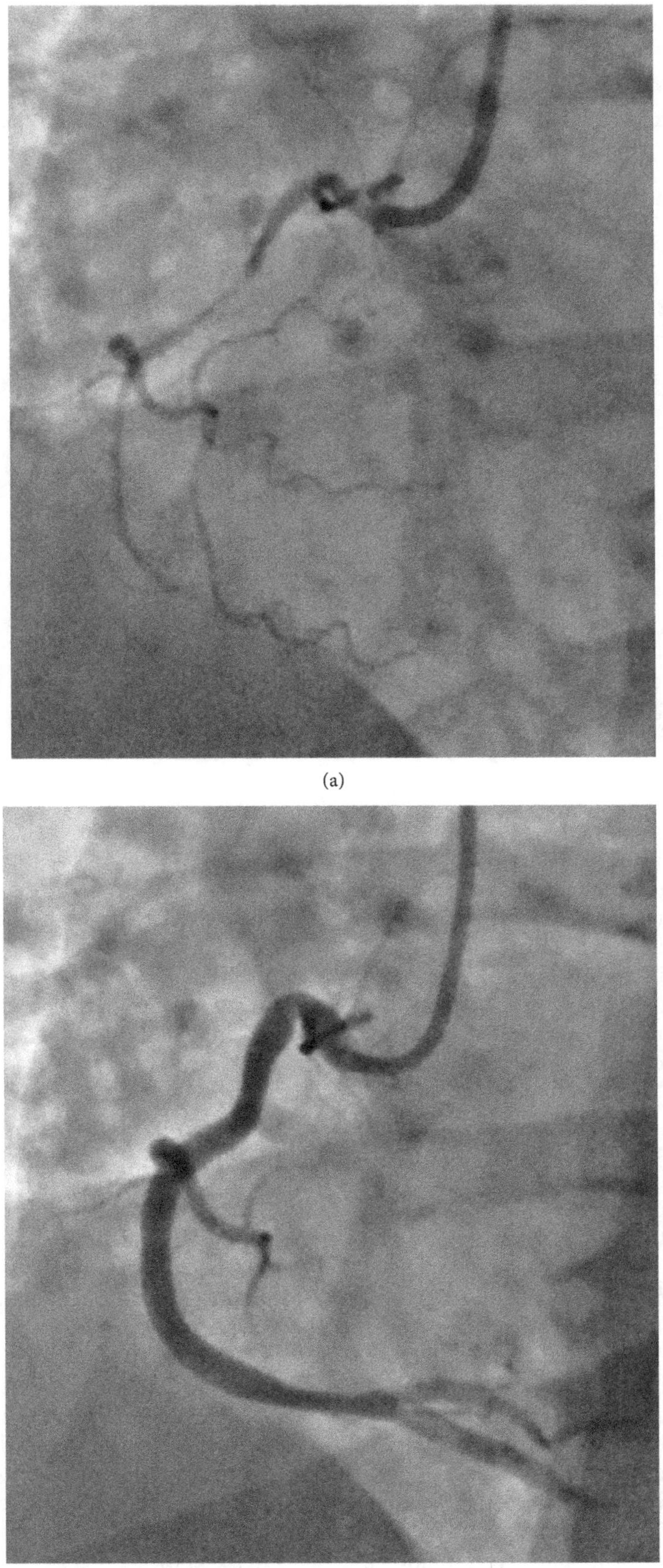

(a)

(b)

FIGURE 2: 'Right coronary artery: before and after.' This figure is a coronary angiogram containing 2 images (a, b). (a) Narrowing of the right coronary artery shortly after cardiac arrest. (b) How the narrowing of the same right coronary artery was almost completely restored immediately after administration of 400 micrograms of intracoronary nitrate.

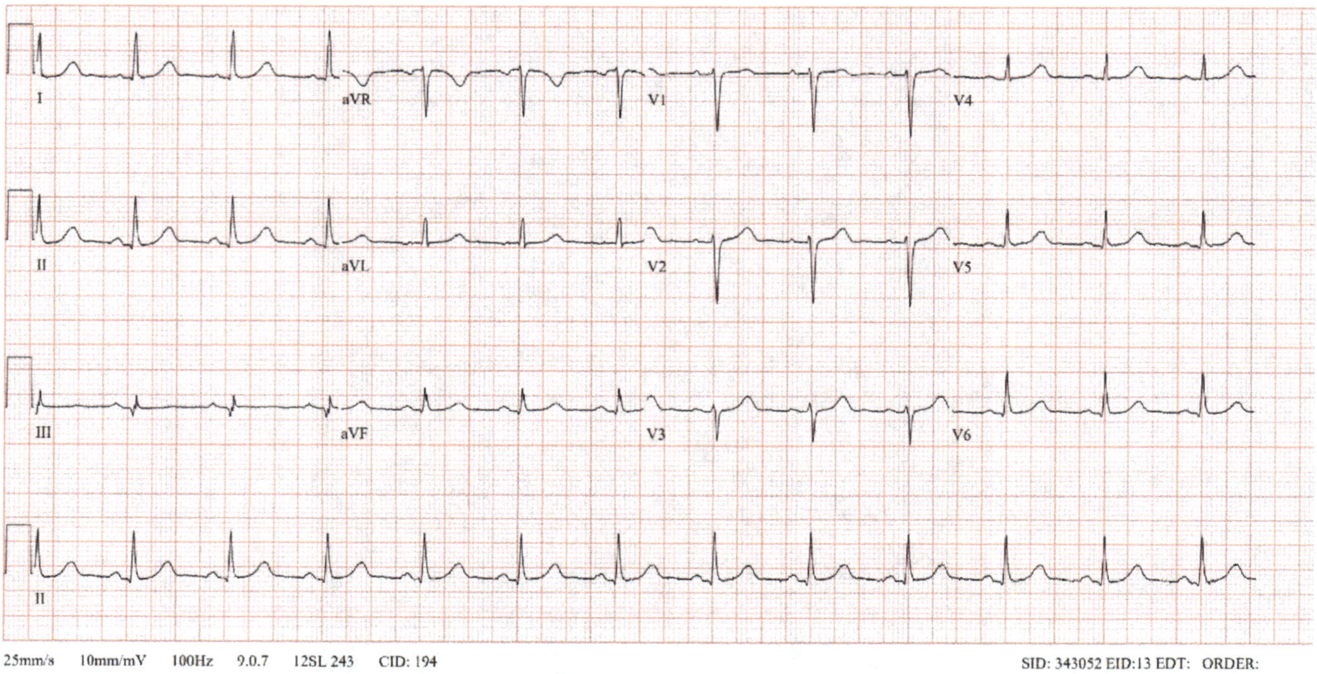

Figure 3: 'Normalized ECG.' This figure is a 12-lead ECG which was taken the day after cardiac arrest. It shows a return to normal sinus rhythm and resolution of the inferior ST-segment elevation.

hypertension, and high cholesterol. She was facing stress at work which is also a known precipitant for vasospasm [5]. She also suffered from lifelong asthma. Previous studies have shown that asthma is associated with a higher incidence of vasospasm [6]. This concoction of hyperlipidemia, hypertension, smoking, and obesity is ordinarily sufficient to induce severe coronary artery disease. An angiogram done two years before this presentation, however, showed only minor plaque disease. The root cause of her symptoms was therefore most likely due to coronary vasospasm and not atherosclerosis.

The striking feature of this case was the many recurrent episodes of rapidly recovering chest pains in the preceding year. These were never fully investigated, but ECG tracings were normal each time. In retrospect, it is highly likely that these were episodes of spasm. Stern and Bayes de Luna documented a similar case whereby a patient presented with multiple episodes of excruciating chest pain over 2 years and a diagnosis of vasospasm was later confirmed. [7]

Due to the increased risk of life-threatening arrhythmias with vasospasm, there is an additional therapeutic option of ICD placement. In similar cases of spasm-induced cardiac arrest, patients have been managed with a combination of medication and ICD [8]. A previous observational study of patients implanted with ICD following spasm-induced arrests showed no further events in the 5-year follow-up period. [9] Currently, there has not been any randomized trials comparing the combination of ICD and medical therapy to medical therapy alone.

Vasospasm is an important differential in the diagnosis of angina or acute coronary syndrome (ACS) as it is easily treated, and if found early, the onset of life-threatening arrhythmias can be prevented.

An Asian study showed that in patients with stable angina or ACS that was not caused by an obstructive atheroma, vasospasm was the cause in 50% and 57%, respectively [10]. A German study similarly performed intracoronary acetylcholine provocation tests in patients with acute chest pain at rest to establish the prevalence of vasospasm as a cause. In 42 out of 86 tested (49%), coronary vasospasm was confirmed as the source of their symptoms. They thus concluded that vasospasm is a frequent cause of ACS and should more regularly be considered as a differential diagnosis [11].

We suggest that healthcare practitioners more frequently consider that while obstructive atheroma is the most common cause of coronary disease, vasospasm could also be a possibility, as this can have implications in management. Diltiazem is very effective in vasospasm but is contraindicated in treatment of ACS patients with reduced left ventricular ejection fraction. In a vasospasm patient misdiagnosed with ACS, diltiazem could be withheld, and the consequences could be detrimental. In cases where acute chest pain is recurrent despite an absence of plaque disease, vasospasm should be highly suspected, and these patients should have coronary angiogram.

Acute chest pain episodes in a relatively young patient, especially if occurring in the early morning (as was the case with our patient and Stern and Bayes de Luna) [7], are warning signs that should raise the suspicion of coronary vasospasm. This characteristic presentation of pain paired with dynamic ECG changes is a key in diagnosis. Calcium channel blockers coupled with the vasodilatory effect of nitroglycerin are extremely effective in the treatment and prevention of vasospastic complications. ICD therapy is effective in preventing recurrence and can be considered if the patient's vasospasm has led to a life-threatening arrhythmia.

Disclosure

This work was performed as part of the employment of the authors by National Health Service Highland.

References

[1] M. Prinzmetal, R. Kennamer, R. Merliss, T. Wada, and N. Bor, "Angina pectoris I. A variant form of angina pectoris: preliminary report," *The American Journal of Medicine*, vol. 27, no. 3, pp. 375–388, 1959.

[2] S. Swarup, S. Patibandla, and S. Grossman, "Coronary artery vasospasm. StatPearls 2021," https://www.ncbi.nlm.nih.gov/books/NBK470181/.

[3] O. Davies, O. Ajayeoba, and D. Kurian, "Coronary artery spasm: an often overlooked diagnosis," *Nigerian Medical Journal*, vol. 55, no. 4, p. 356, 2014.

[4] A. Ishihara, T. Tanaka, Y. Otsu et al., "Prognosis of patients with coronary vasospasm after successful resuscitation from ventricular fibrillation," *Journal of Arrhythmia*, vol. 28, no. 2, pp. 105–110, 2012.

[5] M. Hung, P. Hu, and M. Hung, "Coronary artery spasm: review and update," *International Journal of Medical Sciences*, vol. 11, no. 11, pp. 1161–1171, 2014.

[6] M. Hung, C. Mao, M. Hung, and T. Chen, "Impact of asthma on the development of coronary vasospastic angina," *Medicine (Baltimore)*, vol. 94, no. 42, article e1880, 2015.

[7] S. Stern and A. Bayes de Luna, "Coronary artery spasm," *Circ*, vol. 119, no. 18, pp. 2531–2534, 2009.

[8] V. Rathod, T. Kanitkar, and G. Karamasis, "Out-of-hospital cardiac arrest due to coronary spasm with recurrent ventricular fibrillation," *Case Reports in Cardiology*, vol. 2020, Article ID 8823306, 3 pages, 2020.

[9] Y. Yamashina, T. Yagi, A. Namekawa et al., "Favorable outcomes of patients with vasospastic angina associated with cardiac arrest," *Journal of Cardiology*, vol. 63, no. 1, pp. 41–45, 2014.

[10] M. Hung, C. Cheng, N. Yang, M. Hung, and W. Cherng, "Coronary vasospasm-induced acute coronary syndrome complicated by life- threatening cardiac arrhythmias in patients without hemodynamically significant coronary artery disease," *International Journal of Cardiology*, vol. 117, no. 1, pp. 37–44, 2007.

[11] P. Ong, A. Athanasiadis, S. Hill, H. Vogelsberg, M. Voehringer, and U. Sechtem, "Coronary artery spasm as a frequent cause of acute coronary syndrome: the CASPAR (Coronary Artery Spasm in Patients With Acute Coronary Syndrome) Study," *Journal of the American College of Cardiology*, vol. 52, no. 7, pp. 523–527, 2008.

29

Coronary Embolism despite CHA_2DS_2-VASc Score of Zero: Should we Reconsider Anticoagulation?

Ammar Ahmed,[1] Andrew Assaf,[2] Aditi Shankar,[3] and Marcel Zughaib[2]

[1]*Department of Internal Medicine, Ascension Providence Hospital, Southfield, MI, USA*
[2]*Department of Cardiovascular Disease, Ascension Providence Hospital, Southfield, MI, USA*
[3]*Department of Internal Medicine, Texas Health Presbyterian Dallas, Dallas, TX, USA*

Correspondence should be addressed to Ammar Ahmed; ammar.ahmed@ascension.org
Academic Editor: Yigit Canga

Coronary embolism (CE) is a rare but important cause of acute coronary syndrome. The most common source of emboli is considered to be infective endocarditis and atrial fibrillation. Various studies have estimated the prevalence of coronary embolism; however, diagnosis is challenging. Often, it is difficult to differentiate. Nonetheless, this is an important step as treating the underlying cause of an embolism is essential to limit recurrence. However, while this condition may have fatal consequences, due to its uncommon occurrence, there is no consensus on diagnosis and management. We present a case of a 53-year-old obese male, with a history of paroxysmal atrial fibrillation not on anticoagulation due to a low CHA_2DS_2-VASc score, who presented with chest pain associated with lightheadedness. ECG on admission revealed coarse atrial fibrillation, and troponin was gradually elevating on serial lab workup. Coronary angiography revealed a distal left anterior descending artery occlusion with apical wall akinesis without any evidence of atherosclerotic coronary artery disease. A presumptive diagnosis of coronary embolism secondary to paroxysmal atrial fibrillation was made, and the patient was started on anticoagulation despite a low CHA_2DS_2-VASc score. This case not only highlights coronary embolism but also illustrates that a low CHA_2DS_2-VASc score does not mean there is no risk of emboli. For such patients, it is important to take clinical reasoning into account along with the CHA_2DS_2-VASc score to determine the benefit of anticoagulation.

1. Introduction

Of patients presenting with acute coronary syndrome, a minority will have a coronary embolism (CE) [1]. This is a rare occurrence of nonatherosclerotic coronary artery disease; nonetheless, it can have fatal consequences. Studies conducted in 1978 and 1989 found that 4-7% and 13% of all ACS cases at coronary angiography or autopsy, respectively [2, 3]. The most recent study on prevalence was conducted by Shibata et al. in 2015, who demonstrated 2.9% of patients with ACS were due to CE [4]. The most common sources of emboli are infective endocarditis and nonvalvular atrial fibrillation [4, 5]. Other sources include cardiac tumors, paradoxical emboli through a patent foramen ovale, or iatrogenic [1]. Importantly, Shibata et al. also reported that over 50% of the patients in their study with CE and atrial fibrillation had a $CHADS_2$ less than 2 [4]. While some of these patients would have higher scores using the CHA_2DS_2-VASc score, it is important to note neither scoring system account for a CE event. Currently, optimal therapy has not been established [4]. Patients with a reversible cause of thromboembolism are recommended to receive 3 months of anticoagulation, in line with the management of venous thromboembolism [1]. However, patients with atrial fibrillation as a source of embolism can have recurrence and should receive continuous anticoagulation even with a low CHA_2DS_2-VASc score [1, 4]. This is important as a second CE event can be preventable. Patients who have undergone PCI should also be on antiplatelet therapy [1].

The mechanism of cardiac embolism in atrial fibrillation can be explained by Virchow's triad of endothelial damage, hypercoagulability, and stasis [6, 7]. Due to the anatomy of the left atrial appendage, it constitutes the microenvironment for thrombus formation during and after an episode of atrial

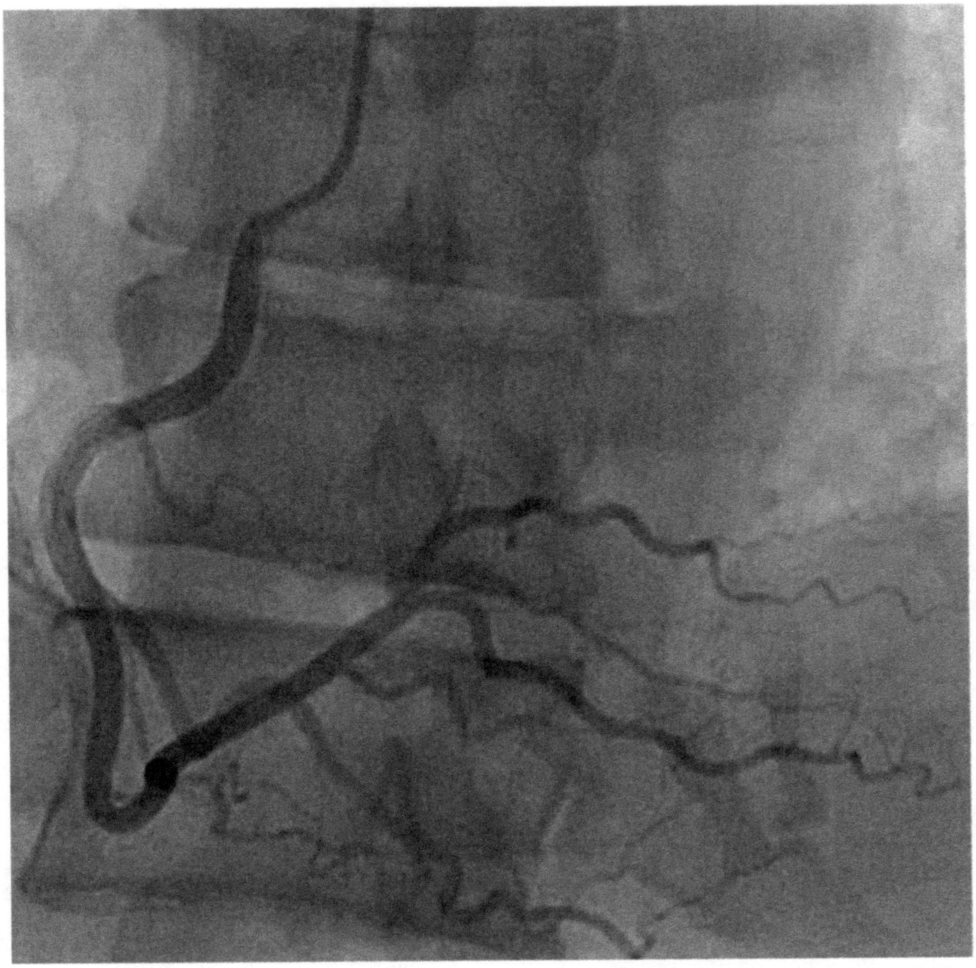

FIGURE 1: Left heart catheterization via the right radial approach. Selective angiograph of the right coronary artery in the left anterior oblique cranial projection revealing a medium caliber vessel angiographically free of any significant atherosclerotic disease.

fibrillation [8]. Therefore, appropriate investigation should be carried out to identify the source of the thrombus.

2. Case Presentation

We report the case of a 53-year-old obese gentleman who presented with acute sudden onset pressure-like chest pain associated with lightheadedness. This was the first time the patient reported having chest pain. He had no exertional symptoms. He called EMS and was immediately transferred to our facility. The patient was reportedly diagnosed with paroxysmal atrial fibrillation in the past year by his primary care physician but was not placed on anticoagulation since his CHA_2DS_2-VASc score was 0. He had never had any stress testing done. He was otherwise a lifelong nonsmoker, and his family history was unremarkable. Vital signs were stable on admission. His physical exam was pertinent for a middle-aged gentleman in no acute distress but with an irregularly irregular rhythm, borderline tachycardic rate, and variables S1 and S2 without any murmurs, rubs, or gallops. ECG on admission revealed coarse atrial fibrillation with a rapid ventricular rate and premature ventricular contractions. Chest X-ray did not reveal any acute abnormality. Pertinent labs on admission included a normal hemoglobin and white blood cell count with mild thrombocytopenia, normal prothrombin time and activated partial thromboplastin time, and normal basic metabolic panel but with mild hyperglycemia. His initial troponin T was 0.02 ng/ml followed by 0.03 ng/ml and finally 0.80 ng/ml (0.10 ng/ml being the upper limit of normal in our lab). ProBNP was 1104 pg/ml (normal range 50–137 pg/ml). His TSH was undetectable, FT4 was 3.79 ng/dl (normal range 0.93–1.7 ng/dl), FT3 was 6.9 pg/ml (normal range 2–4.4 pg/ml), hemoglobin A1c was 5.6%, and LDL was 58 mg/dl. Transthoracic echocardiogram was done with contrast to improve opacification of the left ventricle. It revealed a mildly reduced ejection fraction (EF 45-50%), akinesis of the apical wall, normal right ventricular systolic function, mildly dilated left and right atria, mild to moderate mitral, and tricuspid valve regurgitation along with moderate pulmonary hypertension. The patient was given a full-dose aspirin, high dose statin, and a beta blocker along with a heparin drip. A left heart catheterization was performed and revealed evidence of thrombotic occlusion of the distal left anterior descending artery without any evidence of obstructive epicardial atherosclerotic coronary disease (Figures 1–4). A 6 French EBU 3.0 catheter was used to engage the left main coronary artery, and a BMW wire was used to cross the lesion, and a 2.5 mm × 16 mm balloon

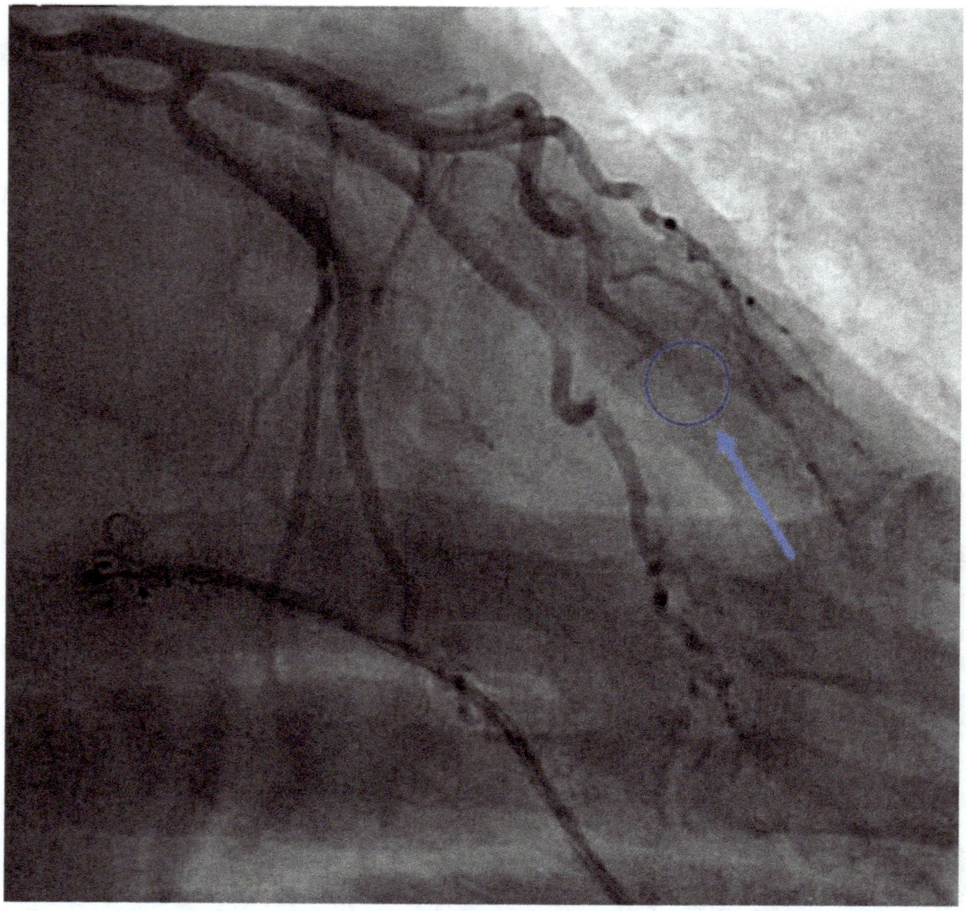

FIGURE 2: Left heart catheterization via the right radial approach. Selective angiograph of the left coronary artery in the right anterior oblique caudal projection revealing a no significant atherosclerotic disease but with a filling defect noted in the distal left anterior descending artery.

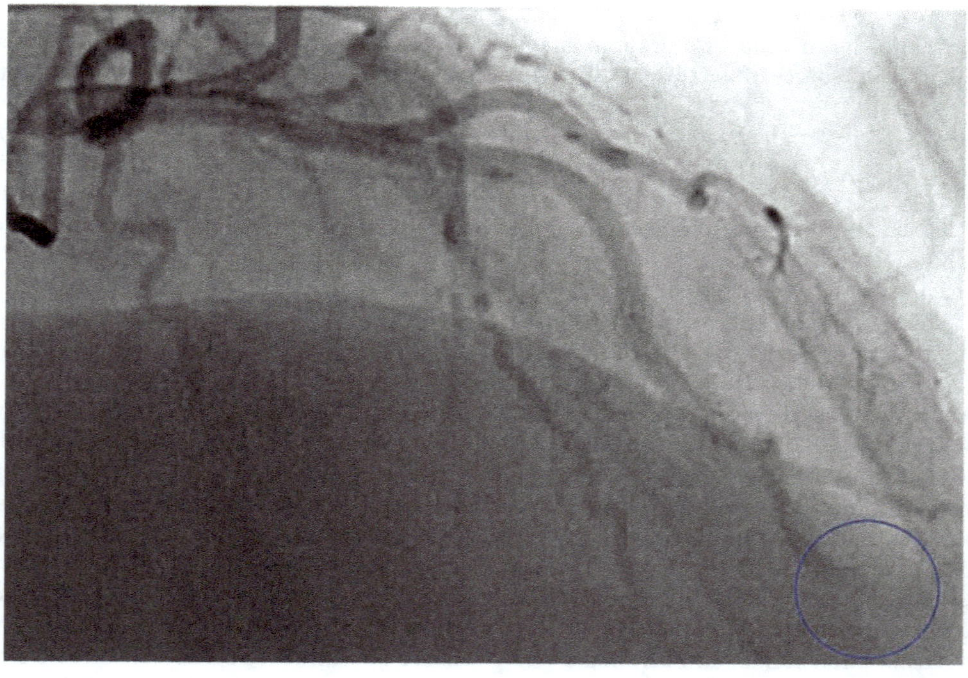

FIGURE 3: Left heart catheterization via the right radial approach. Selective angiograph of the left coronary artery in the right anterior oblique cranial projection revealing a distally occluded left anterior descending artery with thrombus (blue circle).

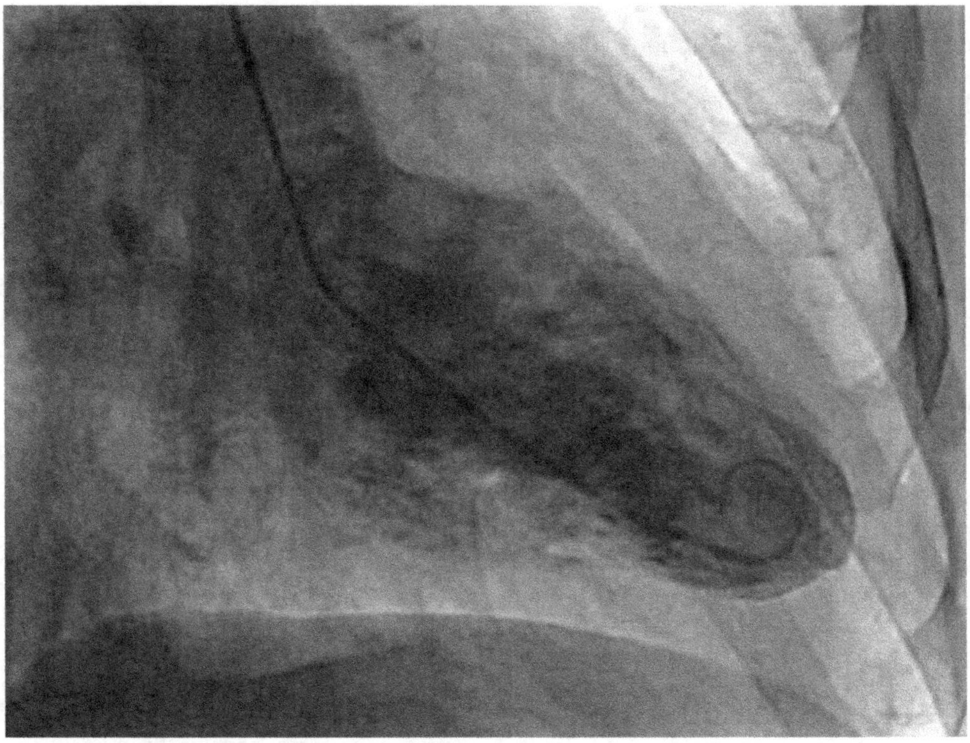

FIGURE 4: Left ventriculogram revealing a mildly reduced ejection fraction (visual estimation of 40%) along with akinesis of the distal anterior, apical anterior, and apical and apical inferior walls without evidence of an apical thrombus.

was used to dilate the lesion with marginal benefit likely due to organized thrombus. The patient was then started on low dose aspirin and clopidogrel for dual antiplatelet therapy. He was also started on rivaroxaban which would allow for one-time daily dosing. As well he was continued on metoprolol which was started on his presentation to the emergency room. He will continue triple therapy for one month and then continue clopidogrel and rivaroxaban. His hospitalization was otherwise uneventful and was later on discharged with close outpatient follow-up.

3. Discussion

Diagnosis of coronary embolism can be challenging. Our patient had no evidence of atherosclerotic disease on heart catheterization; this in the setting of atrial fibrillation greatly swayed our differential towards an embolism. However, had there been a thrombus with concomitant atherosclerotic disease, arriving at a definite diagnosis would be far more difficult. Shibata et al. have proposed criteria for diagnosis, presented in Table 1, of which our patient has met 1 major and 2 minor criteria [4]. Per their proposed method, this would suggest a definite diagnosis of coronary embolism. Nonetheless, no set standard of diagnosis has been established.

TABLE 1: Criteria for diagnosis of coronary embolism (Shibata et al.).

Criteria for diagnosis of coronary embolism
Major criteria
Evidence of coronary embolism or thrombus angiographically without atherosclerosis.
Evidence of coronary emboli to multiple sites concomitantly.
Systemic embolization in the absence of acute myocardial infarction induced left ventricular thrombus.
Minor criteria
Stenosis of nonculprit coronary artery < 25%.
Evidence of embolic sources based on noninvasive imaging.
Presence of risk factors for emboli, cardiomyopathy, rheumatic heart disease, prosthetic valve, PFO, atrial septal defect, history of cardiac surgery, infective endocarditis, or hypercoagulable state.

Patients with 2 or more major criteria, 1 major and 2 minor, or 3 minor criteria were considered to have a definite coronary embolus. Patients with 1 major and 1 minor or 2 minor criteria were considered to have a probable coronary embolus.

An additional challenge is to establish the etiology of the embolism. In a study conducted by Lacey et al., 147 cases of coronary embolism from 1990 to 2017 were reviewed [5]. It was found that the three most common etiologies of coronary embolism were infective endocarditis, atrial fibrillation, and prosthetic valve thrombosis, respectively. Other rare causes that have been documented include left ventricular thrombus, atrial myxoma, and papillary fibroelastoma. However, with the advancement in early diagnosis, atrial fibrillation may have surpassed infective endocarditis as the most common etiology; however, that remains a postulation as of now [5].

Thrombophilia may also be considered in patients with CE; however, the relationship between thrombophilia and arterial thromboembolism is still contested. Little data is available to link these two entities [1, 9]. The decision to pursue a thrombophilia workup should thus be made judiciously. Guiding principles may be derived from stroke management as there are too few cases of CE to establish specific guidelines. Nonetheless, this workup should only be pursued if no other obvious etiology is present, and laboratory testing will result in changes to patient management [1].

The most frequently involved vessel is the left anterior descending artery followed by the left circumflex, right coronary, and left main coronary artery, respectively [5]. This is in agreement with a study by Prizel et al., who found the left anterior descending to be the most commonly involved artery [3].

The infrequent occurrence of coronary embolism is thought to be related to the surrounding anatomy [3, 5]. With a wide aortic orifice relative to the coronary ostia, most emboli leaving the aortic outflow tract would likely continue to further organs. More so, the ostia of the coronary arteries are at sharp angles to the aorta making it further less accessible to an embolism.

Currently, there are no formal guidelines with regard to workup and management of coronary embolism [5]. Treatment must be individualized based on lesion amenability to interventional techniques as well as the underlying etiology. Lacey et al. reported use of thrombectomy in nearly half of the cases that were reviewed along with balloon angioplasty +/- stent placement along with thrombolysis. Upon discharge, a third of patients were prescribed anticoagulation +/- antiplatelet agents [5]. Shibata et al. also note that histological study may aid in diagnosis and is a benefit if the thrombus is aspirated [4]. However, a challenge remains that many emboli lodge in distal segments of culprit vessels, at times beyond what is accessible to a catheter. Such patients should continue to receive medical management. This includes anticoagulation for 6 months or 3 if a reversible risk factor has now resolved, as well as antiplatelet therapy if PCI was done [1]. Studies have not demonstrated significant mortality benefit with aspiration thrombectomy in patients with ST segment elevation myocardial infarction [10].

This case was further complicated by the patients' diagnosis of atrial fibrillation. Atrial fibrillation increases the risk of systemic thromboembolism. Interestingly, in the cohort study by Shibata et al., 18 out of 30 patients who had atrial fibrillation and developed a coronary embolism had a $CHADS_2$ score of 0-1 [4]. However, when reevaluated with the CHA_2DS_2-VASc score, 11 of the 18 patients had a score of 2 or greater [4]. A CHA_2DS_2-VASc score of 2 or above is an indication for use of prophylactic anticoagulation according to the most recent guidelines published in 2019 [11]. There is uncertainty whether anticoagulation is warranted in patients with a CHA_2DS_2-VASc of 0 or 1; however, clinical judgment is recommended. The unadjusted stroke risk for patients with a CHA_2DS_2-VASc of 0, 1, and 2 is 0.2%, 0.6%, and 2.2% per year, respectively [11]. There is no evidence that treatment with aspirin for patients with low CHA_2DS_2-VASc scores (≤ 1) offers any clinical benefit [11]. Of note, hyperthyroidism was not found to be an independent risk factor for thrombosis [12, 13].

Our patient had a CHA_2DS_2-VASc score of 0 and absence of left ventricular and left atrial appendage thrombus on transthoracic echocardiography even though transesophageal echocardiography was not performed. Left atrial appendage occlusion devices can be considered if there is an absolute contraindication to anticoagulation or increased risk of bleeding if indeed the left atrial appendage was the source of embolism [14], but further studies are needed in this regard as the data on the use of devices for coronary embolism is limited. This case clearly illustrates the imperfection of the assumptions underlying a "low" CHA_2DS_2-VASc score and the importance of clinical judgment to guide the decision to anticoagulate such patients.

4. Conclusion

We reported a case of a 53-year-old male who was found to have coronary embolism secondary to atrial fibrillation off anticoagulation because of a CHA_2DS_2-VASc score of zero. Coronary embolism is rare and sometimes a challenge to diagnose. The most reported etiologies of coronary embolism are valvular masses (e.g., infective endocarditis), atrial fibrillation, and prosthetic valve thrombosis. Treatment is individualized and is based on the etiology. Even though our patient did not qualify for anticoagulation because of a low CHA_2DS_2-VASc score, this serves as a reminder of the imperfection of our assumptions which raises the question whether we should have a lower threshold to initiate anticoagulation. This is not to say that anticoagulation is without risks; however, a more individualized approach may be needed.

Abbreviations

CE: Coronary embolism
ACS: Acute coronary syndrome
AF: Atrial fibrillation
PFO: Patent foramen ovale
PCI: Percutaneous coronary intervention.

Disclosure

This case was originally presented in the Michigan Chapter of the American College of Cardiology 2020 ePoster Session by Andrew Assaf, Adidit Shankar, and Marcel Zughaib.

References

[1] C. Raphael, J. Heit, G. Reeder et al., "Coronary embolus: an underappreciated cause of acute coronary syndromes," *JACC. Cardiovascular Interventions*, vol. 11, no. 2, pp. 172–180, 2018.

[2] B. F. Waller, "Atherosclerotic and nonatherosclerotic coronary artery factors in acute myocardial infarction," *Cardiovascular Clinics*, vol. 20, no. 1, pp. 29–104, 1989.

[3] K. Prizel, G. M. Hutchins, and B. Bulkley, "Coronary artery embolism and myocardial infarction," *Annals of Internal Medicine*, vol. 88, no. 2, pp. 155–161, 1978.

[4] T. Shibata, S. Kawakami, T. Noguchi et al., "Prevalence, clinical features, and prognosis of acute myocardial infarction attributable to coronary artery embolism," *Circulation*, vol. 132, no. 4, pp. 241–250, 2015.

[5] M. Lacey, S. Raza, H. Rehman, R. Puri, D. L. Bhatt, and A. Kalra, "Coronary embolism: a systematic review," *Cardiovascular Revascularization Medicine*, vol. 21, no. 3, pp. 367–374, 2020.

[6] T. Watson, E. Shantsila, and G. Lip, "Mechanisms of thrombogenesis in atrial fibrillation: Virchow's triad revisited," *The Lancet*, vol. 373, no. 9658, pp. 155–166, 2009.

[7] F. Kolodgie, R. Virmani, A. Finn, and M. E. Romero, "Embolic myocardial infarction as a consequence of atrial fibrillation," *Circulation*, vol. 132, no. 4, pp. 223–226, 2015.

[8] K. Bartus, R. Litwinowicz, J. Natorska et al., "Coagulation factors and fibrinolytic activity in the left atrial appendage and other heart chambers in patients with atrial fibrillation: is there a local intracardiac prothrombotic state? (HEART-CLOT study)," *International Journal of Cardiology*, vol. 301, pp. 103–107, 2020.

[9] I. Martinelli, P. M. Mannucci, V. de Stefano et al., "Different risks of thrombosis in four coagulation defects associated with inherited thrombophilia: a study of 150 families," *Blood*, vol. 92, no. 7, pp. 2353–2358, 1998.

[10] J. Ge, A. Schäfer, G. Ertl, and P. Nordbeck, "Thrombus aspiration for ST-segment-elevation myocardial infarction in Modern Era: still an issue of debate?," *Circulation. Cardiovascular Interventions*, vol. 10, no. 10, 2017.

[11] C. T. January, L. S. Wann, H. Calkins et al., "2019 AHA/ACC/HRS focused update of the 2014 AHA/ACC/HRS guideline for the management of patients with atrial fibrillation: a report of the American College of Cardiology/American Heart Association Task Force on Clinical Practice Guidelines and the Heart Rhythm Society," *Journal of the American College of Cardiology*, vol. 74, no. 1, pp. 104–132, 2019.

[12] D. Singer, G. Albers, J. Dalen et al., "Antithrombotic therapy in atrial fibrillation: American College of Chest Physicians evidence-based clinical practice guidelines (8th edition)," *Chest*, vol. 133, no. 6, pp. 546S–592S, 2008.

[13] P. Chan, J. Hai, C. Y. Yeung et al., "Benefit of Anticoagulation therapy in hyperthyroidism-related atrial fibrillation," *Clinical Cardiology*, vol. 38, no. 8, pp. 476–482, 2015.

[14] M. Nishimura, S. Sab, R. Reeves, and J. C. Hsu, "Percutaneous left atrial appendage occlusion in atrial fibrillation patients with a contraindication to oral anticoagulation: a focused review," *Europace*, vol. 20, no. 9, pp. 1412–1419, 2018.

Novel Technique of Surgical Management of Scimitar Syndrome

Mary Lark,[1] Amanda Cai,[2] Phillip Rideout,[1] David Gregg,[1] Pal Suranyi,[2,3] Fred A. Crawford,[4] and Valerian L. Fernandes[2]

[1]*College of Medicine, Medical University of South Carolina, Charleston, SC 29425, USA*
[2]*Department of Cardiology, Medical University of South Carolina, Charleston, SC 29425, USA*
[3]*Department of Radiology, Medical University of South Carolina, Charleston, SC 29425, USA*
[4]*Department of Surgery, Medical University of South Carolina, Charleston, SC 29425, USA*

Correspondence should be addressed to Valerian L. Fernandes; fernandv@musc.edu

Academic Editor: Adam Torbicki

Scimitar syndrome is a rare congenital abnormality resulting from right-sided pulmonary venous return to the inferior vena cava rather than to the left atrium. It is usually detected in early childhood with symptoms of recurrent chest infection and finding of pulmonary hypertension due to left to right shunt. We report a case of a 40-year-old woman with scimitar syndrome discovered on chest X-ray during evaluation of recurrent pneumonia. Surgical correction was achieved with a novel technique of using a synthetic graft connecting the scimitar vein across the right atrium to the left atrium along with ligation of the scimitar vein connection to the inferior vena cava. The patient continues to do well 10 years after surgery, and the shunt graft shows good flow on echocardiogram. We present her clinical and imaging data and details of the surgical technique along with a brief review of surgical literature.

1. Introduction

Scimitar syndrome is a variant of partial anomalous pulmonary venous connection (PAPVC), which results in pulmonary venous connection from the right lung to the inferior vena cava (IVC) [1]. The name is derived from a curvilinear (scimitar-shaped) shadow alongside the right heart border on chest X-ray (Figure 1). Scimitar syndrome is usually associated with other cardiac and pulmonary defects, including atrial septal defects (ASD), dextroposition of the heart, right lung hypoplasia, and pulmonary hypertension [2]. Severe cases in childhood result in cyanosis and pulmonary hypertension, requiring surgical correction. However, some cases are not discovered until adulthood, either due to worsening, symptomatic left to right shunt, or incidental discovery on chest X-ray after recurrent pulmonary infections. Surgical repair of these defects is especially difficult, with several methods requiring cardiopulmonary bypass to repair this anomaly. We present a novel surgical technique used in the repair of scimitar syndrome in a middle-aged woman.

2. Case Report

A 40-year-old Caucasian woman presented to her primary physician with recurrent fevers, chills, wheezing, and cough. She was a welder by profession and had a long history of respiratory symptoms and allergies. She was treated with a course of antibiotics for a presumed pneumonia. When her cough and other symptoms persisted, a chest X-ray was performed and showed a curvilinear abnormality alongside her right heart border consistent with scimitar syndrome (Figure 1). Upon further review of history, the patient endorsed worsening shortness of breath over the past year and occasional palpitations with exertion, but denied symptoms with normal activity. She had recurrent pulmonary infections and asthma/allergy episodes throughout childhood and adult life. Physical exam showed normal jugular venous pressure (JVP). She had a parasternal heave but her apex was not localized. The heart sounds were normal and she did not have any murmurs.

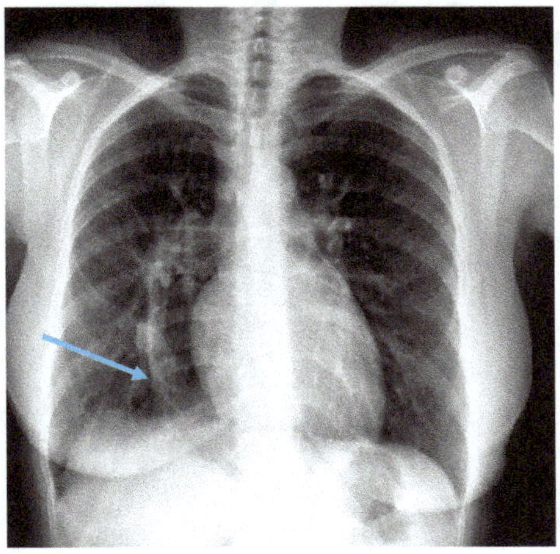

FIGURE 1: Frontal upright PA CXR of patient. Arrow pointing to scimitar vein in the right lower lung.

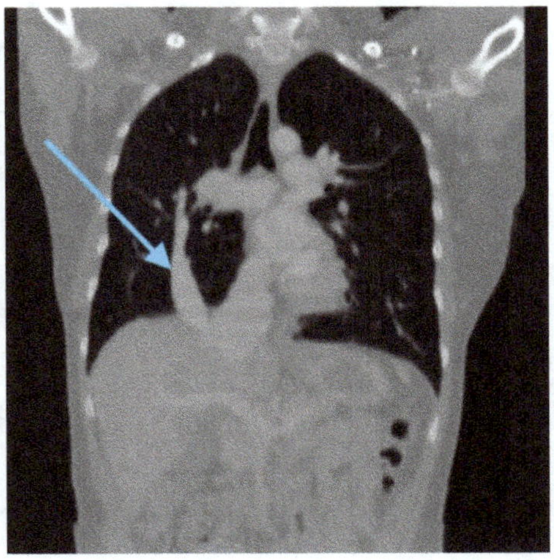

FIGURE 2: Coronal CT with IV contrast. Arrow pointing to scimitar vein in the right lower lobe, which drains into the IVC.

Echocardiogram showed dilatation of the right atrium and right ventricle with and interatrial shunt consistent with a patent foramen ovale (PFO). Ejection fraction was normal.

Computed tomography (CT) of the chest (Figure 2) showed a hypoplastic right upper lobe and compensatory large right lower lobe. There was a large right pulmonary artery with a large arteriovenous malformation (AVM) from the pulmonary artery into the anomalous scimitar vein which attached to the inferior vena cava. The majority of the right lung pulmonary venous return was to the inferior vena cava via the scimitar vein. A single small vestigial inferior pulmonary vein on the right extended to the left atrium. The left pulmonary veins drained normally into the left atrium.

Transthoracic echocardiography (TEE) confirmed right atrial and right ventricular dilatation and normal left pulmonary venous return into the left atrium. There was an atretic right inferior pulmonary vein opening into the right atrium. The right lower pulmonary vein was not visible by echocardiography. A PFO was confirmed by color Doppler and agitated saline injection.

Cardiac catheterization showed normal coronary arteries and normal left ventricular end-diastolic pressure. The PFO allowed easy passage of the multipurpose catheter into the left atrium. Pulmonary angiography, aortogram, and scimitar venography were also performed using a 6F pigtail catheter. Right pulmonary artery angiogram identified partial anomalous pulmonary venous return via scimitar vein to the IVC (Figure 3). The patient was referred for surgical correction due to persistent shunt and recurrent pulmonary infections. Upon multidisciplinary review of the case, the traditional approach of reimplanting the anomalous scimitar vein into the left atrium was deemed to carry excessive risk and was therefore deferred. After review of the patient's CT imaging, a simplified interatrial baffle redirecting the anomalous pulmonary venous blood to the left atrium was pursued.

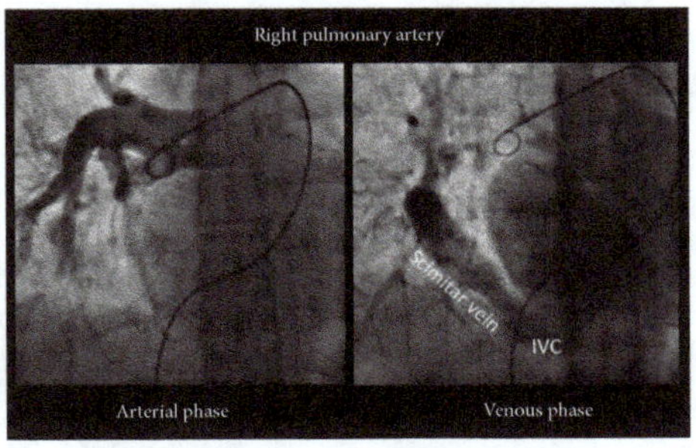

FIGURE 3: Pulmonary angiogram in anterior-posterior projection. The pigtail catheter is in the right pulmonary artery. The arterial phase [left frame] reveals the right pulmonary arteriogram. The right frame shows the venous phase with the scimitar vein from the right upper lobe draining into the IVC.

3. Surgical Technique

After satisfactory general anesthesia, the patient was placed on cardiopulmonary bypass. With the heart completely decompressed, the lung was retracted. The anomalous vein was identified in an oblique fissure of the right lung and demonstrated to drain through the diaphragm. The anomalous vein was dissected for a distance of several centimeters from the diaphragm up and toward the hilum of the lung. The right atrium was opened through a longitudinal incision approximately 1.5 cm away from the AV groove. There was a large fossa ovalis and a small patent foramen ovale. These landmarks were used as guide for excising the entire fossa ovalis to a diameter of approximately 1.6 to 1.8 cm. A ribbed 16 mm Gore-Tex graft was chosen and sutured end-to-side to this newly created atrial septal defect with continuous 5-0 Prolene suture. A linear incision slightly smaller than the graft was made very low in the lateral right atrial wall, and the graft was brought through this defect and then through a defect in the pleura. A linear incision was made in the anomalous pulmonary vein, and the graft was sutured to this vein meticulously with a continuous 5-0 Prolene suture (Figure 4). After confirming both anastomosis and the patency of the graft, the anomalous vein was ligated between the Gore-Tex graft and the diaphragm. The patient tolerated the procedure well and was discharged on warfarin four days after the procedure.

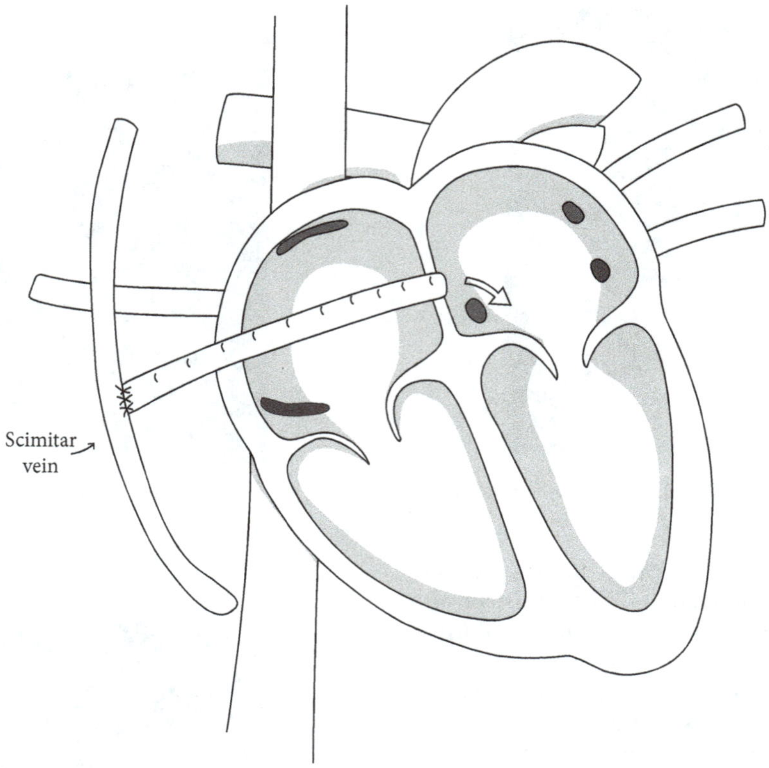

Figure 4: Schematic diagram of the scimitar vein and the surgically created baffle. The baffle connects the scimitar vein to the left atrium via the right atrium. The blue arrow points to the ligated scimitar vein.

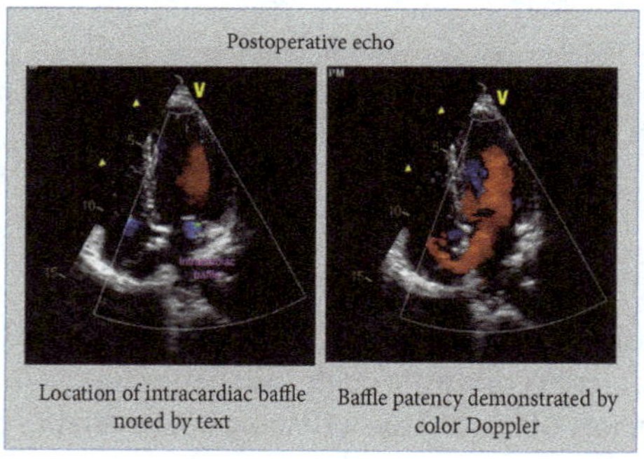

Figure 5: Echocardiogram, apical four chamber view. The left frame shows the baffle traversing the right atrium and opening into the left atrium. The right frame shows color flow through the baffle into the left atrium.

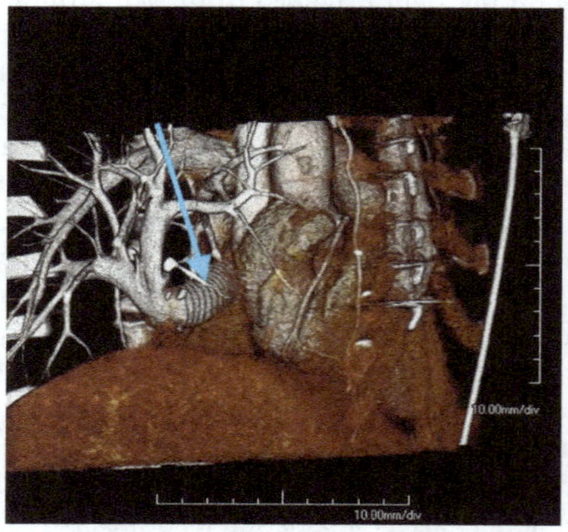

Figure 6: 3D volume rendering of postoperative CT angiogram from a right anterior oblique view. Arrow pointing to the artificial baffle, draining the scimitar vein, aiming posteriorly toward the left atrium.

4. Postoperative

ECHO showed a right ventricular peak systolic pressure of 22 mmHg with no intracardiac shunts. The graft passing through the right atrium was noted to be patent with good flow on Doppler (Figure 5). A pulmonary perfusion scan was performed which showed a differential perfusion of 47.8% to the left lung and 52.2% to the right lung. One-month postoperative cardiac-gated CTA showed that the synthetic graft remained widely patent with no evidence of thrombus (Figures 6–9).

The patient noted an uneventful recovery with less fatigue and improvement in her breathing during follow-up visits. She has continued to do well for 10 years after the procedure. The shunt was well-visualized with good flow on serial follow-up echocardiograms.

5. Discussion

Surgical correction of scimitar syndrome in adults is usually reserved for symptomatic patients with worsening left to right shunt. Numerous surgical techniques have been

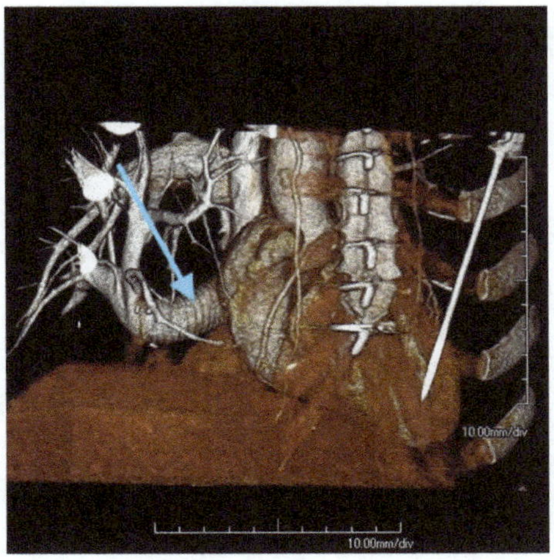

FIGURE 7: 3D volume rendering of postoperative CTA from a less oblique RAO view. Arrow pointing to the artificial baffle diverting the scimitar vein toward the left atrium behind the right atrium.

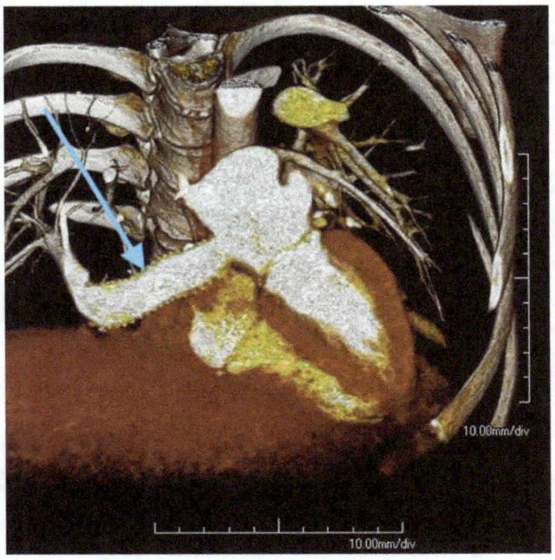

FIGURE 8: 3D volume rendering, cutaway view, of postoperative CTA. Arrow pointing to the artificial baffle connecting the scimitar vein with the left atrium via the posterior aspect of the right atrium.

described, with most requiring deep hypothermia and circulatory arrest. The first corrective operation was performed by Kirklin and associates [3] in 1956 without the use of cardiopulmonary bypass. Shumacker and Judd [4] devised a method using cardiopulmonary bypass, involving direct reimplantation of the anomalous pulmonary vein into the right atrium. This method was modified by Zubiate and Kay [5] in 1962 with the use of an interatrial patch developed to redirect flow into the left atrium through an ASD.

Direct anastomosis of the scimitar vein to the left atrium was first described by Honey [6] in 1977. However, there were frequent complications associated with this method, including inadvertent constriction or occlusion via thrombosis. This thrombosis is attributed to mobilization of the

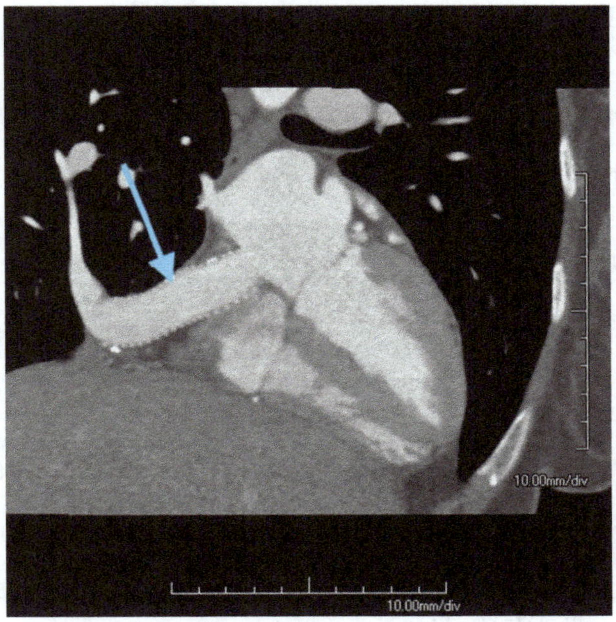

FIGURE 9: Oblique multiplanar reformat of postoperative CTA. Arrow pointing to the widely patent artificial baffle connecting the scimitar vein with the left atrium via the posterior aspect of the right atrium. There is no filling defect inside the graft to suggest thrombus.

scimitar vein with resultant vessel distortion or the tortuous coursing of the scimitar vein resulting in kinking. Dupuis and colleagues [7] described these complications in a series of 37 patients that underwent classical surgical repair. Of these 37 patients, only 12 had acceptable outcomes without evidence of thrombosis. Additional surgical complications include stenosis of the intracardiac baffle, pulmonary hypertension, and hemoptysis [8].

Our method is based upon the approach described by Harrison and colleagues [9]. We used a Gore-Tex graft penetrating through the walls of the right atrium to connect the scimitar vein to the left atrium via a newly created ASD. This method prevents the complications associated with moving the scimitar vein itself, while successfully correcting the left-to-right shunt through a more direct path than the traditional method. The ease and success of this technique should make it the preferred surgical strategy for surgical repair of symptomatic scimitar syndrome in adults.

6. Conclusion

Traditional surgical repair of scimitar syndrome is difficult and complicated. The technique described using synthetic graft baffle provides a more direct path for right-sided pulmonary venous return to the left atrium. The ease and success of this technique and the long-term graft patency should make it the preferred surgical strategy for surgical repair of symptomatic scimitar syndrome in adults.

Consent

The patient was informed of the nature of the surgical procedure, the associated risks and benefits, and their rights as a patient. The patient expressed informed consent to the procedure.

References

[1] U. Gudjonsson and J. W. Brown, "Scimitar syndrome," *Seminars in Thoracic and Cardiovascular Surgery: Pediatric Cardiac Surgery Annual*, vol. 9, no. 1, pp. 56–62, 2006.

[2] G. Cooper, "Case of malformation of the thoracic viscera: consisting of imperfect development of the right lung and transposition of the heart," *London Medical Gazette*, vol. 18, pp. 600-601, 1836.

[3] J. W. Kirklin, F. H. Ellis Jr., and E. H. Wood, "Treatment of anomalous pulmonary venous connections in association with interatrial communications," *Surgery*, vol. 39, no. 3, pp. 389–398, 1956.

[4] H. B. Shumacker Jr. and D. Judd, "Partial anomalous pulmonary venous return with reference to drainage into the inferior vena cava and to an intact atrial septum," *The Journal of Cardiovascular Surgery*, vol. 5, pp. 271–278, 1964.

[5] P. Zubiate and J. H. Kay, "Surgical correction of anomalous pulmonary venous connection," *Annals of Surgery*, vol. 156, no. 2, pp. 234–250, 1962.

[6] M. Honey, "Anomalous Pulmonary Venous Drainage of Right Lung to Inferior Vena Cava ('Scimitar Syndrome'): Clinical Spectrum in Older Patients and Role of Surgery," *QJM: An International Journal of Medicine*, vol. 46, no. 4, pp. 463–483, 1977.

[7] C. Dupuis, L. A. C. Charaf, G. M. Brevière, P. Abou, M. Rémy-Jardin, and G. Helmius, "The "adult" form of the scimitar syndrome," *The American Journal of Cardiology*, vol. 70, no. 4, pp. 502–507, 1992.

[8] R. Reddy, R. Shah, J. Thorpe, and J. Gibbs, "Scimitar syndrome: a rare cause of haemoptysis," *European Journal of Cardio-Thoracic Surgery*, vol. 22, no. 5, p. 821, 2002.

[9] L. H. Harrison Jr., S. K. Tam, and C. P. Mueller, "Partial anomalous pulmonary venous connection in adults: a simplified approach," *The Annals of Thoracic Surgery*, vol. 89, no. 1, pp. 283–285, 2010.

31

Management of Pacemaker Implantation during COVID-19 Infection

Luigi Rivetti, Roberto Mantovan, Nadir Sitta, Ricarda Marinigh, Giuseppe Allocca, Moemen Mohammed, Fausto Pizzino, and Giuseppe Nucifora

Department of Cardiology, "S. Maria dei Battuti" Hospital, AULSS 2 Veneto, Via Brigata Bisagno, Conegliano (TV), Italy

Correspondence should be addressed to Luigi Rivetti; dott.luigirivetti@virgilio.it

Academic Editor: Kathleen Ngu

The management of device implantation during the COVID-19 infection has not well defined yet. This is the first case of complete atrioventricular block in a symptomatic patient affected by the COVID-19 infection treated with early pacemaker implantation to minimize the risk of virus contagion.

1. Introduction

Heart disease patients with the concomitant COVID-19 infection could have higher risk of mortality, and their management could be particularly challenging [1].

Recently, the European Society of Cardiology (ESC) Guidance [2] and Italian position paper [3] about the treatment of cardiovascular (CV) disease in COVID 19 infection patients have been published; however, the suggested management of atrioventricular (AV) conduction disorder patients is not matching between the two proposed guidelines. This is the first report about an AV block patient affected by the COVID-19 infection treated with early permanent pacemaker (pPM) implantation.

On March 12th 2020, a 75-year-old female, with no previous cardiovascular history or previous drugs taking, was admitted to our Emergency Department because of a traumatic syncope during fever. Five days prior to her admission, she had myalgia, cough, dyspnea, and fevers up to 39.5°C. At the electrocardiogram (ECG), the patient showed complete AV block with ventricular escape rhythm and atrial fibrillation. The laboratory tests revealed normal high-sensitivity troponin and ionemia, but high C-reactive protein (11 mg/l; n.v.<1 mg/L). The echocardiogram showed normal biventricular function, while the chest X-ray revealed bilateral consolidations. The moderate hypoxia (PO2 = 64 mmHg) at the blood gas confirmed the hypothesis of a pneumonia; thus, a nasopharyngeal swab was performed, with a positive result for SARS-CoV-2 on the real-time reverse transcriptase–polymerase chain reaction assay.

Although the consensus to prevent cardiac implantable electronic device (CIED) infections recommends to delay the procedure until a patient has afebrile for at least 24 hours [4], a single chamber PM (Medtronic-Advisa SR MRI™) was implanted in the same day of the admission (Figure 1), two hours after the positive result for the SARS-CoV-2 swab infection. The procedure was performed in thirty minutes using resorbable sutures to avoid further surgical wound checks. The medical staff wore FPP2-masks, while the patient had a surgical mask according to the World Health Organization recommendation [5]. At last, the patient has been transferred in a COVID 19 dedicated hospital to continue the appropriate medical therapy. There, the patient was treated with antiviral drugs (lopinavir/ritonavir 200/100 bis in die (BID) for 14 days), hydroxychloroquine (400 mg BID for the day 1 followed by 200 mg BID for four days), azythromycin (500 mg on day 1, followed by 250 mg for seven days), and enoxaparin (4000 units/day subcutaneously). After two weeks from the pPM implantation, the COVID-19 infection was effectively treated, and the patient was discharged home. No pPM-related complications were reported, as far as no other viral contagion episodes were documented among the noninfected staff. Moreover, the home-remote monitoring was preferred to check the pPM parameters after the

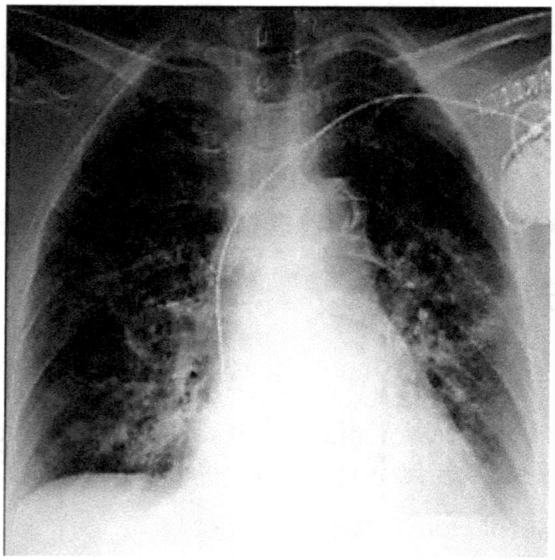

FIGURE 1: The chest X-ray of the COVID-19 patient after the pPM implantation.

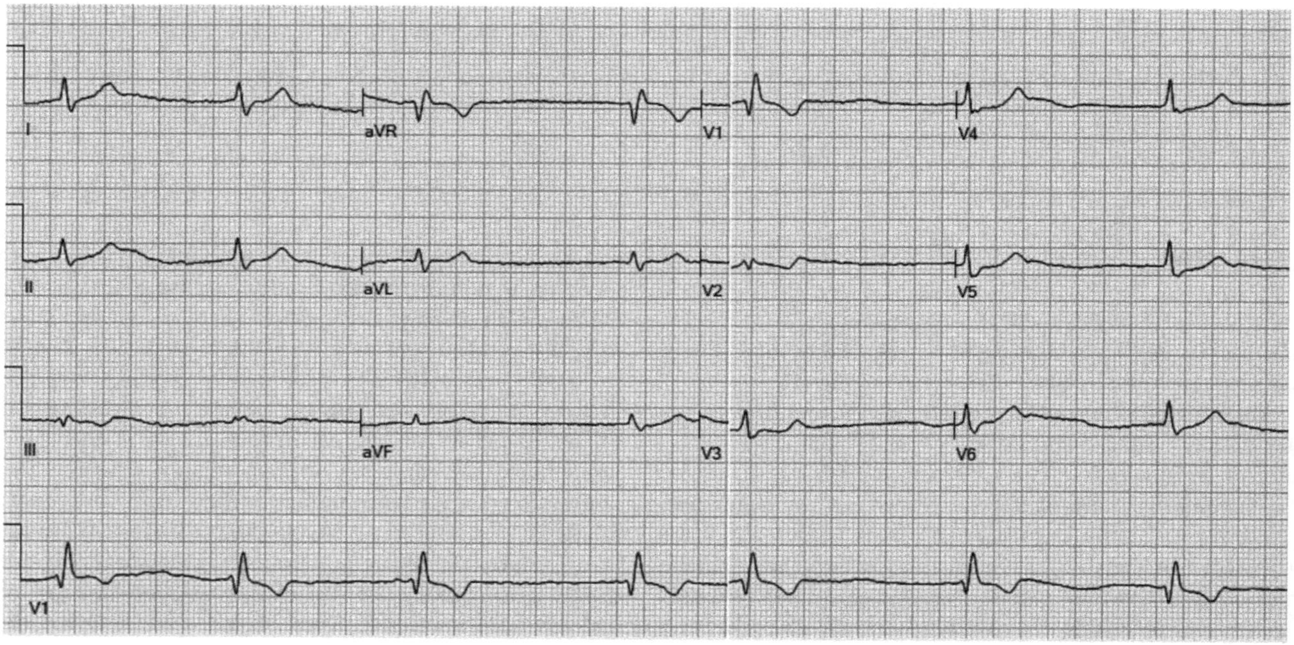

FIGURE 2: The ECG of the patient before the pPM implantation.

discharge avoiding any potential favourable condition of the virus hospital reinfection. Nowadays, the patient is asymptomatic, her clinical general conditions are satisfactory, and the pPM parameters are in range. Figures 2 and 3 showed the ECG before the pPM implantation and after the COVID 19 infection. It confirmed that no change in the conduction disturbance happened when the infection was solved; moreover, the pacing rate was 100% at the PM check after 3 months.

2. Discussion

In the era of COVID-19, the management of heart disease patients with the concomitant virus infection has not been completely defined yet. Moreover, as other known cardiotropic virus in case of myocardial involvement [6], the hypothesis that COVID-19 could lead to the exacerbation of conduction system disorders, or sinus node disease or new-onset high degree AV block, is actually under study, albeit no cases have been already described. The hypothesis of myocarditis has been considered unlikely in this case, as far as both the high-sensitivity troponin and the biventricular function were normal, although exclusive involvement of the conduction tissue cannot be excluded. Conversely, the hypoxia due to the pneumonia has probably leaded to the demonstration of a preexisting conduction disorder in this patient.

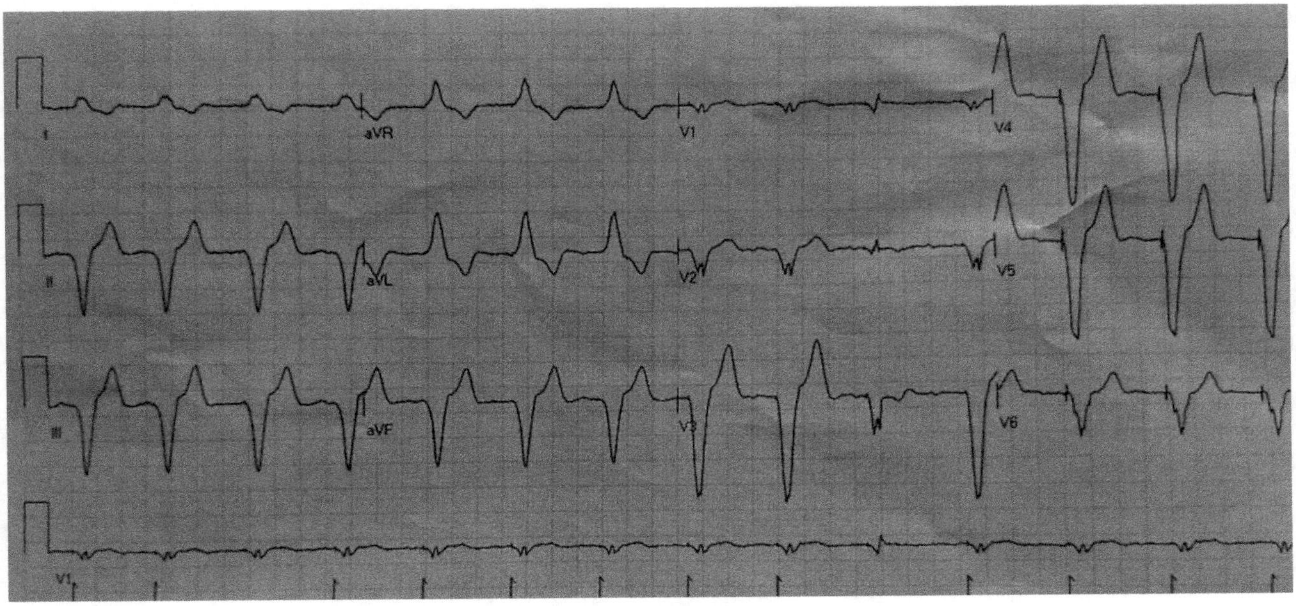

FIGURE 3: The ECG of the patient after the pPM implantation.

Several guidelines have already proposed different approaches about the management of AV conduction disorders patients; however, no real-world data are available until now in this specific setting. Hence, the ESC recommendation [2] suggested a medical drug approach with isoprenaline and atropine and the implantation of temporary PM (tPM), leading the potential pPM after recovery from the COVID-19 infection. Conversely, the Italian position paper [3] recommends avoiding in any cases the tPM for risk infection, thus preferring early pPM implantation. In this controversial field, at least three reasons could explain the approach that we chose of implanting early a pPM: first of all, the early pPM implantation has reduced the time of exposure of the potential viral contagion for the medical staff, allowing us to transfer the patient to a dedicated COVID-19 hospital where continuing the appropriate drug treatment. Secondly, the early implantation of a pPM has reduced the risk of potential hemodynamic consequences for the patient, as bradycardia and cardiogenic shock, frequently due to the AV block. Thirdly, although the consensus to prevent CIED infections recommend generally to wait for 24 hours since an afebrile patient [4], it is needful to evaluate case by case, especially in viral diseases that rarely have been associated to the CIED infection yet.

Interestingly, it is known that tPM patients are up to 2.5 times more prone to develop an infection before the pPM implantation [7], with higher mean reported complication rates [8], such as lead's dislodgement with malsensing/malpacing, pneumothorax, and cardiac perforation. Moreover, it has been documented that in survivors, the duration of COVID-19 viral shedding was in media 20 days, up to a maximum of 37 days [9]. Based on these considerations, the choice of a tPM would expose not only the patient to a higher risk of complications for such a long time but also the entire staff to a higher risk of viral contagion, not allowing the immediate transfer of the patient to the dedicated COVID-19 hospital. Furthermore, in our region, the management of COVID-19 patients in dedicated areas has been also assigned to general medical doctors [10]; thus, it would have been hard for them if the specific management of a tPM is without any previous experience.

To our knowledge, this is the first report of a COVID-19 infection patient symptomatic for AV block treated with early pPM implantation. This approach allowed us to preserve all the medical equipment and the other patients from the potential viral contagion in a no COVID-19 hospital and to obtain the best outcome for the patient, transferring her to a dedicated COVID-19 area to continue the appropriate medical treatment.

References

[1] S. Shi, M. Qin, B. Shen et al., "Association of cardiac injury with mortality in hospitalized patients with COVID-19 in Wuhan, China," *JAMA Cardiology*, vol. 5, no. 7, pp. 802–810, 2020.

[2] "2020 ESC Guidance for the diagnosis and management of CV disease during the COVID-19 pandemic," May 2020 https://www.escardio.org/Education/COVID-19-and-Cardiology/ESC-COVID-19-Guidance.

[3] M. M. Gulizia, M. Zecchin, F. Colivicchi et al., "ANMCO position paper: guidance for the management of suspected or confirmed COVID-19 patients requiring urgent electrophysiological procedures," *Giornale Italiano di Cardiologia*, vol. 5, pp. 336–340, 2020.

[4] C. Blomström-Lundqvist, V. Traykov, P. A. Erba et al., "European Heart Rhythm Association (EHRA) international consensus document on how to prevent, diagnose, and treat cardiac implantable electronic device infections," *European Heart Journal*, vol. 22, 2020.

[5] "Coronavirus disease (COVID-19) advice for the public: when and how to use masks–WHO Raccomandations 2020," https://www.who.int/emergencies/diseases/novel-coronavirus-2019/advice-for-public/when-and-how-to-use-masks.

[6] S. H. Rezkalla and R. A. Kloner, "Influenza-related viral myocarditis," *Wisconsin Medical Journal*, vol. 109, no. 4, p. 209, 2010.

[7] M. Brignole, A. Auricchio, G. Baron-Esquivias et al., "2013 ESC Guidelines on cardiac pacing and cardiac resynchronization therapy: the task force on cardiac pacing and resynchronization therapy of the European Society of Cardiology (ESC)," *European Heart Journal*, vol. 29, pp. 2281–2329, 2013.

[8] F. V. Tjong, U. W. de Ruijter, N. E. G. Beurskens, and R. E. Knops, "A comprehensive scoping review on transvenous temporary pacing therapy," *Netherlands Heart Journal*, vol. 10, pp. 462–473, 2019.

[9] F. Zhou, T. Yu, R. du et al., "Clinical course and risk factors for mortality of adult inpatients with COVID-19 in Wuhan, China: a retrospective cohort study," *Lancet*, vol. 395, no. 10229, pp. 1054–1062, 2020.

[10] C. Di Nora, G. Cioffi, A. Iorio et al., "Systolic blood pressure target in systemic arterial hypertension: is lower ever better? Results from a community-based Caucasian cohort," *European Journal of Internal Medicine*, vol. 48, pp. 57–63, 2018.

32

An Unusual Case of Left Atrial Mural Thrombus following Aortic Valve Replacement

Mohamed E. Taha[1] **Ammar Eljack**[2] **Hisham Ibrahim,**[3] **and Chanwit Roongsritong**[4]

[1]*Department of Internal Medicine, University of Nevada, Reno, NV, USA*
[2]*Department of Internal Medicine, Beaumont Health, Detroit, MI, USA*
[3]*Department of Internal Medicine, University of Iowa, IA, USA*
[4]*Department of Heart and Vascular Health, Renown Regional Medical Center, Reno, NV, USA*

Correspondence should be addressed to Mohamed E. Taha; m_tahir1985@yahoo.com

Academic Editor: Alfredo E. Rodriguez

The left atrial thrombus is a well-known complication of atrial fibrillation and rheumatic mitral valve disease and carries a high risk for systemic thromboembolism. They are generally dissolved after a certain period of optimal anticoagulation. A large thrombus, on the other hand, may persist even with adequate anticoagulation. The surgical removal of a thrombus theoretically poses some risk of systemic embolization, making its management a clinical dilemma. Furthermore, a refractory thrombus is uncommon. Thus, an evidence-based guideline in selecting the optimal therapy is needed. We report a case of a 74-year-old male with atrial fibrillation and a history of unprovoked pulmonary embolism who was incidentally found to have a massive left atrial thrombus shortly after discontinuing warfarin about 4 months following bioprosthetic aortic valve replacement. The thrombus was refractory to anticoagulation posing a clinical management dilemma. This case is interesting in terms of presentation and the approach to diagnosis and treatment.

1. Introduction

Left atrial thrombus (LAT) formation is a well-known complication of atrial fibrillation and rheumatic mitral valve disease. They carry a high risk for systemic thromboembolism; therefore, early detection and treatment should be established with a high index of suspicion [1]. The left atrial appendage is the most common location of the LAT; therefore, the appendage is usually ligated during open heart surgery. In terms of treatment, anticoagulation remains the preferred approach once LAT has been detected. We present a case of a 74-year-old male who developed a massive LAT shortly after discontinuing warfarin about 4 months following bioprosthetic aortic valve replacement. The thrombus was also refractory to anticoagulation posing a clinical management dilemma.

2. Case Description

The patient is a 74-year-old Caucasian male with a history of atrial fibrillation, CHA2DS2-VASc score of 6, unprovoked deep venous thrombosis, and pulmonary embolism on long-term warfarin, who was initially found to have aortic stenosis (AS) in 2015 during preoperative cardiovascular evaluation for surgery on his right foot. His echocardiography at the time revealed moderate aortic stenosis (peak gradient of 32 mmHg, mean gradient of 22 mmHg), an ascending aorta diameter of 3.7 cm, and a severely enlarged left atrium (left atrial volume index of 66 mL/m^2). His atrial fibrillation was controlled with propafenone and warfarin. Subsequently, his AS was followed clinically and echocardiographically every 6-12 months according to the guidelines.

By the end of 2017, he developed a worsening dyspnea on exertion and persistent atrial fibrillation along with episodes of symptomatic bradycardia (heart rate in 30-40 s) for which he underwent pacemaker implantation. His echocardiography revealed worsening aortic stenosis; the calculated valve area was 0.8 cm^2 with a peak gradient of 45 mmHg and a mean gradient of 27 mmHg. The left ventricular systolic function was mildly reduced with an ejection fraction (LVEF) of 40%.

Upon further evaluation which included transesophageal echocardiography (TEE) and dobutamine stress echocardiography (DSE), it was felt that his clinical features were consistent with a low-flow, low-gradient severe AS. He was subsequently referred for evaluation for transcatheter aortic valve replacement (TAVR).

While awaiting TAVR, his symptoms continued to progress as he developed syncopal episodes. Furthermore, as part of his pre-TAVR evaluation, he underwent CT angiography of his chest which revealed a worsening of his ascending aortic aneurysm with an aortic root diameter measuring 4.6 cm (Figure 1). A shared decision was made to let him undergo open heart surgery to repair both pathologies. By February 2018, he underwent a successful complex surgical procedure with bioprosthetic AVR (27 mm Edwards Perimount Magna pericardial valve), ascending aortic aneurysmal repair (30 mm Hemashield tube graft), mitral valve repair (36 mm Edwards flexible annuloplasty), left-sided maze procedure, and left atrial appendage excision and ligation (the LAA was ligated at its base and excised, and the stump was oversewn in 2 layers using #4-0 prolene sutures). He was placed back on warfarin and aspirin. He was discharged after an uneventful hospital course with referral to our outpatient anticoagulation clinic and cardiac rehabilitation program.

His anticoagulation was closely monitored. Four months later, however, he presented with persistent frank hematuria. A shared decision was made to stop his warfarin since it had been more than 3 months from his bioprosthetic valve replacement and more than 10 years from the onset of his lone PE. He was subsequently referred for further urological workup. Two months later, while his hematuria had resolved, it was accidentally discovered that he had a sizable left atrial thrombus upon undergoing surveillance CT chest imaging for his ascending aorta, which was further delineated using TEE (Figure 2). Subsequently, he was restarted back on warfarin with a heparin bridge, while no decision was made to pursue surgery.

He had a follow-up TEE 4 months later which showed a very little to no change in the size of the thrombus despite adequate anticoagulation. Fortunately, there has not been any thromboembolic event up to date.

3. Discussion

A refractory left atrial thrombus is a clinical dilemma because of its risk of systemic complications and a lack of an evidence-based guideline in selecting optimal therapies. LAT is often associated with atrial fibrillation or rheumatic mitral valve stenosis. They account for >45% of cardiogenic

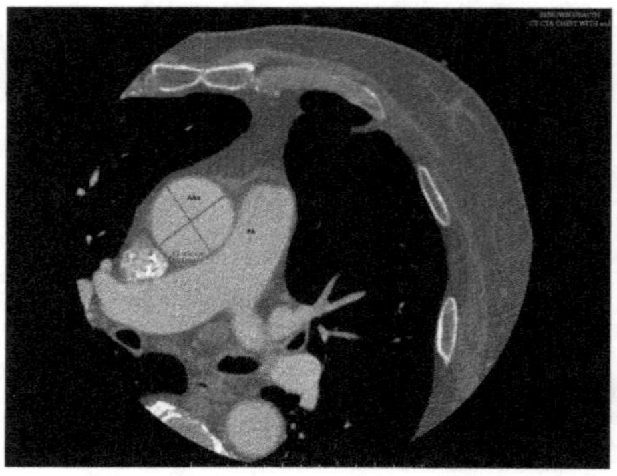

Figure 1: Computed tomography (CT) of the chest showing the enlarged ascending aorta measuring 4.6 × 4.3 cm. AAo, ascending aorta; PA, pulmonary artery.

thromboembolic events [1]. LAT often forms in the left atrial appendage (LAA) because of its shape and the presence of trabeculations. However, it can arise around the free atrial wall especially in cases of a dilated atrium. In our presented case, his left atrium was severely dilated; however, the left appendage was already excised. Based on the interrogation of his pacemaker, he had also been in sinus rhythm since the day of his pacemaker implantation.

Thrombus formation in the left atrium after LAA exclusion has been previously reported with endocardial occlusion devices (Watchman, Boston Scientific, Marlborough, Massachusetts or Amplatzer Cardiac Plug (ACP), St. Jude Medical, St. Paul, Minnesota). Its mechanism was mainly attributed to platelet aggregation in the setting of a foreign body in the left atrium [2, 3]. In the study by Lakkireddy et al., the risk for LA thrombus formation using a lariat device was discovered to be as low as 2%, mostly occurring within 90 days [4]. There are no published data regarding LA thrombus formation at postsurgical excision and ligation of the LAA as in our case.

Our patient developed a massive thrombus despite taking both warfarin and aspirin. He had a history of atrial fibrillation but was in sinus rhythm for at least 6 months before the thrombus was detected (since the maze procedure). He is 74 years old, but he has no history of hypertension or diabetes mellitus. He did have one episode of DVT and pulmonary embolism along with a severely dilated left atrium which may have partly contributed to the development of the thrombus [5].

In terms of management, various options including anticoagulation, thrombolytic treatment, endovascular intervention, and open surgery exist. Anticoagulation is generally considered as the first-line therapy. Even with the failure of medical management, there is little evidence either in favor of or against aggressive management to remove the thrombus [6]. In our patient, he was restarted on warfarin and surgical consultation was made; however, the latter was deferred.

4. Conclusion

The left atrial thrombus is a known complication of atrial fibrillation and rheumatic mitral valve disease, especially in the setting of an enlarged left atrium. If not detected and

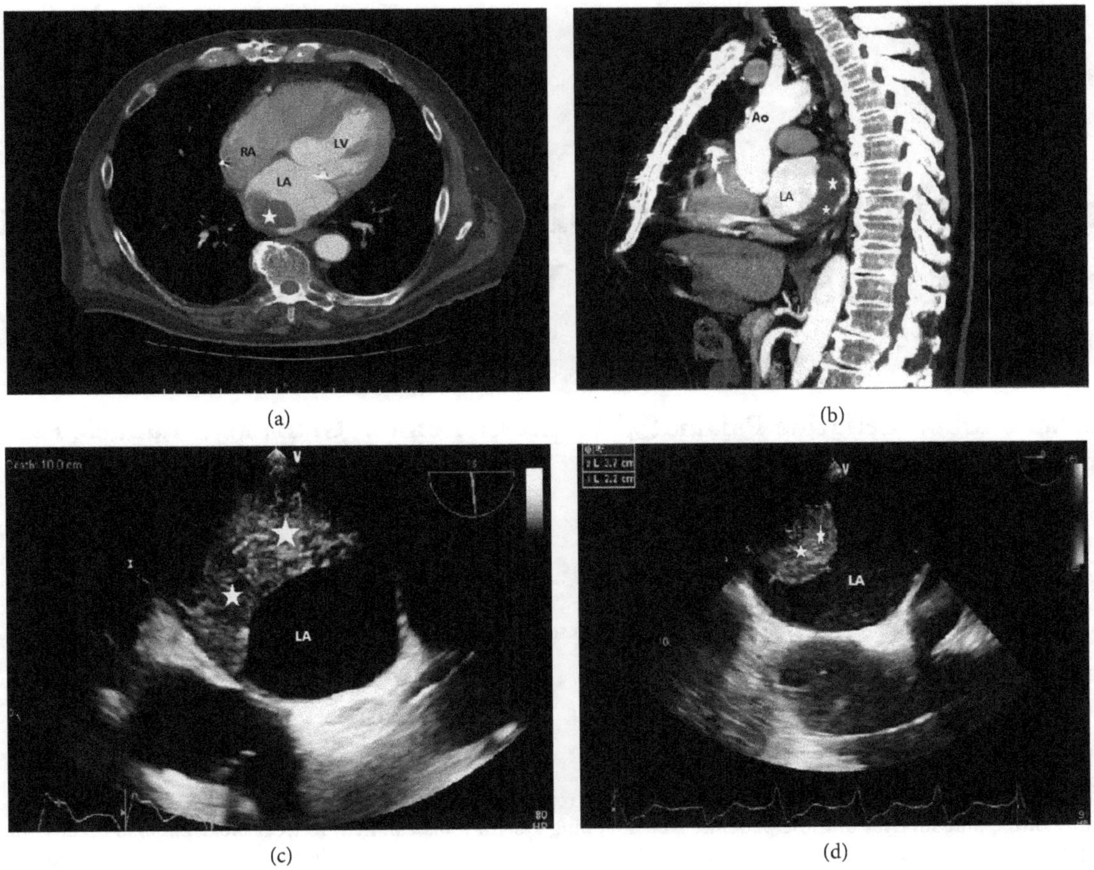

Figure 2: (a and b) Computed tomography (CT) of the chest showing a thrombus (stars) in the left atrium of the heart (LA). (c and d) Transesophageal echocardiogram (TEE) showing the thrombus in the left atrium of the heart (LA). Ao, aorta; LA, left atrium; LV, left ventricle; and RA: right atrium.

properly treated, it can lead to devastating thromboembolic complications. Anticoagulation is usually the treatment of choice which usually results in the desolation of the thrombus; however, in some cases, LAT might be refractory to anticoagulation creating a decisional dilemma as in our presented case. More cases and effort are needed to have a standardized approach to treat this category of patients.

References

[1] N. M. Al-Saady, O. A. Obel, and A. J. Camm, "Left atrial appendage: structure, function, and role in thromboembolism," *Heart*, vol. 82, no. 5, pp. 547–554, 1999.

[2] M. Gasparini, C. Ceriotti, and R. Bragato, "Huge left atrial thrombus after left atrial appendage occlusion with a Watchman device," *European Heart Journal*, vol. 33, no. 16, p. 1998, 2012.

[3] I. Cruz-Gonzalez, J. Martín Moreiras, and E. García, "Thrombus formation after left atrial appendage exclusion using an Amplatzer cardiac plug device," *Catheterization and Cardiovascular Interventions*, vol. 78, no. 6, pp. 970–973, 2011.

[4] D. Lakkireddy, A. Vallakati, A. Kanmanthareddy et al., "Left atrial thrombus formation after successful left atrial appendage ligation: case series from a nationwide survey," *Journal of the American College of Cardiology*, vol. 65, no. 15, pp. 1595-1596, 2015.

[5] A. Kristiansen, L. Brandt, T. Agoritsas et al., "Applying new strategies for the national adaptation, updating, and dissemination of trustworthy guidelines: results from the Norwegian adaptation of the Antithrombotic Therapy and the Prevention of Thrombosis, 9th Ed: American College of Chest Physicians Evidence-Based Clinical Practice Guidelines," *Chest*, vol. 146, no. 3, pp. 735–761, 2014.

[6] U. O. Egolum, D. G. Stover, D. Lenihan et al., "Intracardiac thrombus: diagnosis, complications and management," *The American Journal of the Medical Sciences*, vol. 345, no. 5, pp. 391–395, 2013.

33

Octogenarian Atrial Fibrillation Ablation with New NavX EnSite "Live View" Tool

Mariano Rillo,[1] Zefferino Palamà,[1] Francesco Zonno,[2] Giulia My,[1] Raffaele Punzi,[1] Luigi My,[1] and Luigi Sciarra[3]

[1]*Cardiology Unit "Villa Verde", Taranto, Italy*
[2]*Abbott Medical Italia, Sesto San Giovanni, Italy*
[3]*Cardiology Unit "Policlinico Casilino", Rome, Italy*

Correspondence should be addressed to Luigi Sciarra; lui.sciarra@libero.it

Academic Editor: Ertugrul Ercan

Background. Atrial Fibrillation ablation in older patients represents a challenge to be addressed to ensure the improvement of the quality of life and survival of these patients. New mapping system tools can help to treat older patients because of its ability to simplify and reduce procedural risks. The new NavX EnSite "Live view" tool allows dynamic "beat to beat" activation and voltage mapping visualization in order to instantly recognize vein disconnection and minimize RF deliveries. *Methods.* An 81-year old patient with paroxysmal AF and well-documented firing focus trigger underwent pulmonary veins isolation using NavX EnSite Precision, HD Grid multipolar catheter, and the new "Live view" tool. *Results.* All pulmonary veins were successfully isolated with no procedural complications. "Live view" tool allows to perform shorter and safer procedure (total procedural time: 90 minutes, left atrium dwell time: 60 minutes, total RF delivery number: 78). *Conclusion.* "Live view tool" allows dynamic activation and voltage mapping in order to perform a safe and tailored approach to ablation, especially in older patients.

1. Introduction

In recent years, we have witnessed a generational shift in patients undergoing atrial fibrillation (AF) ablation [1]. Therefore, AF ablation in older patients represents a challenge to be addressed to ensure the improvement of the quality of life and survival of these patients.

2. Case Presentation

We report the case of an 81-year old patient with a strongly symptomatic paroxysmal AF (mEHRA score 2b) [2], resistant to multiple drug therapy attempts, with a good functional state, and well documented to be a pulmonary vein focal firing AF ("P on T" phenomena as shown in Figure 1). The patient was highly motivated to solve his arrhythmia problem. We performed AF ablation with pulmonary veins isolation using NavX EnSite Precision, HD Grid multipolar catheter, and the new "Live view" tool that allow dynamic "beat to beat" activation and voltage mapping visualization.

As we can see in Figure 2, the new "Live view" tool allows to instantly view the presence of conductive gaps in vein isolation and their disappearance.

All pulmonary veins were successfully isolated, and no procedural complications were observed. Total procedural time was 90 minutes, left atrium dwell time was 60 minutes, and total RF delivery number was 78.

3. Discussion

A tailored ablation strategy can target specific triggers and drivers of atrial fibrillation [3]. When atrial fibrillation mechanism is well identified, as in our case, ablation procedure should not be denied only for the age factor. In fact, a successful atrial fibrillation ablation significantly and persistently improves quality of life, with a significant reduction in arrhythmia symptoms frequency and severity [4]. Key to the success of a tailored ablation strategy is an accurate identification of AF triggers and their treatment. In terms of efficacy, durable pulmonary vein isolation represents the

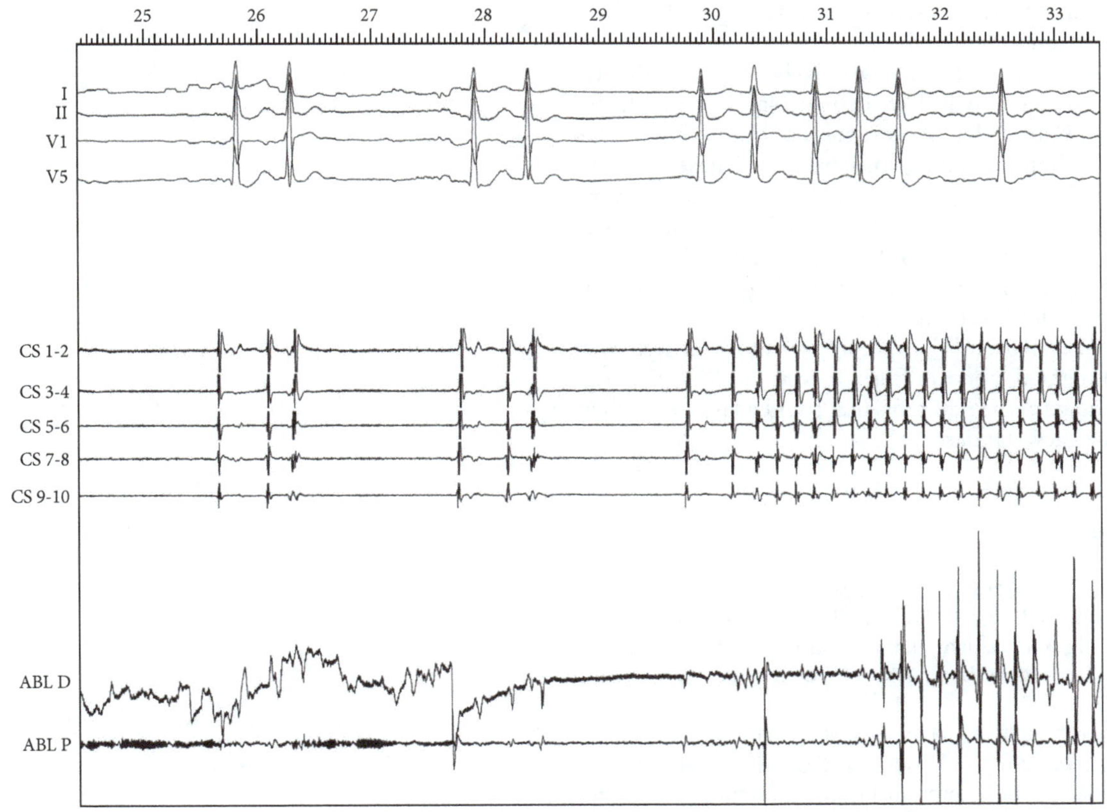

Figure 1: "P on T" phenomena as AF trigger during catheter positioning (I-II-V1-V6: ECG lead; CS: coronary sinus decapolar diagnostic catheter tracings; ABL: bipolar ablation catheter tracings).

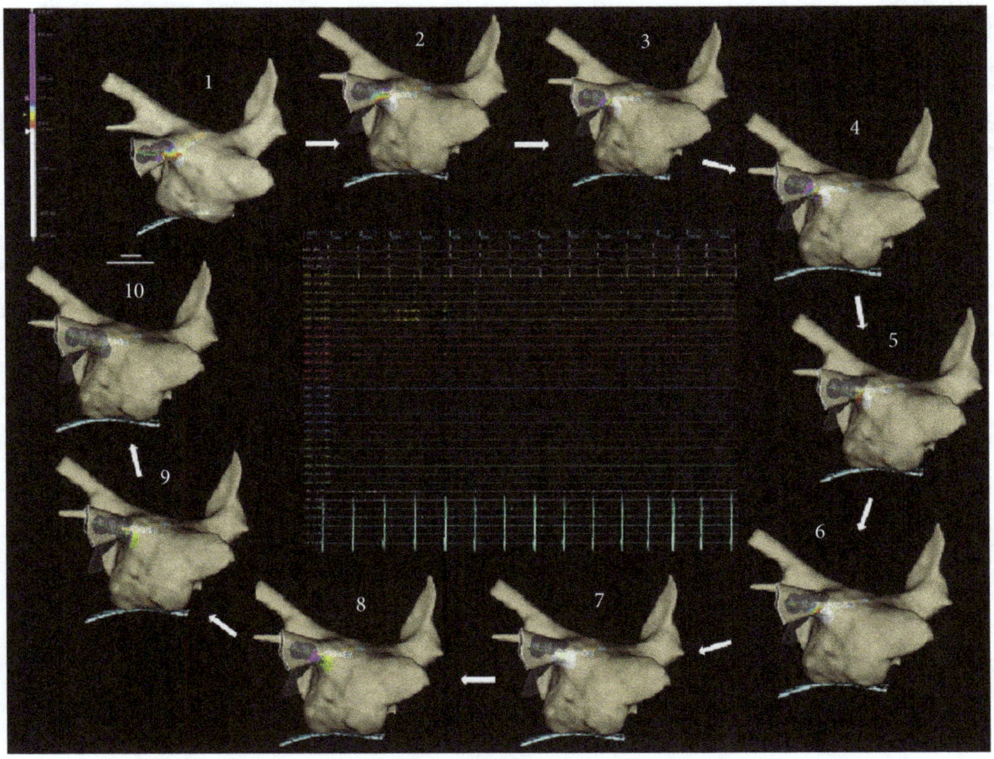

Figure 2: "Live view" tool allows to instantly view the presence of conductive gaps in vein isolation and their disappearance. Beat to beat activation map visualization (1 to 10), EGMs recordings show PV signal disappearance during ablation (HD grid in vein ostium during ablation).

cornerstone of any AF ablation procedure, especially when PV firing focus was identified.

The limits in terms of safety can also be overcome thanks to the use of the new tools, like the new NavX EnSite Precision "Live view" tool, that allow dynamic "beat to beat" activation and voltage mapping visualization. These features turn into a reduction of unnecessary radiofrequency deliveries, of left atrium dwell time, and of total procedural time. Indeed, this tool allows to instantly recognize vein disconnection during RF application, without having to redo a new voltage map to check vein deconnection.

A tailored approach [5], especially when the arrhythmia is well documented, appears feasible even in older patients, taking advantage of the new tools that could guarantee higher safety and efficacy standards.

References

[1] C. Teunissen, N. Clappers, R. J. Hassink, J. F. van der Heijden, F. H. Wittkampf, and P. Loh, "A decade of atrial fibrillation ablation: shifts in patient characteristics and procedural outcomes," *Netherlands Heart Journal*, vol. 25, no. 10, pp. 559–566, 2017.

[2] G. J. Wynn, D. M. Todd, M. Webber et al., "The European Heart Rhythm Association symptom classification for atrial fibrillation: validation and improvement through a simple modification," *Europace*, vol. 16, no. 7, pp. 965–972, 2014.

[3] H. Ghanbari and H. Oral, "Atrial fibrillation ablation strategy: "ready made" or "tailored"?," *Card Electrophysiol Clin*, vol. 4, no. 3, pp. 353–361, 2012.

[4] R. Weerasooriya, P. Jais, M. Hocini et al., "Effect of catheter ablation on quality of life of patients with paroxysmal atrial fibrillation," *Heart Rhythm*, vol. 2, no. 6, pp. 619–623, 2005.

[5] L. Sciarra, Z. Palamà, and M. Nesti, "Catheter ablation for atrial fibrillation - the tailored approach," *Biomedical Journal of Scientific & Technical Research*, vol. 18, no. 5, pp. 13928–13931, 2019.

A Unique Compensatory Mechanism for Total Pulmonary Vein Occlusion Post Atrial Fibrillation Catheter Ablation Visualized by Multimodality Imaging

Ayman R. Fath,[1] Amro Aglan,[2] Luis R. Scott,[1] Clinton E. Jokerst,[3] Hemalatha Narayanasamy,[1] Farouk Mookadam,[1] Nawfal Mihyawi,[4] Nithin R. Venepally,[1] Sudheer Konduru,[1] and Reza Arsanjani[1]

[1]*Department of Cardiovascular Diseases, Mayo Clinic Arizona, USA*
[2]*Beth Israel Deaconess Medical Center, Harvard Medical School, Boston, MA, USA*
[3]*Department of Radiology, Mayo Clinic Arizona, USA*
[4]*Department of Internal Medicine, Creighton University Arizona Health Alliance, USA*

Correspondence should be addressed to Reza Arsanjani; arsanjani.reza@mayo.edu

Academic Editor: Panagiotis Korantzopoulos

Pulmonary vein (PV) stenosis is a rare and serious complication of radiofrequency catheter ablation (RFCA) for atrial fibrillation. However, it can be asymptomatic or mildly symptomatic depending on the severity of the stenosis and the development of compensatory mechanisms. This study provides a detailed description and visualization of a unique type of venous collaterals that bypass the PV stenosis and drain directly in the left atrium alleviating PV stenosis sequelae. This study reports a case of a 61-year-old male who presented with mild dyspnea and fatigue 3 years post atrial fibrillation RFCA. After a thorough evaluation of the case, a redo-ablation was planned. As a part of the preablation workup, a transesophageal echocardiography (TEE), a ventilation-perfusion (V/Q) scan of the lungs, and a chest computed tomography angiogram (CTA) were performed. The TEE revealed total obstruction of the left superior PV, with no color Doppler flow detected. It also showed evidence of multiple collateral flows at the os of the left superior PV. The V/Q scan showed a large perfusion defect involving the entire left upper lobe consistent with a compromised left upper PV flow. The CTA with 3D volume rendering revealed the total occlusion of the left superior PV at its ostium. Moreover, the scan confirmed the pulmonary venous drainage via small collateral channels that was suggested by the TEE.

1. Introduction

Atrial fibrillation (AF) is the commonest atrial arrhythmia resulting from one or multiple wavelets propagating in different directions [1]. Pulmonary veins (PVs) and PV ostia are the primary foci of these wavelets that trigger AF [1]. Radiofrequency catheter ablation (RFCA) with pulmonary vein isolation is recommended for eligible patients with symptomatic atrial fibrillation [1, 2]. Severe PV stenosis is a rare complication of RFCA with PV isolation (~1%), and the incidence of symptomatic severe PV stenosis requiring treatment is even less common [3]. Symptomatic total PV occlusion may develop over years and has been reported in the literature. We present a case of total PV occlusion following RFCA that remained mildly symptomatic due to partial compensation from collateral circulation formation which bypassed the occluded segment of PV. The collateral circulation flows were identified with transesophageal echocardiography (TEE) and confirmed with chest computed tomography angiogram (CTA).

2. Case Report

A 61-year-old gentleman presented with mild dyspnea and fatigue. He was noted to be in AF on pacemaker interrogation and ECG. His history was significant for paroxysmal AF

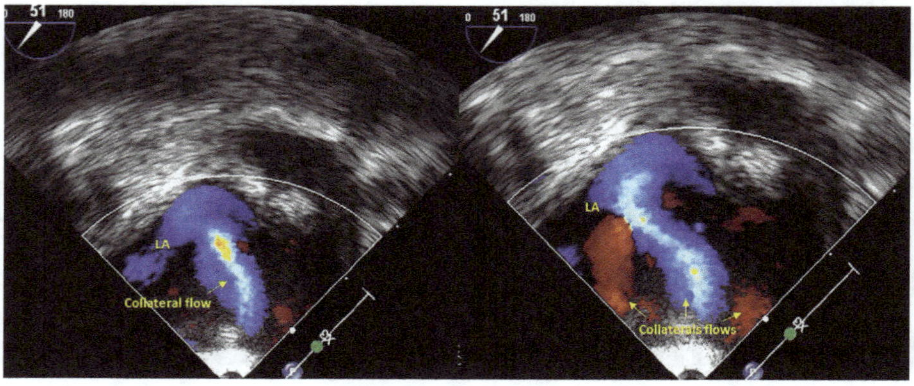

FIGURE 1: TEE shows multiple collateral flows at the os of the left superior PV with peak velocity of the predominant flow of 45 cm/s.

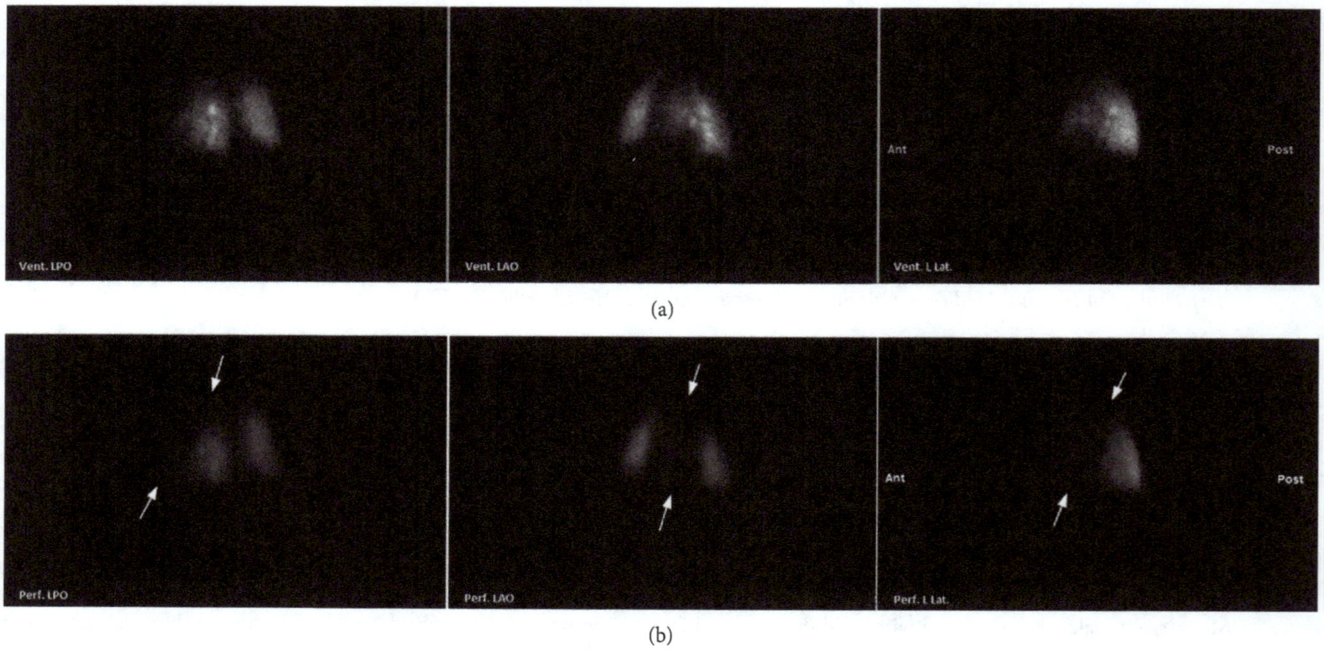

FIGURE 2: Lung V/Q scan showing absent perfusion of the left upper pulmonary lobe and lingula (arrows) based on the comparison of the relatively (a) normal ventilation to the (b) abnormal perfusion in the left posterior oblique (LPO), left anterior oblique (LAO), and left lateral (L lat.) projections.

diagnosed three years prior when he was admitted to the hospital with embolic stroke. The AF was initially managed with a rate-lowering calcium channel blocker and flecainide coupled with a direct oral anticoagulant. Despite optimized medical therapy, he continued to be symptomatic; therefore, he underwent antral RFCA two months later. The ablation consisted of PV isolation using radiofrequency catheter ablation. Complete isolation with entrance and exit block of the left side PV was achieved. Due to the rise in esophageal temperature during radiofrequency application, the right-sided veins were not completely isolated. Complex fractionated atrial electrogram ablations were targeted for ablation in both the left and right atria, as well as the ostium of the coronary sinus. The patient had postablation prolonged sinus pause that required dual-chamber pacemaker implantation. At presentation, his device interrogation revealed an AF burden of 60% with several periods of rapid ventricular response. In light of the ongoing symptoms, a redo-ablation was planned. The patient has no pertinent past medical, social, or family history. Physical examination showed irregular heart rhythm but was otherwise unremarkable.

As a part of the preablation workup, a TEE, a ventilation-perfusion (V/Q) scan, and a chest CTA were performed. The TEE revealed total obstruction of the left superior PV, with no color Doppler flow detected. It also interestingly showed evidence of multiple collateral flows at the os of the left superior PV with a peak velocity of the predominant flow of 45 cm/s (Figure 1).

The V/Q scan of the lungs showed a large mismatched perfusion defect involving the entire left upper lobe and lingula and relatively decreased but preserved ventilation in the left upper lung, consistent with a compromised left upper PV flow (Figure 2).

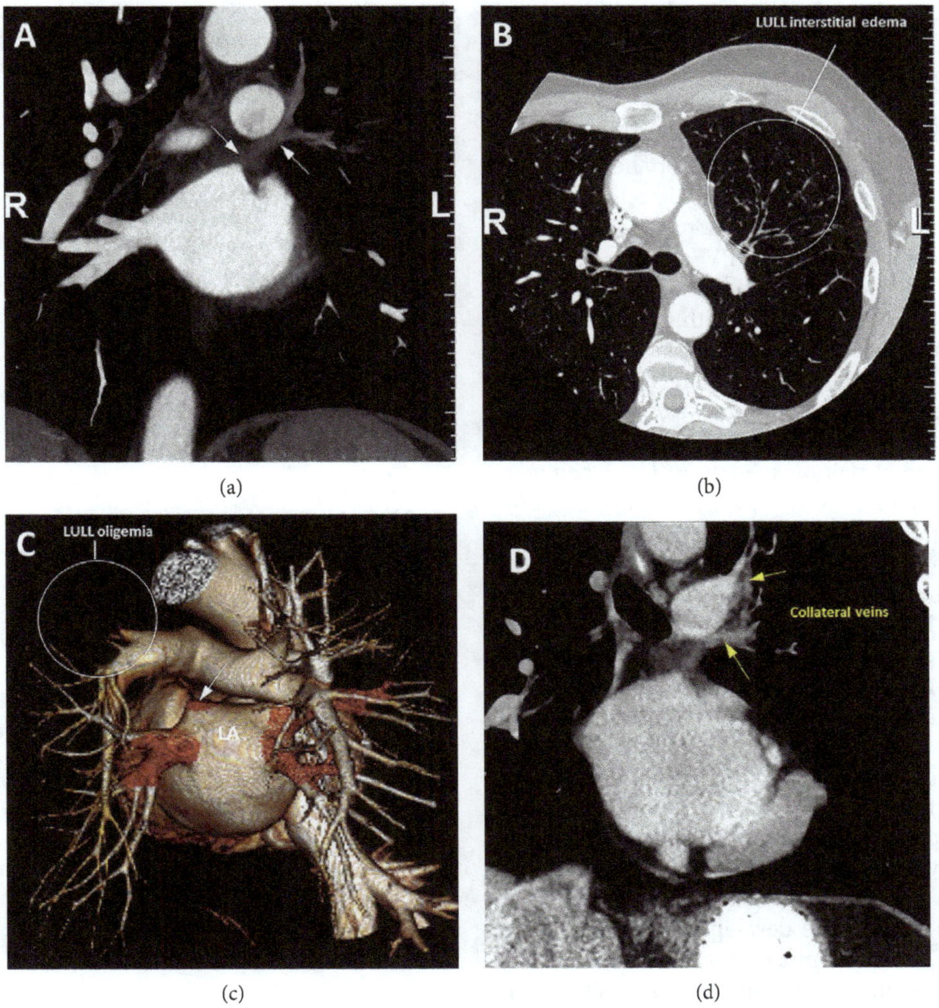

Figure 3: Coronal oblique view (a), axial view (b), and volume-rendered 3D reconstruction (c) from an arterial phase CT angiogram demonstrate absence or stump of the left superior pulmonary vein (white arrows) and left upper lobe oligemia ((c), circled) and chronic interstitial edema ((b), circled). Coronal oblique vascular reconstruction from a delayed venous phase CT angiogram (d) demonstrates small collateral draining veins (yellow arrows). LULL = left upper lung lobe.

The CTA of the chest with 3D volume rendering showed the total occlusion of the left superior PV at its ostium and confirmed residual pulmonary venous drainage via small collateral channels. It also showed chronic interstitial edema, fibrosis, and oligemia within the left upper lobe. The remainder of the lungs appeared clear (Figure 3).

3. Discussion

Treatment of AF includes pharmacologic therapy with rate control, rhythm control, and/or invasive therapy with catheter ablation. Cryoablation and RFCA are approved treatment modalities for patients with symptomatic paroxysmal or persistent AF refractory or intolerant to medical treatment [2, 4]. Most of the ectopic beats in AF arise from PVs and PV ostia; therefore, PV isolation is the main focus of ablation procedures [1, 4]. Pulmonary vein stenosis is the most frequently reported long-term complication post-RFCA. The mechanism of such is likely due to endocardial injury causing scar and cicatrization with intimal hyperplasia and fibrosis associated with the healing process [5]. However, its incidence has been getting lower over time due to increased awareness and improvement in ablation techniques [3].

Symptoms of PV stenosis depend on the ipsilateral lung perfusion reflecting the ability to develop compensatory mechanisms [6]. These compensatory mechanisms include alteration of pulmonary hemodynamics and redistribution of blood flow with neovascularization of the ipsilateral lung. This makes the venous drainage of the affected area mostly dependent on the ipsilateral veins draining the healthy lobes [6]. Di Biase et al. [6] completed a physiologic evaluation with V/Q scanning of 18 patients with PV occlusion among 1780 patients who underwent AF ablation from 1999 to 2004. The study showed that all patients with severe symptoms had relative perfusion $< 25\%$ of the ipsilateral lung, whereas all asymptomatic patients and those with mild symptoms were above this value. Our case supports this study findings; the patient was mildly symptomatic with relative perfusion of 50% of the ipsilateral lung, which was likely due to compensatory changes as described above. Furthermore, our patient has developed additional compensatory collateral veins bypassing the occluded PV and draining directly in the left atrium. These collateral veins are believed to contribute to more symptom relief.

Yun et al. [7] discussed the spontaneous improvement in most cases of PV stenosis due to compensatory hemodynamics. They reported hemodynamic changes detected by time-resolved contrast-enhanced magnetic resonance angiography (TR-MRA) in a patient with right PV stenosis following RFCA of AF. TR-MRA demonstrated prominent systemic arteries in the right thorax connected with the right pulmonary artery, suggesting pulmonary to systemic arterial collaterals. In addition, on a velocity-encoded cine image, the flow direction of the right pulmonary artery was reversed in the diastolic phase resulting in drainage of oxygen-rich blood back to the contralateral pulmonary artery. These hemodynamic changes were similar to those seen in congenital unilateral PV atresia [8]. Our study shows a different type of collateral flow that developed on the venous side, detected by TEE and confirmed with CTA.

In conclusion, PV stenosis is a serious complication of RFCA. Its incidence has been reported to range from 3% to 42% depending on the technique used and assessment method [9]. It is associated with significant morbidity and complications that may require revascularization or even partial lobectomy. Diagnosis of PVS can be challenging due to its nonspecific symptoms; therefore, it requires a low index of suspicion. The spectrum of symptoms can vary from persistent cough to severe dyspnea and significant hemoptysis. Nonetheless, some patients may remain asymptomatic or mildly symptomatic due to the development of compensatory mechanisms. Different compensatory mechanisms have been well documented in the literature including alterations of pulmonary hemodynamics and redistribution of blood flow. In our case report, we demonstrate another compensatory drainage mechanism via collateral veins connected directly to the left atrium. We also illustrate the utility of a detailed TEE and CTA with 3D volume rendering in identifying these collateral veins.

Supplementary Materials

The following supplementary material is available online. Movie Clips: Video 1: TEE shows total obstruction of the left superior pulmonary vein (LSPV), with no color Doppler flow detected. It also shows collateral flow at the os of the LSVP (yellow arrow). *(Supplementary Materials)*

References

[1] M. Haïssaguerre, P. Jaïs, D. C. Shah et al., "Spontaneous initiation of atrial fibrillation by ectopic beats originating in the pulmonary veins," *The New England Journal of Medicine*, vol. 339, no. 10, pp. 659–666, 1998.

[2] C. T. January, L. S. Wann, J. S. Alpert et al., "2014 AHA/ACC/HRS guideline for the management of patients with atrial fibrillation: executive summary," *Circulation*, vol. 130, no. 23, pp. 2071–2104, 2014.

[3] C. Teunissen, B. K. Velthuis, R. J. Hassink et al., "Incidence of pulmonary vein stenosis after radiofrequency catheter ablation of atrial fibrillation," *JACC. Clinical electrophysiology*, vol. 3, no. 6, pp. 589–598, 2017.

[4] H. Calkins, G. Hindricks, R. Cappato et al., "2017 HRS/EHRA/ECAS/APHRS/SOLAECE expert consensus statement on catheter and surgical ablation of atrial fibrillation," *Heart Rhythm*, vol. 14, no. 10, pp. e275–e444, 2017.

[5] G. W. Taylor, G. N. Kay, X. Zheng, S. Bishop, and R. E. Ideker, "Pathological effects of extensive radiofrequency energy applications in the pulmonary veins in dogs," *Circulation*, vol. 101, no. 14, pp. 1736–1742, 2000.

[6] L. Di Biase, T. S. Fahmy, O. M. Wazni et al., "Pulmonary vein total occlusion following catheter ablation for atrial fibrillation," *Journal of the American College of Cardiology*, vol. 48, no. 12, pp. 2493–2499, 2006.

[7] D. Yun, J. I. Jung, Y. S. Oh, and H. J. Youn, "Hemodynamic change in pulmonary vein stenosis after radiofrequency ablation: assessment with magnetic resonance angiography," *Korean Journal of Radiology*, vol. 13, no. 6, pp. 816–819, 2012.

[8] K. S. Roman, C. J. Kellenberger, C. K. Macgowan et al., "How is pulmonary arterial blood flow affected by pulmonary venous obstruction in children? A phase-contrast magnetic resonance study," *Pediatric Radiology*, vol. 35, no. 6, pp. 580–586, 2005.

[9] E. B. Saad, N. F. Marrouche, C. P. Saad et al., "Pulmonary vein stenosis after catheter ablation of atrial fibrillation: emergence of a new clinical syndrome," *Annals of Internal Medicine*, vol. 138, no. 8, pp. 634–638, 2003.

35

Not your Common Athletic Heart Problem: Using Coronary CTA to Visualize Spontaneous Coronary Artery Dissection

Padma Shenoy, Taher Tayeb, Pedro Covas, Nardos Temesgen, and Cynthia Tracy

The George Washington University Hospital, Washington, DC, USA

Correspondence should be addressed to Padma Shenoy; pshenoy@gwu.edu

Academic Editor: Assad Movahed

A 19-year-old healthy male collegiate athlete presented with typical anginal symptoms after running a 5K race. He had complained of similar symptoms off and on for the past month. On presentation, troponin was 0.12 ng/ml (reference value < 0.01 ng/ml), which peaked at 17.7 ng/ml and CK-MB was 28.71 IU/L (reference value < 25 IU/L). ECG showed diffuse biphasic T-waves. Coronary computed tomography angiogram (cCTA) demonstrated a 1.5 cm dissection in the left anterior descending artery and a 1.9 × 1.8 cm attenuation defect in the left ventricular apex consistent with thrombus. Subsequent coronary catheterization confirmed dissection of the left anterior descending artery. Spontaneous coronary artery dissection (SCAD) is a rare phenomenon. Diagnosis can be made through noninvasive measures but is usually done through left heart catheterization. In young patients who present with an NSTEMI, clinical suspicion for SCAD among other conditions should be raised. Additionally, recognizing that complications such as intracardiac thrombi can occur in SCAD is critical in ensuring appropriate therapy.

1. Background

SCAD is a rare, nonatherosclerotic condition known to affect predominantly women with a mean age of 42-53 years [1, 2]. It can cause acute coronary syndrome in patients who do not have typical risk factors such as hypertension, hyperlipidemia, diabetes mellitus, or tobacco use. Risk factors for SCAD include female sex, pregnancy, connective tissue disorders, fibromuscular dysplasia, physical exertion, and cocaine abuse. In some cases, cannabis use has been associated with coronary artery dissection [3]. Additionally, complications from SCAD including left ventricular thrombus have been documented [4].

In this case, the patient is a young active male who may have had a cannabis use history prior to his coronary artery dissection. It is important to include SCAD in the differential diagnosis for otherwise healthy, young, and/or male patients, especially in the setting of suspected or documented cannabis use. Patients should be evaluated for additional complications in all cases of SCAD such as mural thrombi, so that adequate therapy can be provided.

2. Case Presentation

A 19-year-old male collegiate athlete with no chronic illnesses presented to the Emergency Department with typical anginal symptoms after running a 5K race. He had chest tightness and sharp pain localized to his center and left chest. Associated symptoms included mild back pain and left arm tingling. He had similar symptoms for the month prior to presentation, which he would experience 15-20 minutes following a strenuous workout and lasting up to 2 hours. He presented to the hospital after his race because his pain was persistent and unremitting through the day.

His family history includes hypertension and type 2 diabetes mellitus in his parents. The patient denied history of tobacco, alcohol, or illicit drug use including cannabis and cocaine.

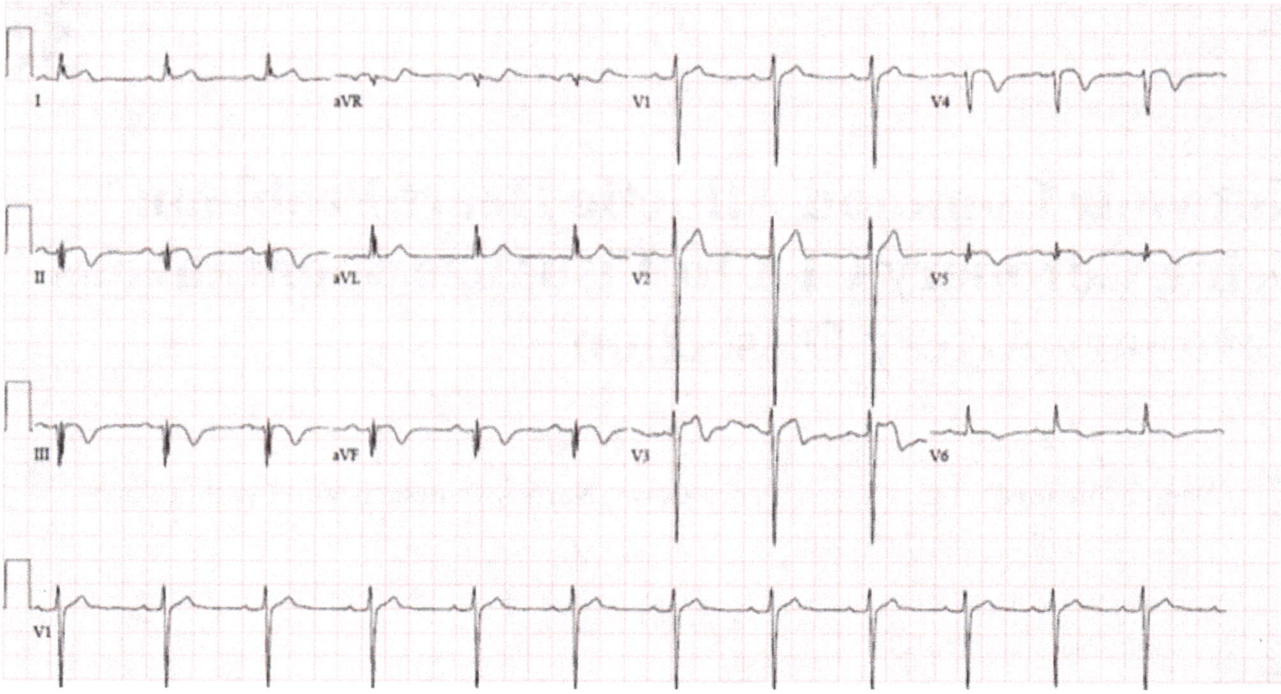

Figure 1: 12-lead ECG showing ischemic changes.

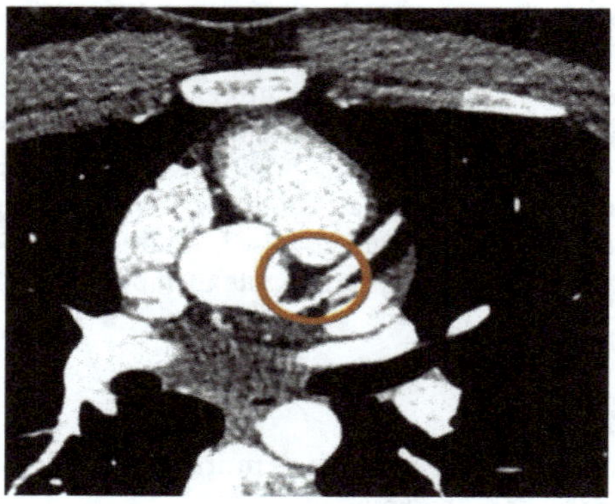

Figure 2: cCTA showing focal dissection in proximal LAD.

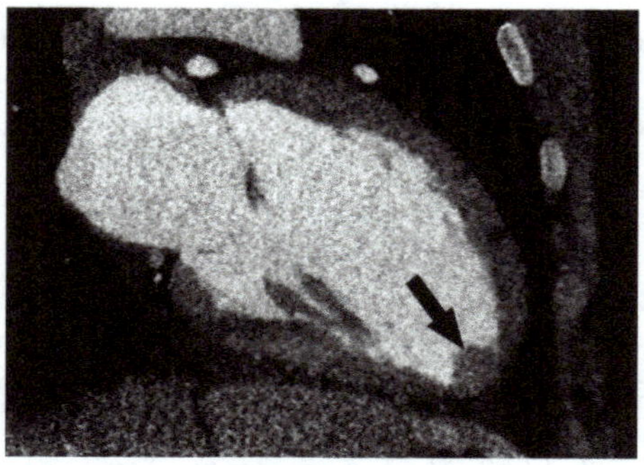

Figure 3: cCTA showing left ventricular apical thrombus.

On arrival to the hospital, vital signs were stable with blood pressure 143/87 mmHg and heart rate of 81 beats per minute. Physical exam was unremarkable. The patient's ECG showed diffuse ST-segment changes and T-wave inversions. Troponin was 0.12 ng/ml on presentation and peaked at 17.7 ng/ml. CK-MB was 28.1 IU/L.

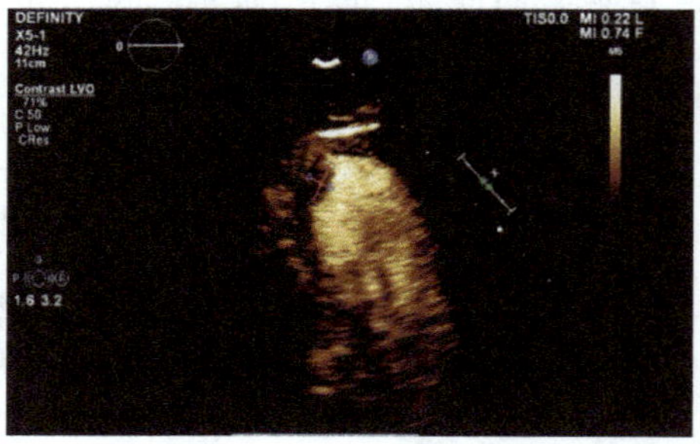

Figure 4: Transthoracic echocardiogram with left ventricular thrombus.

The patient was given aspirin, morphine, and metoprolol and admitted for workup and treatment of NSTEMI.

3. Investigation

The patient had no known conditions prior to presentation, and there had been no pre-existing workup. As mentioned above, the patient had elevated troponin levels and CK-MB on presentation. ECG showed diffuse ST changes and T-wave inversions (Figure 1).

In addition to cardiac enzymes, laboratory tests were significant for elevated C-reactive protein (CRP) of 17.4 mg/L (reference value < 3 mg/L) and urine toxicology positive for cannabinoids and opiates. Of note, patient had been administered morphine in the hospital but did not admit to cannabis use on history.

Lipid panel was grossly unremarkable with a total cholesterol of 145 mg/dL (reference value < 200 mg/dL).

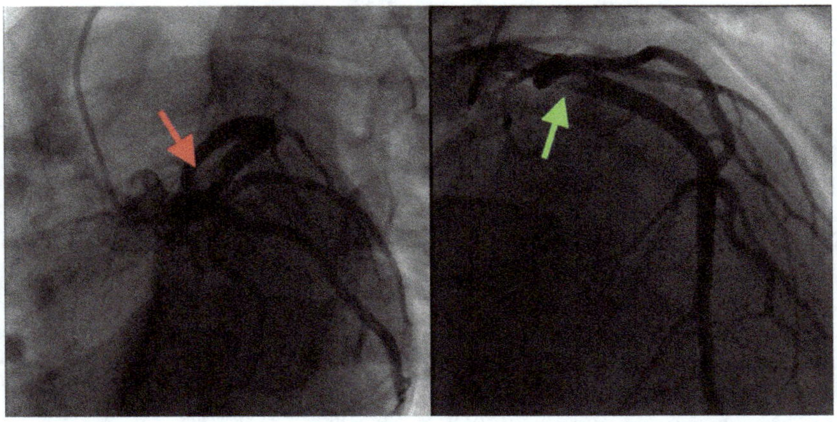

FIGURE 5: LAO caudal (red arrow) and RAO (green arrow) catheterization views of intramural filling defect of LAD.

Hemoglobin A1c was within normal range at 5.1%. Thyroid function tests were within the normal range. Viral panel was undetectable and HIV screening was negative. Screening for connective tissue disorders with ANA and rheumatoid factor was negative.

Coronary CTA showed a 1.5 cm linear low-density defect in the proximal left anterior descending (LAD) artery representing a focal dissection with intramural hematoma versus adherent thrombus (Figure 2). A 1.9 × 1.8 cm thrombus was seen in the left ventricular apex (Figure 3). There was no evidence of coronary atherosclerosis.

Transthoracic echocardiogram showed akinesis of apical septal, anterior, and inferior wall segments, consistent with the proximal LAD lesion. Coronary arteries were otherwise normal and without tortuosity, with an ejection fraction of 45-50%. There was a mildly decreased left ventricular systolic function with a mildly dilated left ventricle. The left ventricular thrombus was visualized and measured 1.4 × 0.7 cm (Figure 4).

Carotid ultrasound was negative for stenosis and evidence of fibromuscular dysplasia.

Cardiac catheterization showed a "large caliber LAD with intraluminal filling defect in the proximal segment with residual 50% lumen. Brisk antegrade flow noted distally. There is also evidence of linear filling defect noted near the LV apex" (Figure 5).

4. Treatment

After imaging demonstrated an LV mural thrombus, the patient was started on a therapeutic heparin drip and subsequently transitioned to enoxaparin bridge to coumadin. For cardiomyopathy, he was treated with metoprolol, high-intensity statin, and aspirin. Troponin level trended down, and the patient was discharged with enoxaparin/coumadin, metoprolol, atorvastatin, and aspirin, as well as referral for cardiac rehabilitation and close outpatient follow-up with cardiology.

5. Outcome and Follow-Up

The patient was discharged 2 days after admission with no additional episodes of chest pain and reported feeling well. He was scheduled for regular cardiology follow-up, INR monitoring, and repeat cCTA after discharge.

An outpatient abdominal CTA showed no high-grade renal artery stenosis or evidence of fibromuscular dysplasia.

At his follow-up appointment with cardiology two days after discharge, lisinopril was added to the patient's regimen for treatment of cardiomyopathy. ECG showed Q waves in inferior leads and T-wave inversions in anterolateral leads.

His INR was monitored twice weekly until the patient was in therapeutic range of 2-3, at which point he discontinued enoxaparin.

Repeat cCTA 12 days after NSTEMI showed near-complete resolution of the previously seen low-density focal dissection with intramural hematoma of the proximal LAD. The narrowing of the LAD had completely resolved, and no new defects were seen in the LAD. The LV mural thrombus had decreased in size, measuring 0.5 × 0.6 cm.

At the patient's two-month follow-up with cardiology, ECG showed less pronounced T-wave inversions in anterolateral leads. Echocardiogram showed mild apical wall motion abnormality attributed to the recent infarct and no thrombus was seen. He had not experienced chest pain. Lisinopril and atorvastatin were discontinued, and metoprolol dose was decreased.

Three months post-MI, a cardiac MRI showed "apical aneurysm with apical and apical inferior dyskinesis. The LV function is mildly reduced with a calculated LVEF of 49%," and coumadin therapy was discontinued.

6. Discussion

Coronary angiography remains the cornerstone in diagnosis of SCAD. With or without the aid of invasive imaging, the role of cCTA in diagnosis of SCAD has not been fully established. We report a case where cCTA aided in the diagnosing of SCAD in a patient presenting with typical ACS symptoms.

SCAD is a disease in which there is separation of the tunica intima and tunica media of the vessel wall which creates a false lumen leading to infarction. SCAD is a rare cause of ACS with an incidence in the general population of 0.1-0.4% [5, 6]. The first reported case was in a postmortem autopsy of a 43-year-old female. SCAD accounts for almost 25% of cases of infarction in women younger than the age

40 years and many cases go undiagnosed until autopsy [6–8]. Risk factors include physical and emotional stressors, pregnancy, fibromuscular dysplasia, and connective tissue disease [9–11].

Coronary angiography remains the gold standard in diagnosing SCAD with or without invasive imaging [12, 13]. Catheterization is associated with less desirable outcome in some cases with SCAD, most likely due to worsening of the dissection and difficulty accessing the lesion [5]. Currently, medical management is preferred [10, 14] unless the dissection is associated with the left main artery, continues to infarct, or causes hemodynamic instability [12, 15]. This encourages the use of noninvasive diagnostic modalities such as cCTA in stable patient to prevent risks associated with PCI such as bleeding, hematoma, and intracardiac injury. Additionally, it has been suggested that there is no difference in long-term outcomes between conservative therapy and PCI in patients with non-high-risk anatomy [16]. High-risk anatomy is defined as dissection in the left main artery or the development of dissection in two vessels.

Another consideration in this case was the use of anticoagulation for treatment of LV mural thrombus with concomitant coronary dissection. Risks of anticoagulation in this setting were extension of the LAD dissection and size of intramural hematoma; however, the benefit of preventing embolism of the thrombus causing a potentially devastating CVA in a young patient was considered as well. The patient was discharged with anticoagulation and antihypertensives with close follow-up to monitor the dissection flap and LV thrombus.

We present a case in which cCTA accurately diagnosed SCAD and LV thrombus, which was then confirmed by coronary angiogram and repeat cCTA showed resolution of thrombus and healing dissection. Given the uncommon incidence of SCAD, there are no studies done that show cCTA can be reliably used for diagnosing coronary dissection, but these would be of utility for diagnosis.

Additional Points

Learning Points/Take Home Messages. (1) Current indication for stent placement in a case diagnosed with SCAD, which are left main disease, unstable patient, or ongoing infarct. (2) The role of cCTA as a potential diagnostic tool. (3) Recognizing SCAD as a case of ACS especially in a population below the age of 50.

Disclosure

The above abstract and corresponding poster were presented at the 2020 Annual Meeting of the Society of General Internal Medicine.

References

[1] C. Krittanawong, A. Kumar, H. U. H. Virk, B. Yue, Z. Wang, and D. L. Bhatt, "Trends in incidence, characteristics, and in-hospital outcomes of patients presenting with spontaneous coronary artery dissection (from a National Population-Based Cohort Study between 2004 and 2015)," *The American Journal of Cardiology*, vol. 122, no. 10, pp. 1617–1623, 2018.

[2] T. Filali, D. Lahidheb, M. Gommidh et al., "Spontaneous multivessel coronary artery dissection associated with cannabis use," *Journal of Cardiology Cases*, vol. 7, no. 1, pp. e4–e7, 2013.

[3] J. H. Joo, A. E. Caldera, and V. G. Divakaran, "Spontaneous coronary artery dissection with left ventricular thrombus," *Proceedings (Baylor University Medical Center)*, vol. 32, no. 1, pp. 99-100, 2019.

[4] H. Gunes, Z. Kucukdurmaz, E. Seker, R. Kurt, I. Salk, and H. Karapınar, "Spontaneous coronary artery dissection diagnosed by multislice computed tomography," *Postepy w Kardiologii Interwencyjnej*, vol. 1, no. 1, pp. 111–113, 2013.

[5] T. Waterbury, M. Tweet, S. Hayes et al., "Early natural history of spontaneous coronary artery dissection | circulation: cardiovascular interventions," 2020, http://Ahajournals.org.

[6] B. J. S. Branco, C. Sanchez, C. Mendoza, M. Magarakis, A. E. Macias, and T. A. Salerno, "Challenges in diagnosis and management of spontaneous coronary artery dissection in a young patient," *Brazilian Journal of Cardiovascular Surgery*, vol. 34, no. 6, pp. 779–782, 2020.

[7] S. Thumma, J. Bathina, S. Madiraju, D. Spodick, and P. Maddukuri, "An unusual case presentation of spontaneous coronary artery dissection," *World Journal of Cardiovascular Diseases*, vol. 2, no. 4, pp. 313–315, 2012.

[8] J. Saw, A. Starovoytov, J. Mancini, and C. E. Buller, "Non-atherosclerotic coronary artery disease in young women," *Journal of the American College of Cardiology*, vol. 58, p. B113, 2011.

[9] E. Verlaeckt, L. Van de Bruaene, M. Coeman, and S. Gevaert, "Spontaneous coronary artery dissection in a patient with hereditary polycystic kidney disease and a recent liver transplant: a case report," *European Heart Journal*, vol. 3, no. 4, pp. 1–5, 2019.

[10] S. N. Hayes, E. S. H. Kim, J. Saw et al., "Spontaneous coronary artery dissection: current state of the science: a scientific statement from the American Heart Association," *Circulation*, vol. 137, no. 19, pp. e523–e557, 2018.

[11] J. Saw, R. Poulter, A. Fung, D. Wood, J. Hamburger, and C. E. Buller, "Spontaneous coronary artery dissection in patients with fibromuscular dysplasia: a case series," *Circulation Cardiovascular Interventions*, vol. 5, no. 1, pp. 134–137, 2012.

[12] H. Sharma, V. Vetrugno, and S. Q. Khan, "Successful treatment of a spontaneous right coronary artery dissection with a 4-mm diameter cutting balloon: a case report," *European Heart Journal - Case Reports*, vol. 3, no. 4, pp. 1–6, 2019.

[13] D. Adlam, F. Alfonso, and A. Maas, "European Society of Cardiology, acute cardiovascular care association, SCAD study group: a position paper on spontaneous coronary artery dissection," *European Heart Journal*, vol. 39, no. 36, pp. 3353–3368, 2018.

[14] M. S. Tweet, M. F. Eleid, P. J. M. Best et al., "Spontaneous coronary artery dissection: revascularization versus conservative

therapy," *Circulation Cardiovascular Interventions*, vol. 7, no. 6, pp. 777–786, 2014.

[15] K. Matsushita, J. Ristorto, O. Morel, and P. Ohlmann, "Progression of left anterior descending artery dissection due to stent implantation for spontaneous coronary artery dissection of left circumflex artery: a case report," *European Heart Journal - Case Reports*, vol. 3, no. 4, pp. 1–6, 2019.

[16] A. Jamil, F. Z. Tajrishi, F. Kahe et al., "Spontaneous coronary artery dissection managed with a conservative or revascularization approach," *Journal of Cardiovascular Medicine (Hagerstown, Md.)*, vol. 21, no. 1, pp. 42–50, 2020.

36

STEMI after Dobutamine Stress Echocardiography in Hyperthyroid State

Mahmood Mubasher, Ashfaq Patel, Mohamed Magdi, and Tahir Hamid

Hamad Medical Corporation, Qatar

Correspondence should be addressed to Mahmood Mubasher; dr.mahmood357@gmail.com

Academic Editor: Antonio de Padua Mansur

Uncontrolled hyperthyroidism has been associated with significant changes in cardiovascular hemodynamics. We report a case of a 39-year-old male who has been recently diagnosed with severe hyperthyroidism. He was undergoing dobutamine stress echocardiography (DSE) for evaluation of symptoms suggestive of stable angina. The exam was complicated by ST-segment elevation myocardial infarction- (STEMI-) required coronary angiography that showed mild coronary artery disease.

1. Introduction

It is known that hyperthyroidism alters the hemodynamics of the cardiovascular system through increasing the oxygen demand [1]. Dobutamine stress echocardiography (DSE) is an effective and safe test to detect coronary artery disease (CAD) with low risk of adverse events [2–4]. STEMI was reported in patients undergoing DSE in about 0.1% of cases; most of them had underlying significant coronary arteries [5, 6]. We detail a case of a 39-year-old male who recently had severe hyperthyroidism. He developed chest pain, significant ST elevation, and raised cardiac enzymes following DSE for angina-type chest pain. Coronary angiography showed CAD with mild luminal stenosis.

2. Case

A 39-year-old Asian male, with a recent diagnosis of severe hyperthyroidism and family history of coronary artery disease but no other cardiovascular risk factors, presented with intermittent angina-type chest pain of 8-month duration. He also reported heat intolerance, recurrent palpitation, sweating, watery diarrhea, and weight loss of 10 kg over a 3-month duration. Methimazole and propranolol were initiated two days before the actual presentation. On examination, he had normal heart sounds, no gallop, murmur, or rub tachycardia but with regular and synchronous heart rate, and no clinical signs of heart failure. Neck exam revealed diffuse mild thyroid enlargement and general exam showed fine hand tremors. Electrocardiography on presentation showed biphasic T waves in V1 and V2 (Figure 1). Three sets of cardiac enzymes were negative; TSH was <0.005 mIU/L (0.45-4.5) and T4 was 48.3 pmol/L (9-20) reference and units. Transthoracic echocardiography was normal with good left ventricular function (ejection fraction (EF): 70%) and no regional wall motion abnormalities. As the patient did not tolerate exercise treadmill stress test, he underwent a dobutamine stress echo. Dobutamine was infused at 3-minute intervals, starting with 10 μg/kg and increasing to 20 μg/kg, 30 μg/kg, and 40 μg/kg in addition to 0.5 mg atropine IV until a target heart rate of 153 bpm accounting for 95% of his maximal predicted heart rate. The patient developed severe chest pain and systemic hypotension with a blood pressure of 80/50 mmHg. ST elevation in the anterolateral leads, new RBBB, and short runs of nonsustained ventricular tachycardia (VT) on continuous ECG monitoring were noted (Figure 2).

Echocardiography showed new regional wall motion abnormalities in the form of akinesia of the apical, mid anteroseptal, and mid anterior walls and hypokinesia of the mid anterolateral and mid posterolateral walls with a drop of EF to 30%. The patient was transferred to the intensive

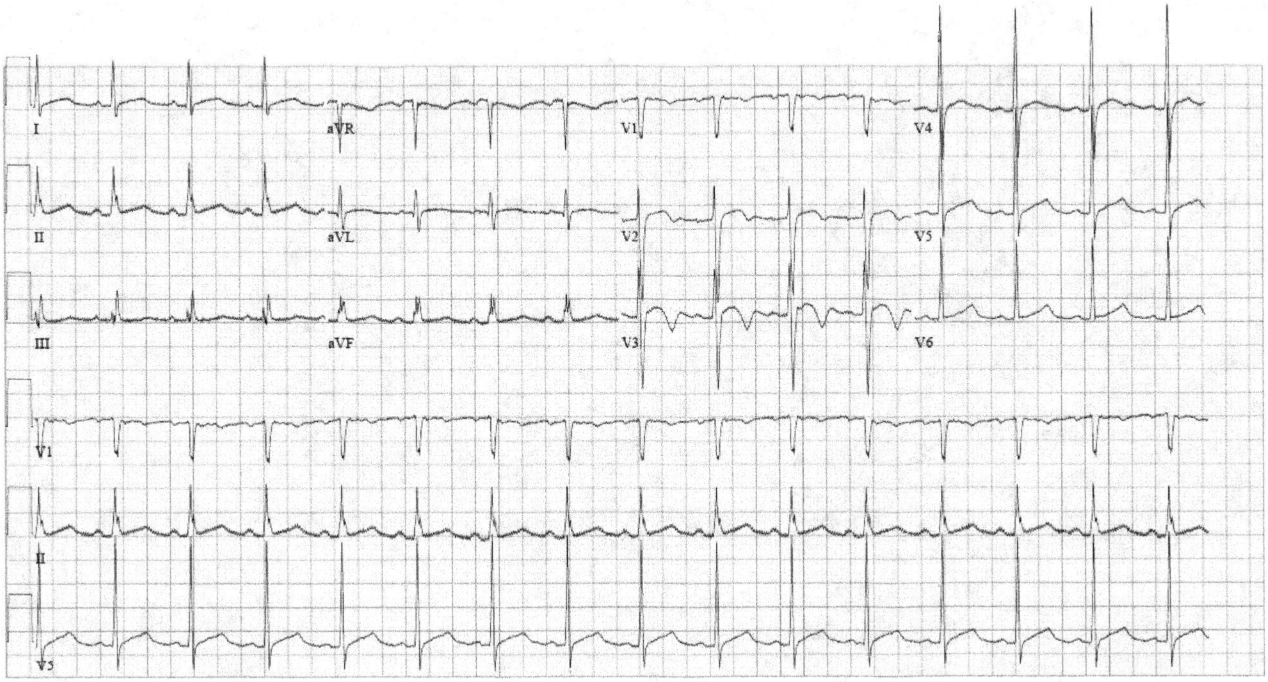

FIGURE 1

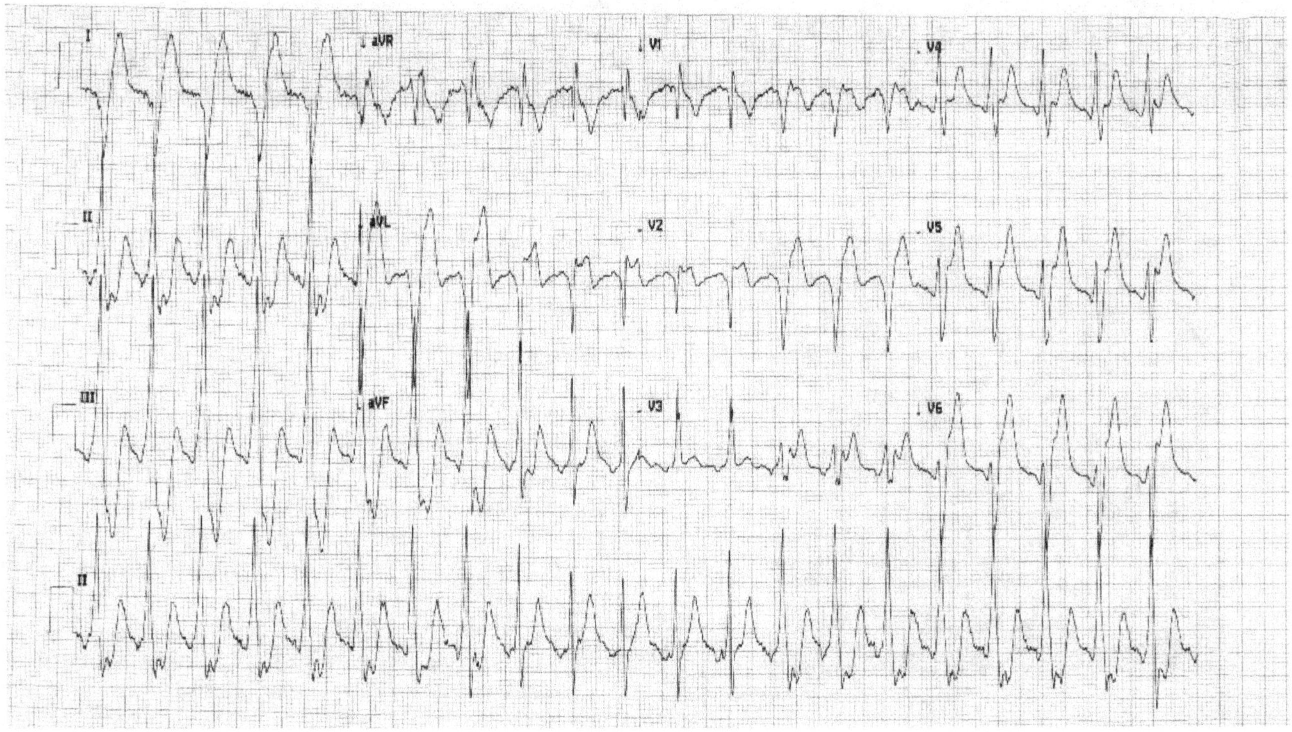

FIGURE 2

care unit, and resuscitation with IV fluids led to improvement in his blood pressure and propranolol was uptitrated till heart rate became controlled. Chest pain and ST elevation normalized spontaneously resolved. Cardiac troponin T reached a peak of 1900 ng/L but serial troponins showed progressive improvement. Global longitudinal strain measures (Figure 3) were abnormal in the left anterior descending (LAD) territory (Figure 4). Dual antiplatelets, heparin infusion along with propranolol and statin, started and kept on IV hydrocortisone 100 mg three times daily for 3 days to decrease the possibility of thyroid storm with coronary angiography (CAG). CAG was done 3 days later and showed

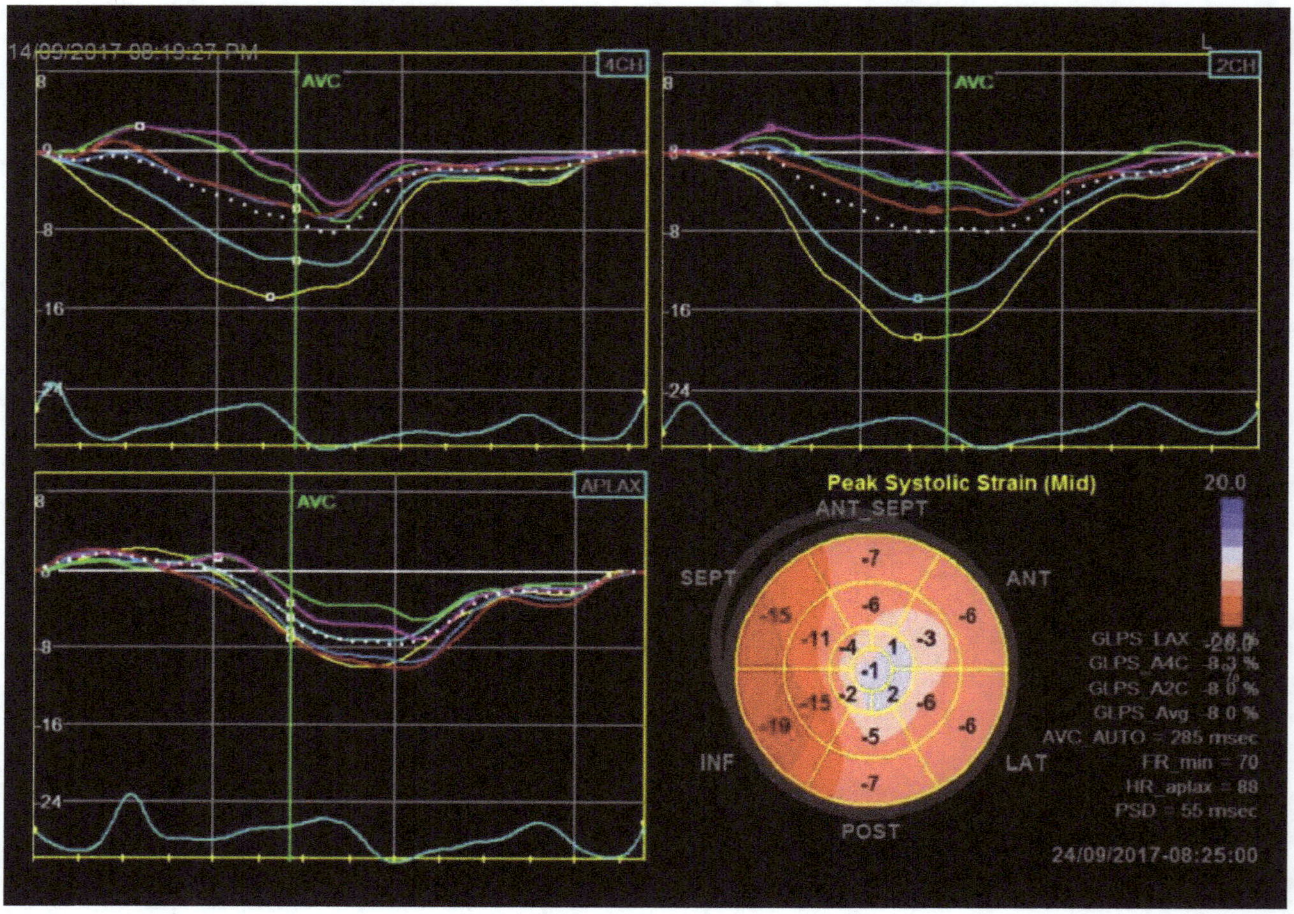

Figure 3

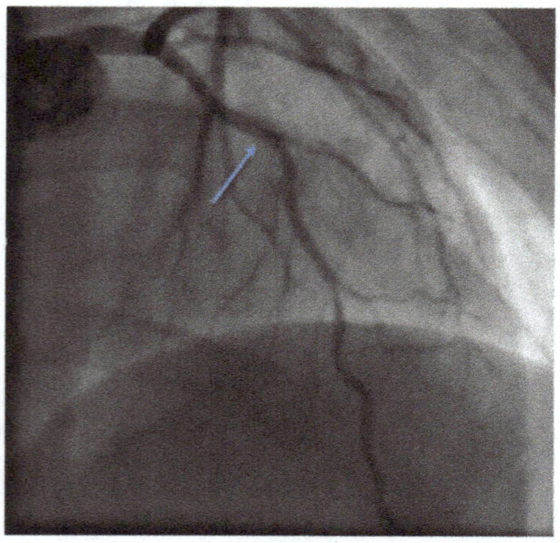

Figure 4

40% LAD stenosis proximal to D1 with no evidence of thrombus, myocardial bridging, or coronary vasospasm. Left circumflex artery (LCX) and right coronary artery (RCA) were normal. No provocation test was done and the patient was discharged home in a stable condition on full medications.

The patient showed dramatic improvement of symptoms over the next few days with improvement of the hyperthyroid state and was discharged successfully with minimal symptoms.

3. Discussion

Cardiovascular symptoms are the most prominent in patients with hyperthyroidism. The features of angina-type chest pain may be present in about 20% of these patients [7]. The possible mechanism includes underlying atheroma, metabolic effect of thyroxin on the myocardium, secondary arrhythmias [7], and transient coronary artery spasm [8, 9]. Similarly, coronary artery vasospasm with DSE has been reported in about 0.14%-0.4% [5, 10]. Studies [11] have shown that stress echocardiography in hyperthyroidism might lead to the hyperdynamic cardiac state, including worse exercise capacity and impaired vasodilatory and contractile reserves. However, the association between hyperthyroidism and myocardial infarction during DSE has never been reported.

In our patient, there was no history suggestive of coronary vasospasm, and coronary angiogram did not show any significant coronary artery disease. The possible mechanism in our case could be an exaggerated response to dobutamine, in the presence of severe hyperthyroidism and moderate coronary artery lesion.

Similarly, studies [10, 12, 13] have shown STEMI due to oxygen supply-demand mismatch, vasospasm, coronary artery dissection, or coronary artery plaque rupture with subsequent thrombus formation.

B-blockade may leave α-adrenergic vasoconstriction unopposed. Whether administration of propranolol enhances coronary spasm is not well established. Alvarez et al. [14] reported coronary vasospasm after administration of propranolol; however, other studies did not support this theory [15]. Other studies found no advantage of propranolol over diltiazem in preventing coronary spasms [16]. Keeping in mind those previous studies done on euthyroid patients, it may be not applicable to our patient which showed dramatic improvement of symptoms after increasing the propranolol doses.

In our case, we did not see any coronary artery dissection or plaque rupture. It is difficult to rule out a plaque rupture with superimposed thrombus formation, but the transient nature of ST elevation will go against this possibility. Similarly, the coronary angiogram procedure was delayed in order to control his hyperthyroid state firstly, and therefore, the thrombus if present might have been resolved during this time.

4. Conclusion

We believe our patient had transient ST-elevation myocardial infarction, secondary to DSE in a poorly controlled hyperthyroid state and moderated coronary artery disease. We would suggest treating hyperthyroidism prior to requesting noninvasive stress test and avoiding invasive coronary angiogram due to thyroid storm risk, based on the clinical picture. Our case also suggests that propranolol may be beneficial in controlling cardiac symptoms and possibly vasospasms in patients with hyperthyroidism.

References

[1] I. Klein and K. Ojamaa, "Thyroid hormone and the cardiovascular system," *The New England Journal of Medicine*, vol. 344, no. 7, pp. 501–509, 2001.

[2] M. L. Geleijnse, P. M. Fioretti, and J. R. T. C. Roelandt, "Methodology, feasibility, safety and diagnostic accuracy of dobutamine stress echocardiography," *Journal of the American College of Cardiology*, vol. 30, no. 3, pp. 595–606, 1997.

[3] F. Lattanzi, E. Picano, E. Adamo, and A. Varga, "Dobutamine stress echocardiography: safety in diagnosing coronary artery disease," *Drug Safety*, vol. 22, no. 4, pp. 251–262, 2000.

[4] B. M. Gordon, V. Mohan, A. T. Chapekis et al., "An analysis of the safety of performing dobutamine stress echocardiography in an ambulatory setting," *Journal of the American Society of Echocardiography*, vol. 8, no. 1, pp. 15–20, 1995.

[5] N. Lamisse, A. Cohen, C. Chauvel et al., "Dobutamine stress echocardiography; a monocentric experience on consecutive patients. Effect of age," *Archives des maladies du coeur et des vaisseaux*, vol. 90, no. 11, pp. 1455–1461, 1997.

[6] M. Fineschi, V. Zaca, M. Padeletti, T. Gori, and P. Aitiani, "Transmural myocardial ischaemia complicating recovery after dobutamine-atropine stress echocardiography in patients with non-significant coronary artery disease: insights from invasive assessment of coronary physiology," *European Journal of Echocardiography*, vol. 12, no. 7, article E34, 2011.

[7] L. Resnekov and R. E. Falicov, "Thyrotoxicosis and lactate producing angina pectoris with normal coronary arteries," *Heart*, vol. 39, no. 10, pp. 1051–1057, 1977.

[8] J. A. Jaber, S. Haque, H. Noor, B. Ibrahim, and J. al Suwaidi, "Thyrotoxicosis and coronary artery spasm: case report and review of the literature," *Angiology*, vol. 61, no. 8, pp. 807–812, 2010.

[9] J. H. Kim, "A case of myocardial ischemia and myocardial injury caused by coronary vasospasm associated with hyperthyroidism," *Korean Circulation Journal*, vol. 30, no. 3, pp. 369–372, 2000.

[10] N. Masencal, I. El Hajjaji, R. El Mahnoud, F. Digne, and O. Dubourg, "Prevalence of coronary artery spasm during dobutamine stress echocardiography," *The American Journal of Cardiology*, vol. 109, no. 6, pp. 800–804, 2012.

[11] G. J. Kahaly, S. Wagner, J. Nieswandt, S. Mohr-Kahaly, and T. J. Ryan, "Stress echocardiography in hyperthyroidism," *The Journal of Clinical Endocrinology & Metabolism*, vol. 84, no. 7, pp. 2308–2313, 1999.

[12] A. Elhendy, W. Ginete, S. Shurmur, and T. R. Porter, "Acute myocardial infarction after a negative dobutamine stress echocardiogram," *European Journal of Echocardiography*, vol. 5, no. 6, pp. 469–471, 2004.

[13] I. Karabinos, A. Papadopoulos, S. Koulouris, A. Kranidis, S. Korovesis, and D. Katritsis, "Spontaneous coronary artery dissection during a dobutamine stress echocardiography," *Echocardiography*, vol. 23, no. 3, pp. 232–234, 2006.

[14] L. Alvarez, J. Zamorano, L. Mataix, C. Almeria, R. Moreno, and J. L. Rodrigo, "Coronary spasm after administration of propranolol during dobutamine stress echocardiography," *Revista Española de Cardiología*, vol. 55, no. 7, pp. 778–781, 2002.

[15] N. De Cesare, S. Cozzi, A. Apostolo et al., *Coronary Artery Disease*, Lippincott-Raven Publishers, 1994.

[16] P. Y. Tilmant, J. M. Lablanche, F. A. Thieuleux, B. A. Dupuis, and M. E. Bertrand, "Detrimental effect of propranolol in patients with coronary arterial spasm countered by combination with diltiazem," *The American Journal of Cardiology*, vol. 52, no. 3, pp. 230–233, 1983.

37

Delayed Diagnosis of Non-ST Segment Elevation Myocardial Infarction in a Young Patient with Multivessel Disease and Familial Hypercholesterolemia Complicated by Cardiogenic Shock Finally Treated with Intra-Aortic Balloon Pump as a Bridge to Extra Corporeal Membrane Oxygenation

Rafał Januszek,[1] Magdalena Jędrychowska,[1] Piotr Jankowski,[2] Dariusz Dudek,[1,3] and Stanisław Bartuś[1,3]

[1] *2nd Department of Cardiology and Cardiovascular Interventions, University Hospital, Krakow, Poland*
[2] *1st Department of Cardiology, Jagiellonian University Medical College, Krakow, Poland*
[3] *Department of Interventional Cardiology, Jagiellonian University Medical College, Krakow, Poland*

Correspondence should be addressed to Rafał Januszek; jaanraf@interia.pl
Academic Editor: Markus Ferrari

Delayed diagnosis of coronary artery disease in young patients after cardiac arrest of unknown origin could increase the risk of death in further diagnostic and therapeutic process. Familial history of premature coronary atherosclerosis and hypercholesterolemia could help in proper diagnosis and treatment. We present a case of a 29-year-old female admitted to the catheterization laboratory with cardiogenic shock and multivessel coronary artery disease treated successfully with multivessel percutaneous coronary intervention and intra-aortic balloon counterpulsation as a bridge to extracorporeal membrane oxygenation.

1. Introduction

Familial hypercholesterolemia (FH) is one of the most common causes of premature coronary atherosclerosis and, in consequence, major cardiovascular events but still very often remains unrecognized early enough and therefore is not treated properly. The risk of coronary heart disease in patients with FH is estimated to be increased at least 10-fold [1]. Based on the presented case of a young woman being treated at our department due to acute myocardial infarction (MI) complicated by cardiogenic shock (CS), we would like to draw attention to several recently discussed problems in cardiology: firstly, severe cardiovascular complications due to undiagnosed FH at a young age; secondly, the cardiac diagnostic process of patients after sudden cardiac arrest; thirdly, the issue of noninfarct related artery (IRA) revascularization in acute MI; and finally, the role of intra-aortic balloon counterpulsation (IABP) in CS as a bridge to extracorporeal membrane oxygenation (ECMO).

2. Case Presentation

A 29-year-old female was admitted to the emergency department (ED) after sudden cardiac arrest at home followed by effective resuscitation. The first recorded heart rhythm was ventricular fibrillation. After effective resuscitation, due to respiratory insufficiency, the patient was intubated and mechanical ventilation was set. Electrocardiography revealed ST-segment depressions up to 1 mm in I, aVL, II, III, and V1-4 leads. The patient was then transported to the ED. At admission to the ED, the patient was hemodynamically stable and preserved systolic blood pressure without inotropes.

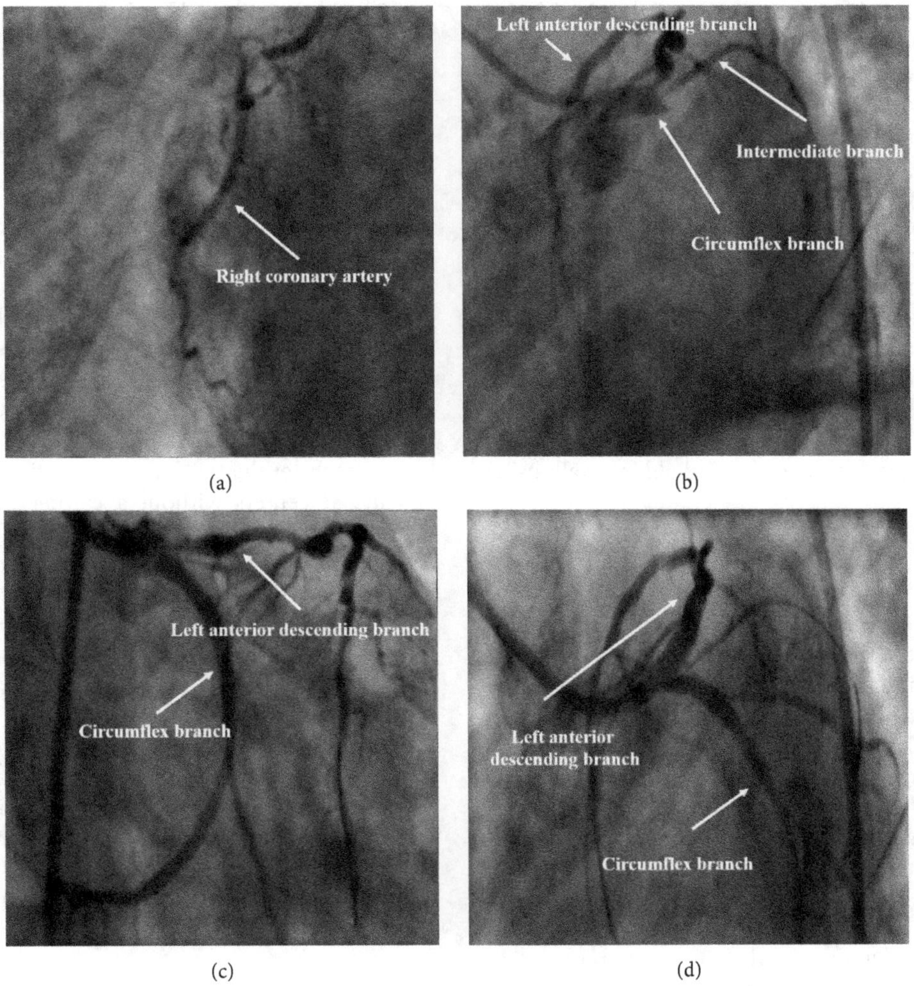

FIGURE 1: (a) Coronary artery angiography: right coronary artery. (b) Coronary artery angiography: left coronary artery. (c) Coronary angiography after percutaneous coronary intervention within circumflex branch. (d) Coronary angiography after percutaneous coronary intervention within the left anterior descending branch.

Considering blood tests, including elevated level of serum D-dimers, at first, computed tomography of the head and chest in pulmonary embolism algorithm was performed. There were signs of cerebral stroke and evident pulmonary embolism. Chest radiograph depicted features of pulmonary edema. At that time, a cardiological consultation was made on the basis of which the cardiac echocardiography was ordered at patient's bedside. Cardiologist consultation and echocardiography revealed impaired left ventricle ejection fraction (LVEF) (approx. 25-30%) with regional contractility impairment (recent akinesis of the lateral, inferior, and posterior walls and hypokinesis of other walls) and moderate mitral regurgitation. The patient was immediately qualified for coronary artery angiography and transferred from ED to the catheterization laboratory (CathLab). During transportation to the CathLab, the first symptoms of CS had developed, and the patient was given first inotrope—noradrenaline. Coronary artery angiography revealed multivessel disease including recessive right coronary artery with 60% stenosis; the left main coronary artery was without significant stenoses, ostial occlusion of the dominant circumflex branch (Cx), left anterior descendent artery (LAD) with multiple significant stenoses: ostial: 80-90%, proximal segment: 70%, medial segment: 80%, and distal segment: 60%, the intermediate branch with 80-90% ostial stenosis. This is presented in Figures 1(a) and 1(b). Percutaneous coronary intervention (PCI) within Cx with thrombectomy and drug-eluting stent (DES) implantation, Onyx 3.5 × 12 mm, 18 atm., was performed and followed by sequential inflation in the intermediate branch (c.b. 1.5 × 12 mm, 20 atm.) and Cx (4.0 × 8 mm, 24 atm.). Due to the progression of CS and no improvement after adding other inotropes (dopamine, dobutamine) at high doses, the decision was made to implant IABP and perform PCI of LAD. Predilation with b.c. 3.0 × 15 mm 20 atm. was performed. Implantation of two DES in the proximal and medial segment was performed: DES Ultimaster (4.0 × 18 mm, 18 atm.) and DES Create (3.0 × 31 mm, 16 atm.). Postdilatation, with b.c. 4.0 × 15 mm, up to 20 atm., was executed using the proximal optimization technique. Then, the patient was then sent to the intensive care cardiology unit in a critical state, with the blood pressure of 40-50 mmHg. Control echocardiography revealed decreased LVEF (around 20%). A fourth inotrope was added (adrenaline) without significant improvement of systolic blood pressure. After consultation at the cardiac surgery department, the patient was qualified for ECMO treatment. The patient was successfully surgically connected to ECMO after transportation to the cardiac surgery unit and surgeons were able to wean from the ECMO, due to the improvement of LVEF after five days. During the long stay at the cardiac surgery unit, several complications developed, including severe bleeding demanding transfusion of more than 16 units of blood products, acute ischemia of the left lower limb, left femoral artery thrombectomy and surgical angioplasty, respiratory tract infections with negative culture (bronchoscopy), pneumonia, pulmonary edema, and recurrent mechanical ventilation necessity. The patient finally survived, was weaned from mechanical ventilation, and was discharged for further rehabilitation after almost 70 days without any neurological deficiencies and able to walk using a walker.

3. Discussion

According to the lack of any previous diagnostic results indicating FH, making the diagnosis at admission was difficult. Correctly collected interviews by rescuers during resuscitation of the patient at her home could shorten the time of transportation to CathLab. The patient's sister's MI performed at a young age and her father's death as a complication of acute MI indicated suspicion of an inherited issue in our patient. All patients following the return of spontaneous circulation who do not have an alternate explanation for cardiac arrest irrespective of the electrocardiography findings may be considered for coronary angiography and possible PCI [2]. It has been demonstrated that direct transport to CathLab was associated with a significant increase in survival rate [3]. Also, the bedside echocardiography should be performed immediately if there is suspicion of underlying cardiac ischemia [4]. Delayed time of reperfusion in MI patients is especially important because it has great impact on mortality rate [5]. In the current case, there was an immediate worsening of clinical state after PCI of IRA at the CathLab. Then, the IABP was inserted and a decision was made to perform non-IRA PCI. The PCI of the IRA and complete revascularization approach were compared in four randomized clinical trials: PRAMI, CvLPRIT, DANAMI-3–PRIMULTI, and Compare-Acute trial. None of them has demonstrated superiority of complete revascularization in mortality reducing to primary PCI of the IRA [6–9]. Another option of left ventricle support device for that patient could be the Impella heart pump. However, first, we did not have this device in CathLab at that time, and secondly, the device is preferred in stable patients with low LVEF undergoing PCIs, although it is also successfully used in acute conditions. Therefore, according to the ESC 2017 consensus, non-IRA PCI during the index procedure is rather not advised in patients with CS [10]. However, in this particular case, we decided to perform PCI of non-IRA due to the young age of the patient. Cardiogenic shock is the main cause of death related to acute MI, with a mortality rate of 40-50% in the absence of aggressive and highly specialized technical care [11–13]. Until 2012, the European and American consensus considered the use of IABP; in the case of post-AMI, cardiogenic shock was rather recommended. Based on the results of recent meta-analyses, the current consensus has changed its recommendations, and now, IABP should be considered in acute MI-related CS and mechanical complications instead of short-term percutaneous mechanical support which is preferred in these patients [3, 14]. Currently, the European consensus does not advocate for the routine usage of IABP due to the results of the large randomized multicenter IABP-SHOCK II trial which showed no survival benefit with IABP support. At 30 days, there was no significant difference in the primary outcome of mortality between IABP and control groups [15]. However, future longer follow-up could modify this approach. On the other hand, the specific use of IABP as a bridge to ECMO in CS has not been closely evaluated. Such a solution may bring special benefits at centers without a cardiac surgery department, without regular access to short-term left ventricle support devices. In this case, additional hemodynamic support is necessary to secure the patient during the time of transportation. In this specific situation, the lack of IABP affects the time for hemodynamic stabilization, length of stay at the ICU, the dose and duration of catecholamine therapy, and renal function. Our main purpose was to maintain the minimal critical organ blood supply and oxygenation until transportation to the cardiac surgery center and then connect the patient to ECMO. It should be noticed that despite the persistent extremely low systolic blood pressure and delay associated with the necessity of organization and transportation to another center, our patient does not have any permanent neurological deficiencies.

4. Conclusions

In conclusion, IABP could serve as bridge therapy to ECMO in young and promising patients with acute MI in the course of multivessel disease complicated by CS. Nationwide screening programs for familial hypercholesterolemia should be conducted to detect patients with FH at the youngest possible age and treat them properly. Young patients after sudden cardiac arrest, and in particular with innate risk factors for premature atherosclerosis, should be first consulted at CathLab to implement the appropriate diagnostic and treatment procedures, which could affect the overall hospital stay length and condition of the patient. Selected patients with cardiogenic shock may benefit from PCI of non-IRA.

References

[1] A. Wiegman, S. S. Gidding, G. F. Watts et al., "Familial hypercholesterolaemia in children and adolescents: gaining decades of life by optimizing detection and treatment," *European Heart Journal*, vol. 36, no. 36, pp. 2425–2437, 2015.

[2] F. Dumas, A. Cariou, S. Manzo-Silberman et al., "Immediate percutaneous coronary intervention is associated with better survival after out-of-hospital cardiac arrest: insights from the PROCAT (Parisian Region Out of Hospital Cardiac Arrest) registry," *Circulation: Cardiovascular Interventions*, vol. 3, no. 3, pp. 200–207, 2010.

[3] A. Cournoyer, É. Notebaert, L. de Montigny et al., "Impact of the direct transfer to percutaneous coronary intervention-capable hospitals on survival to hospital discharge for patients with out-of-hospital cardiac arrest," *Resuscitation*, vol. 125, pp. 28–33, 2018.

[4] C. L. Moore and J. A. Copel, "Point-of-care ultrasonography," *The New England Journal of Medicine*, vol. 364, no. 8, pp. 749 757, 2011.

[5] C. B. Fordyce, H. R. al-Khalidi, J. G. Jollis et al., "Association of rapid care process implementation on reperfusion times across multiple ST-segment–elevation myocardial infarction networks," *Circulation: Cardiovascular Interventions*, vol. 10, no. 1, 2017.

[6] D. S. Wald, J. K. Morris, N. J. Wald et al., "Randomized trial of preventive angioplasty in myocardial infarction," *The New England Journal of Medicine*, vol. 369, no. 12, pp. 1115–1123, 2013.

[7] A. H. Gershlick, J. N. Khan, D. J. Kelly et al., "Randomized trial of complete versus lesion-only revascularization in patients undergoing primary percutaneous coronary intervention for STEMI and multivessel disease: the CvLPRIT trial," *Journal of the American College of Cardiology*, vol. 65, no. 10, pp. 963 972, 2015.

[8] T. Engstrøm, H. Kelbæk, S. Helqvist et al., "Complete revascularisation versus treatment of the culprit lesion only in patients with ST-segment elevation myocardial infarction and multivessel disease (DANAMI-3—PRIMULTI): an open-label, randomised controlled trial," *The Lancet*, vol. 386, no. 9994, pp. 665–671, 2015.

[9] P. C. Smits, M. Abdel-Wahab, F. J. Neumann et al., "Fractional flow reserve-guided multivessel angioplasty in myocardial infarction," *The New England Journal of Medicine*, vol. 376, no. 13, pp. 1234–1244, 2017.

[10] B. Ibanez, S. James, S. Agewall et al., "2017 ESC Guidelines for the management of acute myocardial infarction in patients presenting with ST-segment elevation: the Task Force for the management of acute myocardial infarction in patients presenting with ST-segment elevation of the European Society of Cardiology (ESC)," *European Heart Journal*, vol. 39, no. 2, pp. 119–177, 2018.

[11] N. Aissaoui, E. Puymirat, X. Tabone et al., "Improved outcome of cardiogenic shock at the acute stage of myocardial infarction: a report from the USIK 1995, USIC 2000, and FAST-MI French Nationwide Registries," *European Heart Journal*, vol. 33, no. 20, pp. 2535–2543, 2012.

[12] R. J. Goldberg, F. A. Spencer, J. M. Gore, D. Lessard, and J. Yarzebski, "Thirty-year trends (1975 to 2005) in the magnitude of, management of, and hospital death rates associated with cardiogenic shock in patients with acute myocardial infarction: a population based perspective," *Circulation* vol. 119, no. 9, pp. 1211–1219, 2009.

[13] H. Thiele, U. Zeymer, F.-J. Neumann et al., "Intraaortic balloon support for myocardial infarction with cardiogenic shock," *The New England Journal of Medicine*, vol. 367, no. 14, pp. 1287–1296, 2012.

[14] F.-J. Neumann, M. Sousa-Uva, A. Ahlsson et al., "2018 ESC/EACTS Guidelines on myocardial revascularization," *European Heart Journal*, vol. 40, no. 2, pp. 87–165, 2018.

[15] H. Thiele, U. Zeymer, F.-J. Neumann et al., "Intra-aortic balloon counterpulsation in acute myocardial infarction complicated by cardiogenic shock (IABP-SHOCK II): final 12 month results of a randomised, open-label trial," *The Lancet*, vol. 382, no. 9905, pp. 1638–1645, 2013.

38

Hemodynamic Support using Percutaneous Transfemoral Impella 5.0 and Impella RP for Refractory Cardiogenic Shock

Pratik K. Dalal[1], **Amy Mertens**[1], **Dinesh Shah**[1], and **Ivan Hanson**[1,2]

[1]*Department of Cardiovascular Medicine, Beaumont Health System, Royal Oak, MI, USA*
[2]*Oakland University William Beaumont School of Medicine, Royal Oak, MI, USA*

Correspondence should be addressed to Ivan Hanson; ivan.hanson@beaumont.org

Academic Editor: Markus Ferrari

Acute myocardial infarction (AMI) resulting in cardiogenic shock continues to be a substantial source of morbidity and mortality despite advances in recognition and treatment. Prior to the advent of percutaneous and more durable left ventricular support devices, prompt revascularization with the addition of vasopressors and inotropes were the standard of care in the management of this critical population. Recent published studies have shown that in addition to prompt revascularization, unloading of the left ventricle with the placement of the Impella percutaneous axillary flow pump can lead to improvement in mortality. Parameters such as the cardiac power output (CPO) and pulmonary artery pulsatility index (PAPi), obtained through pulmonary artery catheterization, can help ascertain the productivity of right and left ventricular function. Utilization of these parameters can provide the information necessary to escalate support to the right ventricle with the insertion of an Impella RP or the left ventricle with the insertion of larger devices, which provide more forward flow. Herein, we present a case of AMI complicated by cardiogenic shock resulting in biventricular failure treated with the percutaneous insertion of an Impella RP and Impella 5.0 utilizing invasive markers of left and right ventricular function to guide the management and escalation of care.

1. Introduction

Acute myocardial infarction (AMI) complicated by cardiogenic shock (AMI-CS) is associated with in-hospital mortality between 33% and 55% [1]. Rapid hemodynamic evaluation and left ventricular hemodynamic support using the Impella (Abiomed, Danvers, MA) pumps (2.5, CP, and 5.0) improve outcomes in patients with AMI-CS [2]. However, even with the timely insertion of these devices, mortality in AMI-CS remains unacceptably high [1, 3]. We present a case of AMI-CS in which a patient underwent insertion of Impella CP and revascularization of the infarct-related artery, but remained in refractory shock and required the escalation of hemodynamic support utilizing the percutaneous insertion of Impella RP and Impella 5.0. Herein, clinical decision-making and technical challenges of this approach are outlined.

2. Case

A 61-year-old man presented with 2 days of progressively worsening chest pain. Blood pressure was 90/60 mmHg. The 12-lead ECG revealed sinus tachycardia with a rate of 110 bpm and new left bundle branch block. An echocardiogram revealed a left ventricular ejection fraction of 10%, without evidence of mechanical complications. Troponin was 11 ng/mL. In the emergency department, he developed worsening shock and pulmonary edema necessitating mechanical ventilation. He was urgently triaged to the catheterization laboratory.

Femoral angiography revealed no evidence of atherosclerosis and femoral artery diameters of 9 mm. An Impella CP was inserted via the left femoral artery, and coronary angiography/intervention was performed via the right femoral artery. Coronary angiography revealed 70% stenosis of the distal left main coronary artery, chronic total occlusion of the left anterior descending artery, 80% calcific stenosis of the left circumflex, and chronic total occlusion of the right coronary artery (Figure 1). Invasive hemodynamics revealed refractory cardiogenic shock and biventricular failure (Table 1). Right ventricular failure was presumed to be due to collateral insufficiency to the chronically occluded right coronary artery.

Given marginal hemodynamics and the presence of right ventricular failure, an RP Impella was inserted via the right femoral vein. Despite adequate flow from the RP (4.7 L/m) and CP (3.5 L/m), hemodynamics only modestly improved (Table 2). Percutaneous revascularization of the culprit severe stenosis in the distal left main and proximal circumflex arteries was challenging but ultimately successful using rotational atherectomy and implantation of a 4.0 × 38 Promus Premiere (Boston Scientific, Marlborough, MA) drug-eluting stent, guided by intravascular ultrasound.

Despite biventricular Impella support using CP and RP catheters and successful revascularization, the patient had persistent cardiogenic shock. This manifested as a markedly reduced cardiac power output (CPO) (Table 2). It was elected to escalate left ventricular support using Impella 5.0. Given the large caliber of the femoral arteries and lack of calcification, percutaneous femoral insertion was performed.

Anticipating limb ischemia with large bore sheath insertion, an ex vivo bypass circuit was deemed necessary. With ultrasound guidance, an antegrade 5-French sheath was inserted in the right superficial femoral artery. Next, the existing 6-French sheath in the right femoral artery was replaced with progressively larger sheaths to dilate the arteriotomy. Finally, a 23-French sheath (Abiomed, Danvers, MA) was inserted. Via the 23-French sheath, an Impella 5.0 was inserted into the left ventricle and the existing Impella CP was removed through the left femoral artery. Hemodynamics immediately improved (Table 2). Antegrade perfusion of the 14 F left femoral arterial sheath was not undertaken as the caliber of the femoral artery was adequate to accommodate a 4.6 mm sheath. The ex vivo bypass circuit was created by connecting the 14-French left femoral sheath (donor which originally housed the Impella CP) to the 5-French right femoral antegrade sheath (recipient) (Figures 2(a) and 2(b)). Both legs and feet were warm to touch with intact distal pulses.

In the cardiac ICU, Impella 5.0 and RP support was maintained (Figure 3). Vasopressors were not required. On hospital day 2, the patient developed profound intravascular hemolysis, transient complete heart block, and pulseless electrical activity requiring cardiopulmonary resuscitation. A repeat echocardiogram revealed small LV and RV cavity sizes. Taken together, the findings suggested that the high flow rate from the Impella 5.0 had caused suction of endocardial tissue, leading to hemolysis and increased vagotonia. This improved with volume resuscitation and blood transfusions with reduction in Impella flow rate. On hospital day 3, the Impella RP was explanted uneventfully. The Impella 5.0 was explanted in the OR. Surgical repair of the right common femoral artery was uneventful. Despite confirmation of antegrade flow beyond the femoral artery, fasciotomy of

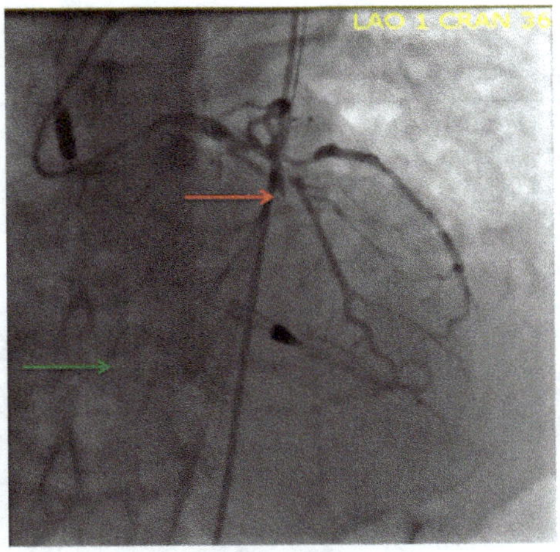

FIGURE 1: Coronary angiography demonstrating an occluded LAD (red arrow) with collaterals to the RCA (green arrow).

TABLE 1

RA: 18 mmHg	CI: 1.69 L/min/m^2
PA: 54/34 mmHg, mean: 31 mmHg	PA Sat: 53%
RV: 54/19 mmHg, EDP: 22 mmHg	FA Sat: 95%
PCWP: 31 mmHg	CPO: 0.74
CO: 3.35 L/min	PAPi: 1.1

the anterior compartment of the right leg was performed because of elevated compartment pressure and clinical evidence of limb ischemia. There was evidence of hematoma and myonecrosis in the right thigh, which was treated with resection of the affected muscle. The patient slowly recovered and was discharged to inpatient rehabilitation on hospital day 30. Left ventricular ejection fraction improved to 40%. He was discharged home from rehabilitation on hospital day 60.

3. Discussion

Early identification of cardiogenic shock and rapid institution of left ventricular mechanical circulatory support prior to primary PCI result in favorable outcomes. The Detroit Cardiogenic Shock Initiative, in which patients with AMI and cardiogenic shock were supported with Impella prior to PCI so as to minimize the "door to unload time," resulted in survival to device explant of 89% and survival to discharge of 84% [2]. This represents substantial improvement compared to the historic survival rate of 50% prior to the institution of such an algorithm. Unfortunately, some patients still have refractory shock despite early mechanical support and successful revascularization. The present case illustrates such a patient, who had refractory shock due to both profound LV failure and concomitant RV failure.

3.1. Refractory Shock in AMI due to LV Failure despite LV Mechanical Circulatory Support. Left ventricular dysfunction is the cause of shock in ~75% of patients with AMI-CS, with the LAD being the most common infarct-related artery in these cases [4, 5]. A retrospective analysis of the SHOCK

Table 2

Pre-RP Impella	Post-RP Impella	Post-Impella 5.0
CPO: 0.52 (normal > 0.6)	CPO: 0.6	CPO: 0.77
PAPi: 0.7 (normal > 0.9)	PAPi: 0.7	PAPi: 1.0
PA saturation: 45%	PA saturation: 43%	PA saturation: 50%

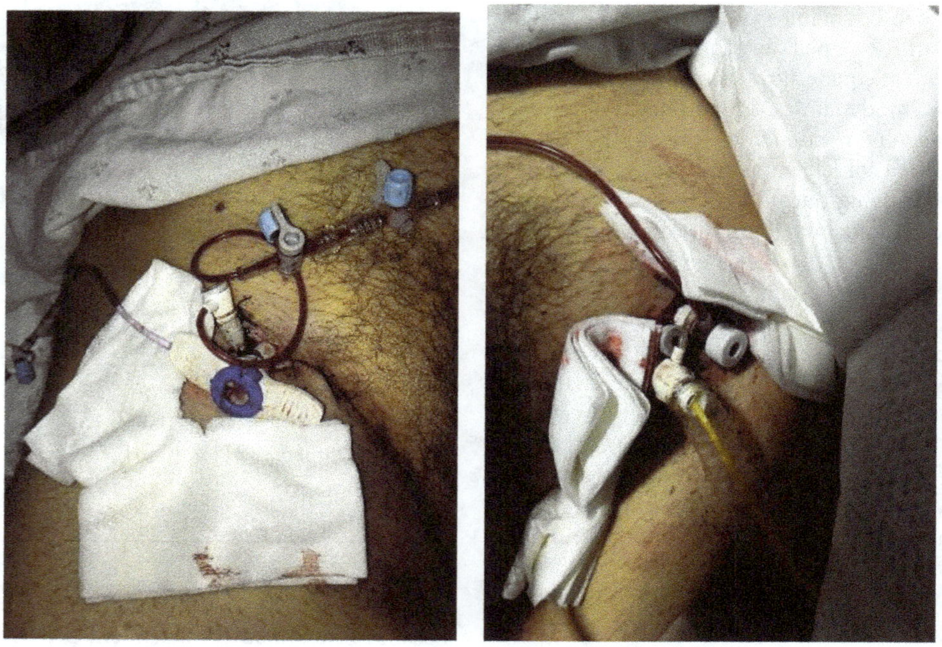

(a) (b)

Figure 2: (a) Receiving limb of the external left femoral artery to right superficial femoral artery bypass. (b) Donor limb of the external left femoral artery to right superficial femoral artery bypass.

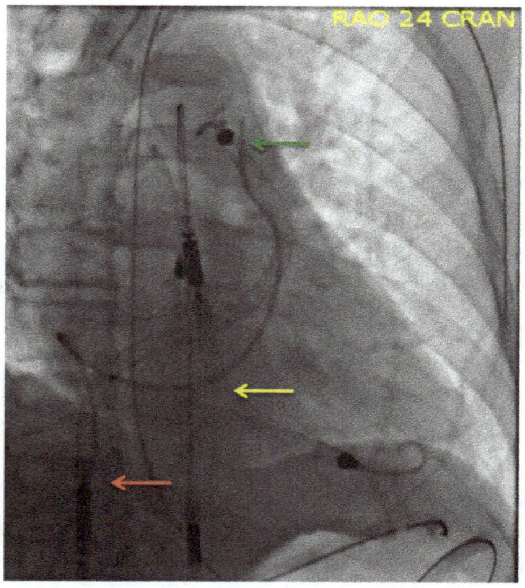

Figure 3: Chest X-ray showing RP Impella with the inlet situated in the inferior vena cava (red arrow) and the outlet in the pulmonary artery (green arrow) and Impella 5.0 with the inlet in the left ventricle and the outlet in the ascending aorta (yellow arrow).

Trial (Should We Emergently Revascularize Occluded Coronaries for Cardiogenic Shock) demonstrated that cardiac power output (CPO, calculated as the product of mean arterial blood pressure and cardiac output, divided by 451) is the most potent predictor of survival in AMI-CS [6]. Furthermore, Impella 2.5 (providing up to 2.5 liters per minute of forward flow) increases CPO to a greater degree than IABP, a device that has not been shown to improve survival in AMI-CS [7]. Therefore, we believe that CPO is a reasonable therapeutic target in AMI-CS, and measures to increase CPO to greater than 0.6 should be undertaken.

Impella CP was designed to provide up to 4.0 liters per minute of forward flow, and is now the standard mechanical circulatory device at our institution for the treatment of AMI-CS. However, some patients have refractory shock despite early use of Impella CP and coronary revascularization. If the cause of refractory shock is LV failure, escalation of LV support should be considered. Options include (1) implantation of a durable left ventricular assist device (LVAD), (2) venoarterial extracorporeal membrane oxygenation (VA-ECMO) with a left ventricular vent, or (3) use of a larger axial flow pump, such as Impella 5.0 [8–10]. Of course, escalation of care assumes that multiorgan failure and anoxic brain injury are not present (in which case, a frank discussion with family members about treatment goals and expectations and terminal weaning of support may be most appropriate).

Impella 5.0 is designed to provide up to 5 liters per minute of forward flow. Full LV support provides complete unloading of the left ventricle, which improves coronary blood flow to the culprit and nonculprit territories [11, 12]. Additional forward flow improves blood pressure and CPO and lessens the requirement of vasopressor agents, which have been shown to worsen survival in AMI-CS [13]. Although the size of the catheter is 9 French, the inflow cage is 21 French. Accordingly, device insertion may not be straightforward, and it usually requires surgical cutdown with anastamosis of a graft conduit to the access artery. Alternatively, a sheathless percutaneous insertion can be performed in the femoral or axillary artery [14]. Transcaval insertion allows for the insertion of a large-bore introducer into the femoral vein, then passage through an iatrogenic fistula from the inferior vena cava into the aorta. When Impella support is no longer needed, the introducer sheath can be removed and the fistula occluded by the insertion of a nitinol occluder device [15]. In our case, the femoral arteries were felt to be large enough to accommodate a 23-French Abiomed sheath. This sheath was selected because it features a softer hemostatic valve to allow the passage of the bulky inflow cage of the Impella 5.0 without kinking the catheter shaft or damaging the internal catheter electronics. It is a peel-away sheath, but it was left in place since removal of the sheath would undoubtedly cause profuse bleeding given the mismatch between the sheath size (23 French) and the catheter size (9 French). Certainly, removal of the peel-away sheath could lead to hematoma formation and compartment syndrome. Ex vivo arterial bypass was needed since the large-bore sheath was flow occlusive to the right lower extremity. Techniques for creating the bypass circuit are described elsewhere [16, 17].

3.2. Refractory Shock in Anterior AMI with Concomitant RV Failure. Pulmonary artery pulsatility index (PAPi, calculated as pulmonary artery systolic pressure – pulmonary artery dia stolic pressure/RA pressure; values < 0.9 suggest RVD) was shown to be a potent predictor of outcome in AMI-CS due to RV failure [18]. In a retrospective analysis of the SHOCK registry, 37% of the patients had hemodynamic evidence of RV dysfunction when presenting with cardiogenic shock. Additionally, in 33% of the patients with RV dysfunction, the infarct-related artery was the LAD [19]. Right ventricular failure in the setting of AWMI could be provoked by collateral insufficiency to a previously occluded right coronary artery, preexisting RV dysfunction from a noncardiac cause, or multivessel coronary occlusion. However, animal models also suggest abnormalities in signaling pathways, such as cell chemotaxis, regulation of endothelial cell proliferation, regulation of apoptosis, and regulation of cytoskeleton organization and cell adhesion in the right ventricle when there is ligation of the left anterior descending artery [20, 21]. Therefore, infarction in one myocardial territory may have additional deleterious effects remotely in distant cardiac tissue. Although the unloading of the left ventricle should reduce pulmonary artery pressure and decrease the work of the RV, there are several mechanisms which lead to a perturbation of RV function. Increased cardiac output from the LVAD increases venous return to the RV, potentially worsening the preexisting RV failure [22]. Excessive leftward shift of the intraventricular septum may also decrease septal contribution to RV contraction, leading to RVF [23, 24]. LV unloading from an LVAD typically reduces tricuspid regurgitation (TR) through decreased RV afterload [25]. In the setting of an incompetent valve, increased RV volume and tethering of valve leaflets to a leftward-shifted septum can intensify TR [25, 26].

Impella RP is a 22-French axial flow pump mounted on an 11-French catheter that is inserted peripherally via the femoral vein and provides up to 4.4 L/min of flow from the inferior vena cava into the pulmonary artery (Figure 3). Results from the Recover Right study showed favorable hemodynamic profiles after insertion, manifested by an improvement in the cardiac index, decrease in central venous pressure, and improved survival at 30 days [27]. In patients who are primarily unloaded with a left-sided mechanical heart pump, a decrease in cardiac power output < 0.6 may suggest poor RV function, especially in cases where the pulmonary artery pulsatility index is <0.9. Several other mechanical circulatory support devices are commercially available for the management of biventricular failure. These include VA-ECMO, biventricular TandemHeart pumps, and various combinations of left-sided Impella and TandemHeart or VA-ECMO pumps [28]. TandemHeart requires a transeptal puncture, a 21 F venous cannula, and a 15-19 F arterial cannula, while VA-ECMO requires an LV "vent" in the form of an Impella to mitigate progressive LV failure due to excessive afterload [29–31].

4. Conclusion

We present a case of biventricular failure complicating anterior wall AMI successfully treated with full hemodynamic support using Impella 5.0 and Impella RP. Refractory cardiogenic shock despite mechanical circulatory support in AMI is a challenging clinical scenario. Two potential mechanisms for refractory shock in this setting include concomitant RV failure and persistent LV pump failure. An understanding of the pathogenesis, diagnosis, and timely management of these hemodynamic conditions is likely to improve survival.

Disclosure

This case was accepted for poster presentation and presented at TCT 2018 in San Diego, California.

References

[1] D. Kolte, S. Khera, W. S. Aronow et al., "Trends in incidence, management, and outcomes of cardiogenic shock complicating ST-elevation myocardial infarction in the United States," *Journal of the American Heart Association*, vol. 3, no. 1, article e000590, 2014.

[2] W. O'Neill, M. Basir, S. Dixon, K. Patel, T. Schreiber, and S. Almany, "Feasibility of early mechanical support during mechanical reperfusion of acute myocardial infarct cardiogenic shock," *JACC: Cardiovascular Interventions*, vol. 10, no. 6, pp. 624-625, 2017.

[3] R. J. Goldberg, J. M. Gore, J. S. Alpert et al., "Cardiogenic shock after acute myocardial infarction: incidence and mortality from a community-wide perspective, 1975–1988," *The New England Journal of Medicine*, vol. 325, no. 16, pp. 1117–1122, 1991.

[4] J. S. Hochman, J. Boland, L. A. Sleeper et al., "Current spectrum of cardiogenic shock and effect of early revascularisation on mortality: results of an international registry," *Circulation*, vol. 91, no. 3, pp. 873–881, 1995.

[5] J. S. Hochman, L. A. Sleeper, J. G. Webb et al., "Early revascularization in acute myocardial infarction complicated by cardiogenic shock," *The New England Journal of Medicine*, vol. 341, no. 9, pp. 625–634, 1999.

[6] R. Fincke, J. S. Hochman, A. M. Lowe et al., "Cardiac power is the strongest hemodynamic correlate of mortality in cardiogenic shock: a report from the SHOCK trial registry," *Journal of the American College of Cardiology*, vol. 44, no. 2, pp. 340–348, 2004.

[7] W. W. O'Neill, N. S. Kleiman, J. Moses et al., "A prospective, randomized clinical trial of hemodynamic support with Impella 2.5 versus intra-aortic balloon pump in patients undergoing high-risk percutaneous coronary intervention: the PROTECT II study," *Circulation*, vol. 126, no. 14, pp. 1717–1727, 2012.

[8] B. G. Leshnower, T. G. Gleason, M. L. O'Hara et al., "Safety and efficacy of left ventricular assist device support in post-myocardial infarction cardiogenic shock," *The Annals of Thoracic Surgery*, vol. 81, no. 4, pp. 1365–1371, 2006.

[9] P. R. Lawler, D. A. Silver, B. M. Scirica, G. S. Couper, G. L. Weinhouse, and P. C. Camp Jr, "Extracorporeal membrane oxygenation in adults with cardiogenic shock," *Circulation*, vol. 131, no. 7, pp. 676–680, 2015.

[10] L. C. Napp, C. Kühn, M. M. Hoeper et al., "Cannulation strategies for percutaneous extracorporeal membrane oxygenation in adults," *Clinical Research in Cardiology*, vol. 105, no. 4, pp. 283–296, 2016.

[11] R. A. Aqel, F. G. Hage, and A. E. Iskandrian, "Improvement of myocardial perfusion with a percutaneously inserted left ventricular assist device," *Journal of Nuclear Cardiology*, vol. 17, no. 1, pp. 158–160, 2010.

[12] M. Remmelink, K. D. Sjauw, J. P. S. Henriques et al., "Effects of left ventricular unloading by Impella recover LP 2.5 on coronary hemodynamics," *Catheterization and Cardiovascular Interventions*, vol. 70, no. 4, pp. 532–537, 2007.

[13] T. Tarvasmaki, J. Lassus, M. Varpula et al., "Current real-life use of vasopressors and inotropes in cardiogenic shock-adrenaline use is associated with excess organ injury and mortality," *Critical Care*, vol. 20, no. 1, p. 208, 2016.

[14] K. Nakamura S. Krishnan et al., "First-in-man percutaneous transaxillary artery placement and removal of the Impella 5.0 mechanical circulatory support device," *The Journal of Invasive Cardiology*, vol. 29, no. 5, pp. E53–E59, 2017.

[15] N. Kamioka, A. Patel, M. A. Burke, A. Greenbaum, and V. Babaliaros, "Biventricular Impella placement via complete venous access," *Catheterization and Cardiovascular Interventions*, 2017.

[16] W. M. Merhi, Z. G. Turi, S. Dixon, and R. D. Safian, "Percutaneous ex-vivo femoral arterial bypass: a novel approach for treatment of acute limb ischemia as a complication of femoral arterial catheterization," *Catheterization and Cardiovascular Interventions*, vol. 68, no. 3, pp. 435–440, 2006.

[17] L. Kizner, C. Flottmann, D. Horstkotte, and J. Gummert, "Bilateral antegrade perfusion of the superficial femoral artery to prevent limb ischaemia during combined use of Impella CP left ventricular assist device and extracorporeal life support," *Interactive Cardiovascular and Thoracic Surgery*, vol. 23, no. 2, pp. 335–337, 2016.

[18] R. Korabathina, K. S. Heffernan, V. Paruchuri et al., "The pulmonary artery pulsatility index identifies severe right ventricular dysfunction in acute inferior myocardial infarction," *Catheterization and Cardiovascular Interventions*, vol. 80, no. 4, pp. 593–600, 2012.

[19] A. Lala, Y. Guo, J. Xu et al., "Right ventricular dysfunction in acute myocardial infarction complicated by cardiogenic shock: a hemodynamic analysis of the Should We Emergently Revascularize Occluded Coronaries for Cardiogenic Shock (SHOCK) Trial and Registry," *Journal of Cardiac Failure*, vol. 24, no. 3, pp. 148–156, 2018.

[20] C. Erdal, G. Karakülah, E. Fermancı et al., "Early biventricular molecular responses to an acute myocardial infarction," *International Journal of Medical Sciences*, vol. 9, no. 1, pp. 74–82, 2012.

[21] R. Bussani, A. Abbate, G. G. L. Biondi-Zoccai et al., "Right ventricular dilatation after left ventricular acute myocardial infarction is predictive of extremely high peri-infarctual apoptosis at postmortem examination in humans," *Journal of Clinical Pathology*, vol. 56, no. 9, pp. 672–676, 2003.

[22] D. J. Farrar, P. G. Compton, J. J. Hershon, J. D. Fonger, and J. D. Hill, "Right heart interaction with the mechanically assisted left heart," *World Journal of Surgery*, vol. 9, no. 1, pp. 89–102, 1985.

[23] M. R. Moon, A. F. Bolger, A. DeAnda et al., "Septal function during left ventricular unloading," *Circulation*, vol. 95, no. 5, pp. 1320–1327, 1997.

[24] J. A. Morgan, G. Paone, H. W. Nemeh et al., "Impact of continuous-flow left ventricular assist device support on right ventricular function," *The Journal of Heart and Lung Transplantation*, vol. 32, no. 4, pp. 398–403, 2013.

[25] K. Krishan, A. Nair, S. Pinney, D. H. Adams, and A. C. Anyanwu, "Liberal use of tricuspid-valve annuloplasty during left-ventricular assist device implantation," *European Journal of Cardio-Thoracic Surgery*, vol. 41, no. 1, pp. 213–217, 2012.

[26] B. C. Lampert and J. J. Teuteberg, "Right ventricular failure after left ventricular assist devices," *The Journal of Heart and Lung Transplantation*, vol. 34, no. 9, pp. 1123–1130, 2015.

[27] M. B. Anderson, J. Goldstein, C. Milano et al., "Benefits of a novel percutaneous ventricular assist device for right heart failure: the prospective RECOVER RIGHT study of the Impella RP device," *The Journal of Heart and Lung Transplantation*, vol. 34, no. 12, pp. 1549–1560, 2015.

[28] S. Kuchibotla, M. L. Esposito, C. Breton et al., "Acute biventricular mechanical circulatory support for cardiogenic shock," *Journal of the American Heart Association*, vol. 6, article e006670, 2017.

[29] M. S. Koeckert, U. P. Jorde, Y. Naka, J. W. Moses, and H. Takayama, "Impella LP 2.5 for left ventricular unloading

during venoarterial extracorporeal membrane oxygenation support," *Journal of Cardiac Surgery*, vol. 26, no. 6, pp. 666–668, 2011.

[30] S. V. Chaparro, A. Badheka, G. R. Marzouka et al., "Combined use of Impella left ventricular assist device and extracorporeal membrane oxygenation as a bridge to recovery in fulminant myocarditis," *ASAIO Journal*, vol. 58, no. 3, pp. 285–287, 2012.

[31] M. Jumean, D. T. Pham, and N. K. Kapur, "Percutaneous bi-atrial extracorporeal membrane oxygenation for acute circulatory support in advanced heart failure," *Catheterization and Cardiovascular Interventions*, vol. 85, no. 6, pp. 1097–1099, 2015.

39

Key Role of Left Atrial Appendage during Redo Ablation in a Case of Long-Standing Persistent Atrial Fibrillation

Shaohui Wu,[1] Guangchen Zou,[2] Xu Liu,[1] Weifeng Jiang,[1] Mu Qin,[1] and Daoliang Zhang[1]

[1]*Shanghai Chest Hospital, Shanghai Jiao Tong University, Shanghai, China*
[2]*Danbury Hospital, Danbury, Connecticut, USA*

Correspondence should be addressed to Guangchen Zou; kenzou@outlook.com

Academic Editor: Assad Movahed

Extrapulmonary vein focal sources have been recognized as the source of atrial fibrillation in some cases, and empiric electric isolation of the left atrial appendage has been proposed for long-standing persistent atrial fibrillation by some. Here, we present a case of redo ablation of long-standing persistent atrial fibrillation in which the left atrial appendage played a key role in maintaining AF during ablation, and atrial fibrillation was terminated by electrical isolation of the LAA. During the ablation, a rare phenomenon of half of the atria in atrial fibrillation while the other half of the atria in atrial flutter was seen.

1. Introduction

The role of focal sources in the initiation and maintenance of atrial fibrillation (AF) have been well recognized, with pulmonary veins (PV) being the most common location of these foci [1]. PV isolation (PVI) is now the cornerstone of catheter ablation for AF [2]. However, PV isolation alone cannot maintain sinus rhythm in many patients, especially in patients with long-standing persistent AF (LSPAF) [3]. So far, extra-PV focal sources maintaining AF have been reported in the superior and inferior vena cava [4, 5], coronary sinus [6], ligament of Marshall [7], crista terminalis, and posterior left atrium [8]. Takashi and colleagues have reported a case of paroxysmal AF originating from a focus localized to the left atrial appendage (LAA) [9]. Here, we present a case of redo ablation of LSPAF in which the LAA played a key role during ablation and AF was terminated by electrical isolation of the LAA.

2. Case Report

A 61-year-old male with LSPAF was referred to our center for repeat catheter ablation. He had previously undergone catheter ablation for persistent AF 12 years ago during which PVI, linear ablations (LA roof line and mitral isthmus line), and complex fractionated atrial electrogram (CFAE) ablations were done. He was in sinus rhythm on follow-up at 3 months and 1 year but was then lost to follow-up. He was again in AF 2 years ago and was referred again to our center for redo ablation.

During the ablation procedure, reconnection sites were ablated and PVI was again achieved. Gaps in the mitral isthmus line were ablated. During CFAE ablation on the LA anterior wall (red circle in Figures 1 and 2), AF terminated to atrial flutter on the coronary sinus (CS) lead (cycle length 330 ms, earliest in CS 9, 10). Activation mapping of the LA and right atrium (RA) showed atrial flutter on the anterior and posterior walls of the LA as well as the RA (cycle length 330 ms, earliest in CS 9,10), but AF in the LAA and surrounding atrial area (marked as pink in Figure 1, average cycle length 150 ms). Activation mapping showed the mechanism of the atrial flutter to be focal (Figure 2. Atrial activation spanning was 145 ms, less than one-half of the cycle length of the atrial flutter, and earliest on the left side of the atrial septum. A line of double potentials (green dots in Figure 2, from the basal LAA to the right PV antrum) with a gap in the middle can be mapped on the anterior wall of the LA. The gap was the area of earliest activation. Radiofrequency energy (35 W, 3 seconds, saline irrigation 25 ml/min) delivery at the gap area terminated the atrial flutter. On repeat mapping of the LA, sinus rhythm

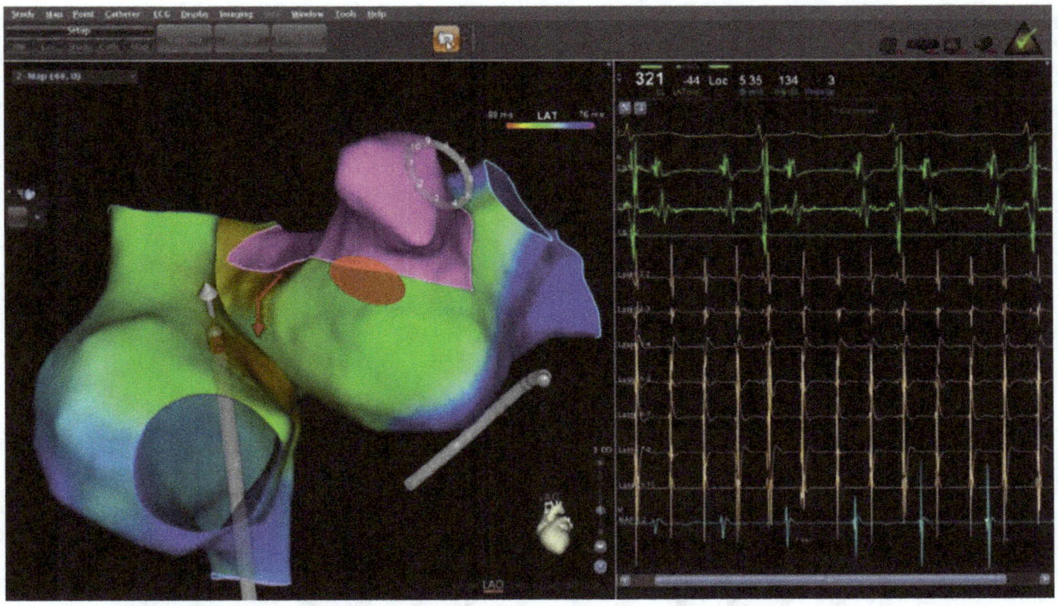

FIGURE 1: Activation mapping of the LA and RA. The LAA and surrounding area is in AF (pink, average cycle length 150 ms); the rest of the atria including the anterior and lateral walls of the LA, the interatrial septum, and the RA are in atrial flutter (cycle length 330 ms, earliest in CS 9, 10). Red circle marked the area ablated during CFAE ablation.

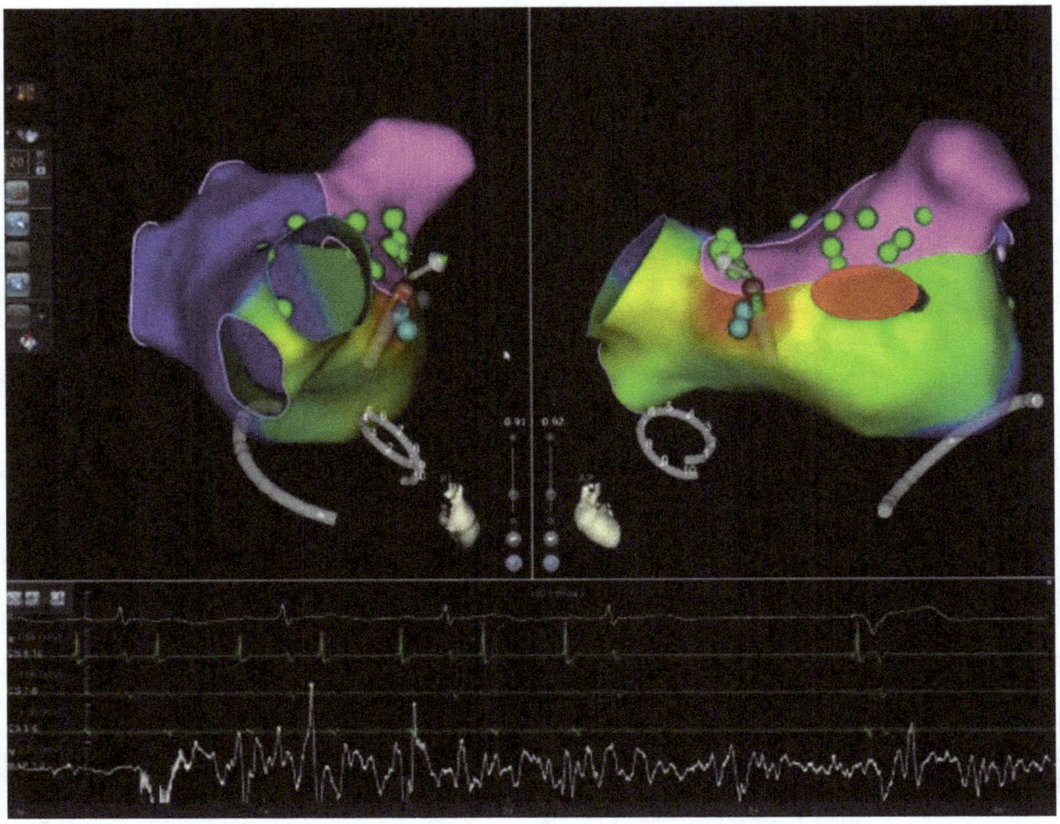

FIGURE 2: Termination of the atrial flutter. Activation mapping showed the mechanism of the atrial flutter to be focal (atrial activation spanning 145 ms, less than one-half of the cycle length of the atrial flutter, which was 330 ms); the earliest point of activation is on the left side of the interatrial septum. A linear area of double potentials with a gap in the middle can be seen from the base of the LAA to the right PV antrum (green dots). The gap is the area of the earliest activation. Radiofrequency energy delivery at the gap (35 W, 3 seconds) terminated the atrial flutter. A paced signal can also be seen from the temporary pacemaker inserted for protection during the procedure. Red circle marked the area ablated during CFAE ablation.

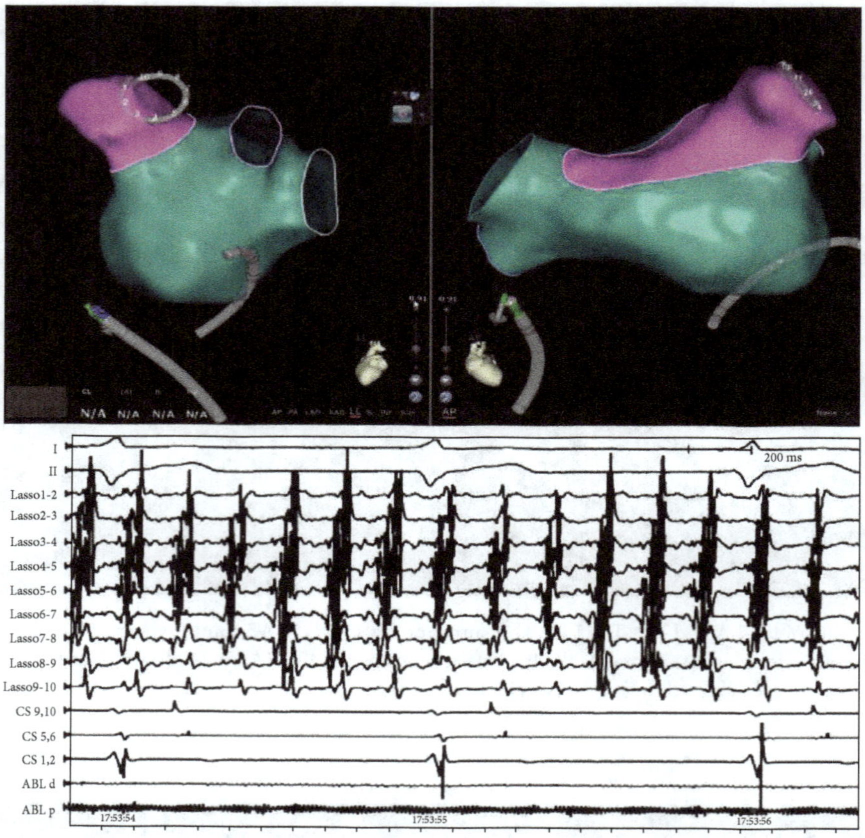

FIGURE 3: Activation mapping and intracardiac electrograms showing the LAA and surrounding area in AF (pink on activation map, lasso in the LAA) while the rest of the atria (green on the activation map) was in sinus rhythm.

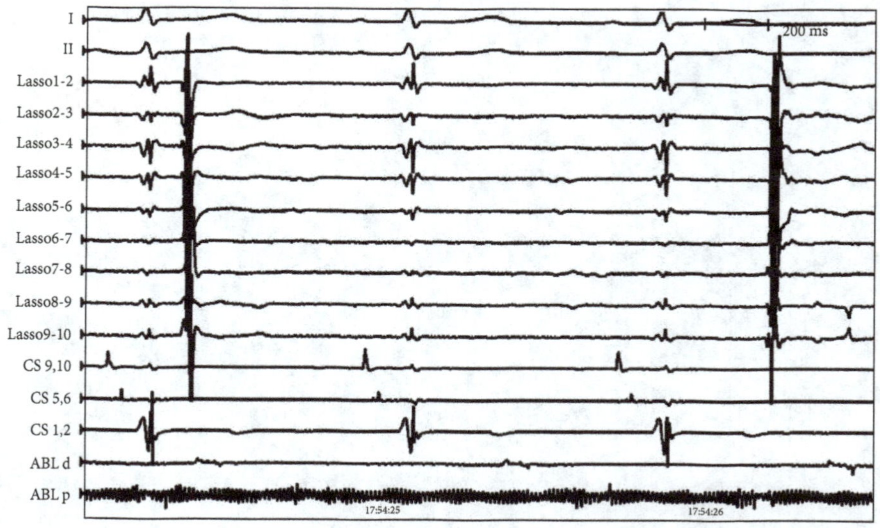

FIGURE 4: Intracardiac electrograms showing slow spontaneous potentials within the LAA after LAA electrical isolation (lasso in the LAA, no cardioversion done).

can be seen in most of the LA while the LAA and its surrounding area remained in AF (pink area in Figure 3). As the anterior LA line was being drawn, with the lasso in the LAA, the potential in the LAA can be observed to slow down and then disconnect from the rest of the atrium (Figure 4). After observation of 30 seconds, there was no reconnection of the LAA to the rest of the LA.

The patient was discharged on no antiarrhythmic medication and was anticoagulated with rivaroxaban. On follow-up, he remained in sinus rhythm 9 months after ablation.

3. Discussion

To our knowledge, this is one of the first detailed reports of a redo ablation of LSPAF in which the LAA played a key role in maintaining the AF during ablation and AF was terminated with LAA electrical isolation. A rare phenomenon of half of the atrium in AF while the other half was in atrial flutter was also seen during the procedure.

PVI is the well-recognized cornerstone for AF catheter ablation, but pulmonary vein isolation alone is often insufficient to maintain sinus rhythm, especially in patients with LSPAF. Various additional ablations including linear and CFAE ablations have not consistently been shown to be superior in clinical trials.

Takashi and colleagues first reported a case of paroxysmal AF treated successfully with LAA isolation in 2005. Di Biase and colleagues then reported in 2010 that LAA firing can be seen in as much as 27% of patients presenting for repeat ablation of AF, and LAA electrical isolation can decrease AF recurrence in these patients [10]. Later in the BELIEF trial, Di Biase and colleagues reported that in patients with LSPAF, empirical electrical isolation of the LAA for both initial ablation, and redo procedure improved long-term freedom from atrial arrhythmias without increasing complications [11].

Though no increase in thrombotic events were seen in the BELIEF study, there are concerns for increased thrombus formation in an electrically isolated LAA and some have reported a higher rate of stroke or TIA after LAA electric isolation [12]. Therefore, long-term anticoagulation is very important if LAA isolation was done during the ablation. Another possible way to mitigate the risk of thrombus formation in an electrically isolated LAA is LAA occlusion. Indeed, the WATCH-Rhythm trial is ongoing to investigate combining AF ablation with LAA electric isolation and LAA closure with a WATCHMAN device in a single procedure.

Other concerns about LAA electric isolation include technical difficulties due to the relative thick tissues at the base of LAA which may cause reconnection after isolation and the thin tissues in some areas of LAA which may make accidental perforation more likely [13, 14].

Our case showed that LAA isolation can be essential for selecting patient presenting for redo ablation of LSPAF. In the era of individualized AF ablation, we feel it is reasonable to do routine careful mapping of the LAA during ablation for LSPAF and isolate the LAA if mapping indicates that LAA is involved in the maintenance of AF.

References

[1] M. Haïssaguerre, P. Jaïs, D. C. Shah et al., "Spontaneous initiation of atrial fibrillation by ectopic beats originating in the pulmonary veins," *The New England Journal of Medicine*, vol. 339, no. 10, pp. 659–666, 1998.

[2] H. Calkins, G. Hindricks, R. Cappato et al., "2017 HRS/EHRA/ECAS/APHRS/SOLAECE expert consensus statement on catheter and surgical ablation of atrial fibrillation: executive summary," *Europace*, vol. 20, no. 1, pp. 157–208, 2018.

[3] A. G. Brooks, M. K. Stiles, J. Laborderie et al., "Outcomes of long-standing persistent atrial fibrillation ablation: a systematic review," *Heart Rhythm*, vol. 7, no. 6, pp. 835–846, 2010.

[4] C. Scavée, P. Jaïs, R. Weerasooriya, and M. Haïssaguerre, "The inferior vena Cava:," *Journal of Cardiovascular Electrophysiology*, vol. 14, no. 6, pp. 659–662, 2003.

[5] C. F. Tsai, C. T. Tai, M. H. Hsieh et al., "Initiation of atrial fibrillation by ectopic beats originating from the superior vena cava: electrophysiological characteristics and results of radiofrequency ablation," *Circulation*, vol. 102, no. 1, pp. 67–74, 2000.

[6] M. Rotter, P. Sanders, Y. Takahashi et al., "Coronary sinus tachycardia driving atrial fibrillation," *Circulation*, vol. 110, no. 6, pp. e59–e60, 2004.

[7] C. Hwang, T. J. Wu, R. N. Doshi, C. T. Peter, and P. S. Chen, "Vein of Marshall cannulation for the analysis of electrical activity in patients with focal atrial fibrillation," *Circulation*, vol. 101, no. 13, pp. 1503–1505, 2000.

[8] W.-S. Lin, C.-T. Tai, M.-H. Hsieh et al., "Catheter ablation of paroxysmal atrial fibrillation initiated by non-pulmonary vein ectopy," *Circulation*, vol. 107, no. 25, pp. 3176–3183, 2003.

[9] Y. Takahashi, P. Sanders, M. Rotter, and M. Haïssaguerre, "Disconnection of the left atrial appendage for elimination of foci maintaining atrial fibrillation," *Journal of Cardiovascular Electrophysiology*, vol. 16, no. 8, pp. 917–919, 2005.

[10] L. Di Biase, J. D. Burkhardt, P. Mohanty et al., "Left atrial Appendage," *Circulation*, vol. 122, no. 2, pp. 109–118, 2010.

[11] L. Di Biase, J. D. Burkhardt, P. Mohanty et al., "Left atrial appendage isolation in patients with longstanding persistent AF undergoing catheter ablation: BELIEF trial," *Journal of the American College of Cardiology*, vol. 68, no. 18, pp. 1929–1940, 2016.

[12] Y. G. Kim, J. Shim, S.-K. Oh, K.-N. Lee, J.-I. Choi, and Y.-H. Kim, "Electrical isolation of the left atrial appendage increases the risk of ischemic stroke and transient ischemic attack regardless of postisolation flow velocity," *Heart Rhythm*, vol. 15, no. 12, pp. 1746–1753, 2018.

[13] J. Whitaker, S. Panikker, T. Fastl et al., "Cardiac CT assessment of tissue thickness at the ostium of the left atrial appendage predicts acute success of radiofrequency ablation," *Pacing and Clinical Electrophysiology*, vol. 40, no. 11, pp. 1218–1226, 2017.

[14] U. Barbero and S. Y. Ho, "Anatomy of the atria," *Herzschrittmachertherapie + Elektrophysiologie*, vol. 28, no. 4, pp. 347–354, 2017.

40

Atrioventricular Conduction Disorders as a Complication of Inferior ST Elevation Myocardial Infarction in Patients with COVID-19 Infection

Yaser Alahmad, Hassan Al-Tamimi, Fadi Khazaal, Mawahib Elhassan, Abdulrahman Arabi, Jassim Al Suwaidi, Awad AlQahtani, and Nidal Asaad

Hamad Medical Corporation, Heart Hospital, Doha, Qatar

Correspondence should be addressed to Yaser Alahmad; yalahmad@hamad.qa

Academic Editor: May Binjumah

This case series demonstrates how COVID-19 infection might affect the heart in the context of acute myocardial infarction. Atrioventricular (AV) block might appear as one of the significant cardiac complications of acute MI in patients who tested COVID-19 PCR positive regardless of the presence of CVOID-19 infection symptoms. In our series, conduction disorders as a complication of acute inferior STEMI are more common in patients who tested positive for the COVID-19 infection. 11 patients out of 18 inferior STEMI patients who have tested positive for the COVID-19 infection have atrioventricular block disorders.

1. Introduction

Coronavirus disease 2019 (COVID-19) is a viral infectious disease caused by severe acute respiratory syndrome coronavirus 2 (SARS-CoV-2). It first emerged in Wuhan, China, in December 2019 [1].

Multiple studies have shown that elders, especially those with chronic underlying diseases, including chronic pulmonary disease, heart diseases, and diabetes mellitus, are more susceptible to COVID-19 complications [2]. Various types of complications with different prevalence have been reported in literature consisting of neurologic [3], hematologic (including coagulative disorders) [4], hepatic [5], renal [6], and finally cardiovascular complications [7].

Multiple studies have shown both increased susceptibility in patients with underlying cardiovascular disease to COVID-19 and severe cardiovascular complications in COVID-19 infected patients, including acute myocardial injury, thrombotic events, arrhythmias, and shock with challenges in acute management [8, 9, 10].

The type and severity of atrioventricular (AV) block associated with COVID-19 have not been described. We aimed to evaluate the incidence of the AV block as a complication, angiographic findings, and clinical outcome in the setting of acute inferior STEMI in patients with COVID-19 infection. We noted that the incidence of atrioventricular block as one of the complications of acute inferior STEMI is higher in patients who were tested as COVID-19 positive versus COVID-19 negative cases.

COVID-19 infection was confirmed with reverse transcription-polymerase chain reaction assays (PCR). Inferior STEMI was defined based on the presence of typical cardiac symptoms associated with at least 1 mm ST-segment elevation in inferior leads.

A total of 44 patients were admitted with acute inferior STEMI between May 1, 2020 and June 15, 2020. All patients met the definition criteria of STEMI with localized ST-elevation, and all were treated in the setting of emergent activation. 18 patients (40.9%) had tested positive for the COVID-19 infection, while 26 patients (59.1%) had tested negative for the COVID-19 infection (59.1%). No complications related to atrioventricular conduction disorders were documented in non-COVID-19 infection patients who presented with acute inferior STEMI (0%). While 11 out of 18 positive COVID-19 infection patients had atrioventricular block (AV) disorders (61%), 8 patients had a high degree of atrioventricular block (44.5%), and 3 patients developed first-degree AV block (16.6%). Although all patients shared the same basic characteristics, including age, gender, race, demographic distribution, and risk factors, conduction disorders were significantly higher in inferior STEMI with positive COVID-19 infection tests.

In this special case series, we are going to present all cases of high-degree atrioventricular block (AV) and one of the three cases of first-degree AV block as the one with the longest PR interval. Table 1 demonstrates the summary of the case series.

This data was collected from Qatar cardiovascular COVID-19 registries. It was approved by the Institutional Review Board in Hamad Medical Corporation, and all performed procedures were following institutional guidelines and recommendations. Due to the nature of the study, written informed consent was not required. The authors declare that all supporting data are available within the article.

2. Case 1

A 48-year-old male complained of chest pain associated with dizziness, subsequently, he shortly lost consciousness and injured his face. He was taken by his colleagues to the peripheral hospital, upon arrival, he was bradycardic and hypotensive, but he was conscious, and both bradycardia and hypotension responded well to IV fluid and atropine. 12 leads electrocardiography (ECG) showed acute inferior STEMI complicated with 3 : 1 high-grade atrioventricular (AV) block (Figure 1(a)). He was transferred by EMS service to the hospital. CT scan of the head revealed no evidence of acute neurologic insult. Urgent coronary angiography showed a heavily thrombotic occlusion of proximal to mid right coronary artery (RCA). Thrombus aspiration was performed, then drug-eluting stent (DES) was deployed successfully. The final TIMI flow was TIMI II flow due to distal microembolization (Figures 2(a) and 2(b)). AV block directly resolved after coronary intervention. COVID-19 PCR testing was initially inconclusive then it came positive without COVID-19 infection related symptoms.

3. Case 2

A 55-year-old male has type 2 diabetes mellitus. He was admitted as case of symptomatic upper urinary tract infection; while he was in the emergency unit, he developed severe chest pain associated with hypotension. ECG showed sinus rhythm with acute inferior STEMI and first-degree AV block, subsequently; he developed complete heart block with signs of RV involvement in serial ECGs (Figure 1(b)).

He underwent thrombus aspiration and successful primary percutaneous coronary intervention (PPCI) to severe thrombotic stenosis from proximal to mid-RCA with DES (Figures 2(c) and 2(d)). Besides DAPT and anti-ischemic medications, he received 24 IV eptifibatide infusion.

Advanced AV block was resolved after IV fluids and inotropes while transferring him to catheterization laboratory. COVID-19 PCR test came positive without COVID-19 infection related symptoms.

4. Case 3

A 57-year-old man without positive cardiac or medical history presented with severe chest pain for 2 hours associated with dizziness and sweating. He has no history of fever or cough, but he has a history of general weakness for one week prior to the current event. On admission, vital signs were remarkable for a blood pressure of 89/56 mmHg, heart rate of 30 bpm, and oxygen saturation at 90% on room air, which improved to 97% with a nonrebreather mask. Initial ECG demonstrated sinus bradycardia with third-degree AV block and ST-segment elevation in inferior leads (Figure 1(c)). Coronary angiography revealed severe three-vessel diseases with significant distal left main stem stenosis. An attempt with balloon angioplasty was done to the thrombotic stenosis in mid-RCA in PPCI setting, but TIMI III flow was not achieved due to severe diffuse disease in distal RCA (Figure 2(e)). A transcutaneous temporary pacemaker wire was inserted. Chest radiography (CXR) demonstrated bilateral pulmonary congestion with infiltration in the left midlung zone. Transthoracic echocardiography showed severe global dysfunction with left ventricle ejection fraction (LVEF) 23%.

The cardiothoracic team was involved in the early stage for possible CABG once his medical condition is allowed, but he developed SARS-CoV-2 pneumonia associated with multiorgan failure in the background of active cardiac ischemia, he was intubated, and he was started on inotropes along with SARS-CoV-2 antiviral agents. COVID-19 pneumonia made his hospital course very challenging with many complications related to SARS-CoV-2 pneumonia like acute respiratory failure, disseminated intravascular coagulation DIC, severe sepsis, and septic shock with a superimposed bacterial infection. AV block was recovered over one week of admission, but due to the significant multiorgan failure, he was arrested and died after 3 weeks of admission.

5. Case 4

A 45-year-old gentleman presented with chest pain for more than 24 hours. Initial ECG showed ST-segment elevation with deep Q waves in inferior leads, which represented late presentation inferior. When he arrived in coronary care unit (CCU), he was hemodynamically stable without chest pain, subsequently, telemetry showed episodes of escape junctional bradycardia, isorhythmic AV dissociation (Figure 1(d)). Subsequently, ECG showed complete heart block (CHB). Coronary angiography showed 100% thrombotic stenosis in distal left coronary circumflex LCX (single vessel disease). Successful PCI to distal LCx with one drug-eluting stent (DES) (Figures 2(f) and 2(g)). COVID-19 PCR test came positive without COVID-19 infection related symptoms.

Table 1: The case series summary including the presentation symptoms, coronary angiography, and ECG findings.

Patient	Presentation	PPCI is done in PPCI setting	Culprit coronary artery	Symptoms related to COVID-19 infection	The peak troponin T (ng/L)	Type of AV block	Specific treatment to AV block	Outcomes
1	Acute inferior STEMI	No	Right coronary artery (RCA)	None	11979	Mobitz 2 type 2 AV block	Atropine and urgent PCI	Recovered
2	Acute inferior STEMI with RV infarction	Yes	RCA	None	9740	Complete heart block	Dopamine and fluid	Recovered
3	Acute inferior STEMI	No	RCA	Severe COVID-19 pneumonia	9704	Complete heart block	Transvenous temporary pacing	Recovered patient died
4	Late inferior STEMI	No	Left coronary circumflex artery (LCX)	None	7226	Accelerated junctional bradycardia, isorhythmic AV dissociation, and complete heart block	Urgent PCI	Recovered
5	Acute inferior STEMI with RV infarction	Yes	RCA	None	3763	Complete heart block	Atropine	Recovered
6	Acute inferolateral STEMI	Yes	RCA	None	11926	Complete heart block	Atropine, transcutaneous temporary pacing, and PPCI	Recovered
7	Acute inferior STEMI	Yes	RCA	None	2320	Complete heart block	PPCI	Recovered
8	Acute inferior STEMI	Yes	RCA	None	12442	Complete heart block	Atropine	Recovered
9	Acute inferior STEMI	Yes	RCA	STEMI happened while he was in the quarantine	1112	First-degree AV block	PPCI	Recovered

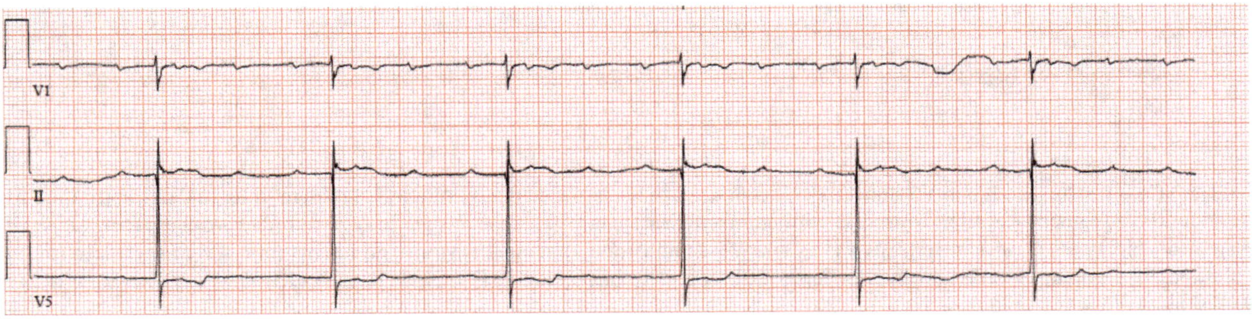

(a)

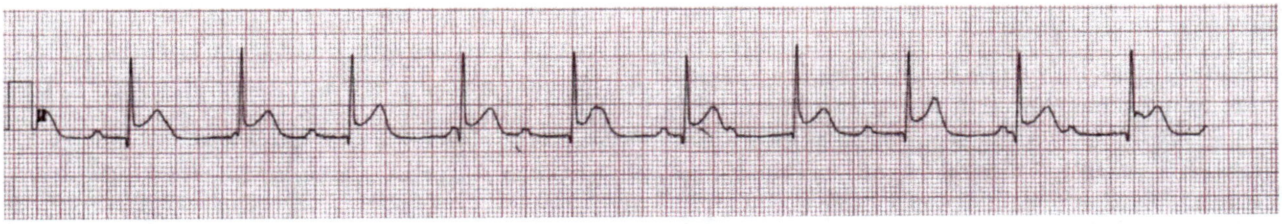

(b)

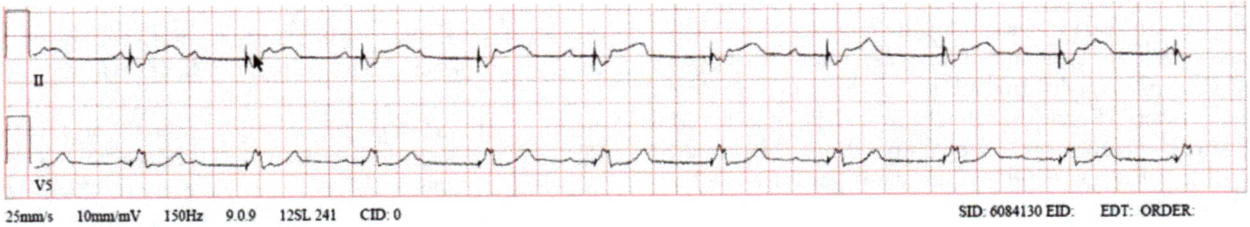

(c)

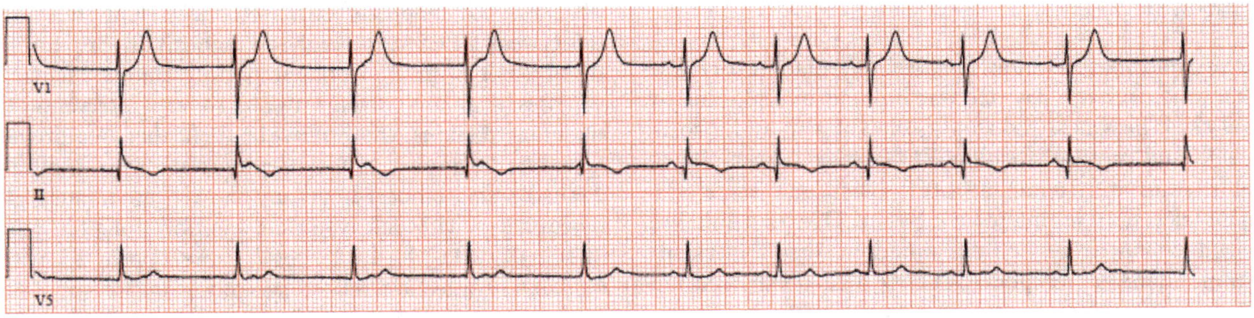

(d)

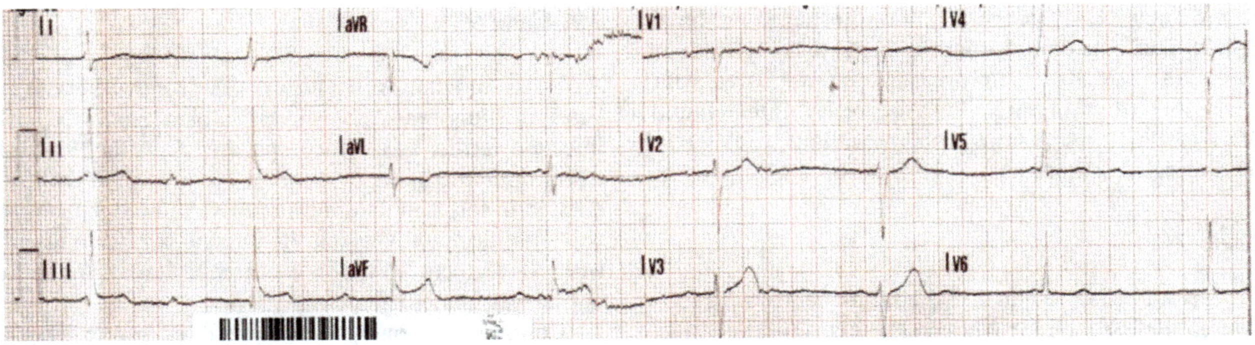

(e)

Figure 1: Continued.

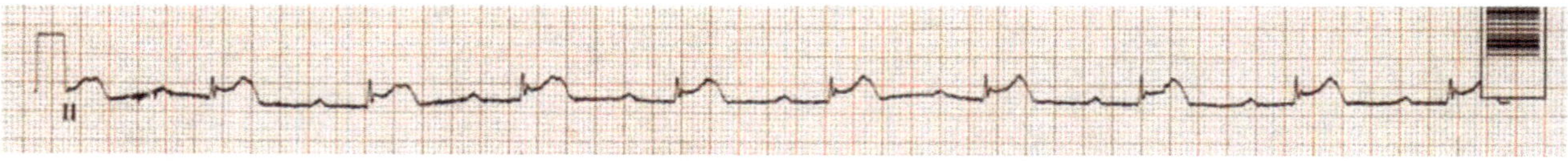

(f)

Figure 1: (a) Case 1: strip lead II and V5 showed significant sinus bradycardia 40 per minute with 3 : 1 high-grade AV block. (b) Case 2: strip lead II showed ST-segment elevation in lead II with complete heart block. (c) Case 3: strip lead II and V5 revealed pacing rhythm with complete heart block. (d) Case 4: strip leads V1, II, and V5 demonstrate junctional rhythm and isorhythmic AV dissociation. (e) Case 7: ECG showed ST-segment elevation in inferior leads with complete heart block. (f) Case 9: strip lead II shows ST segment with first-degree AV block PR = 340 milliseconds.

6. Case 5

A 50-year-old gentleman without significant medical history was brought by EMS with severe chest pain for 5 hours. Initial ECG showed ST-segment elevation in inferior leads with complete heart block which was resolved with 1 mg IV bolus atropine. Repeated ECG at emergency room still showed acute inferior STEMI with new right ventricular infarction.

Urgent coronary angiography demonstrated moderate stenosis in left anterior descending (LAD) and left circumflex (LCX) and totally thrombotic occlusion of midright coronary artery. Successful PPCI to mid-RCA with DES deployment without immediate complications (Figures 2(h) and 2(i)). COVID-19 PCR test came positive without COVID-19 infection related symptoms.

7. Case 6

A 36-year-old male without significant cardiac history is a smoker, one pack per day. He was brought by EMS due to central chest heaviness radiated to the left arm and associated with and profuse sweating. ECG showed escape junctional rhythm with complete heart block and acute ST-segment elevation in inferolateral leads. He was initially managed with atropine, IV fluid, noradrenaline IV infusion, and transcutaneous temporary pacing then transferred for PPCI.

Coronary angiography revealed 100% thrombotic stenosis in proximal RCA. Successful PPCI to ostial to proximal RCA with DES was done without immediate complications (Figures 3(a) and 3(b))). Bradycardia was improved with normal sinus rhythm after RCA coronary intervention. COVID-19 PCR test came positive without COVID-19 infection related symptoms.

8. Case 7

A 52-year-old male presented to the health center with sudden onset of chest pain for 2 hours. He was clinically stable, heart rate at 43 per minute, and blood pressure at 120/80 mmHg. Initial ECG showed sinus bradycardia, and ST-segment elevation in inferior leads associated with third-degree AV block (Figure 1(e)). He was given 300 mg aspirin, 300 mg clopidogrel, 30 mcg IV fentanyl, and 250 ml bolus of normal saline and then transferred to the heart center for PPCI. Coronary angiography revealed severe thrombotic stenosis in the mid-RCA; subsequently, thrombus aspiration was done, followed by successful DES deployment. The final TIMI flow was III (Figures 3(c) and 3(d)). COVID-19 PCR test came positive without COVID-19 infection related symptoms.

9. Case 8

A 49-year-old man with a history of hypertension presented with severe chest pain for 3 hours. He denies any history of fever or cough. Initial ECG demonstrated sinus rhythm with ST-segment elevation in inferior leads. On the way to the cath lab room, he developed hypotension and sinus bradycardia with complete heart block, which was responded to one dose of IV atropine 0.5 mg and IV fluid. Coronary angiography revealed severe three-vessel diseases with moderate distal left main stem stenosis. He underwent PPCI to thrombotic stenosis in proximal and distal RCA with 2 overlapping drug-eluting stents DES (Figures 3(e) and 3(f)). After coronary intervention, he maintained sinus rhythm without further requirements. Chest radiography (CXR) demonstrated no infiltration. Transthoracic echocardiography showed moderately global dysfunction with left ventricle ejection fraction (LVEF) 38%. COVID-19 PCR test came positive without COVID-19 infection related symptoms.

10. Case 9

A 57-year-old man with a history of uncontrolled type 2 diabetes mellitus was recently discharged from COVID-19 infection facility as a noncomplicated COVID-19 infection to continue the home quarantine. He presented with severe chest pain for 3 hours duration. ECG showed sinus rhythm with first-degree AV block PR interval of 340 milliseconds with ST-segment elevation in inferior leads (Figure 1(f)), but he was hemodynamically stable.

Coronary angiography demonstrated severe large burden thrombotic stenosis in mid-RCA, thrombus aspiration was done, followed by successful PPCI to the mid-RCA with 2 overlapping DES without immediate complications (Figures 3(g) and 3(h)).

First-degree AV block showed gradual regression and PR interval normalized during the stay in COVID-19 infection facility.

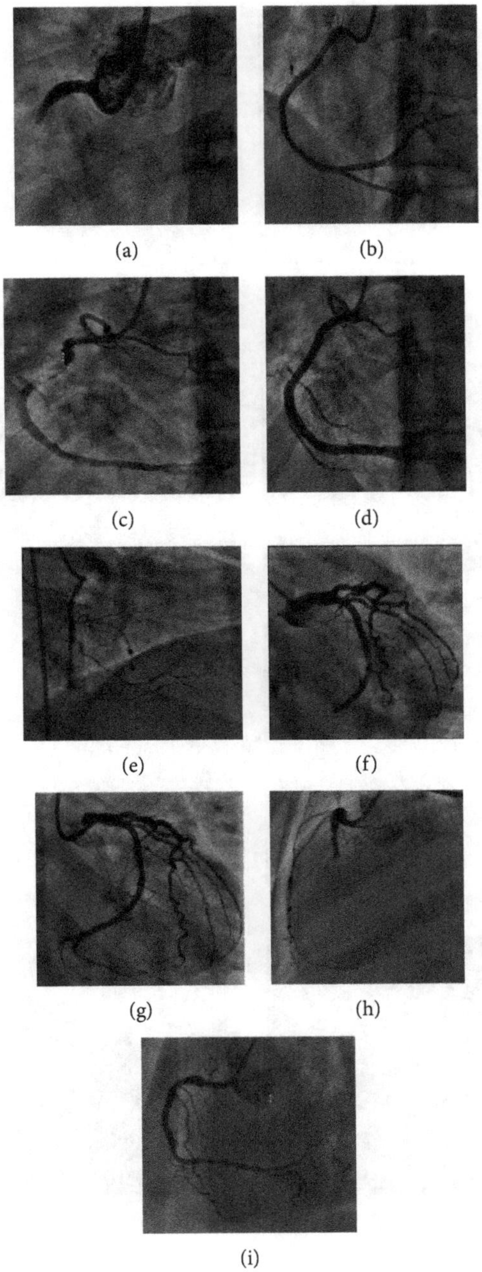

FIGURE 2: Coronary angiography to the culprit lesion. Case 1: (a) left anterior oblique (LAO) projection for right coronary artery (RCA), a thrombotic occlusion to proximal segment; (b) successful PCI to RCA with drug-eluting stent DES, and distal microembolization to very distal RCA happened with TIMI II flow distally. Case 2: (c) left anterior oblique (LAO) projection for right coronary artery (RCA) severe thrombotic stenosis in the proximal segment with TIMI II flow; (d) successful thrombus aspiration and PCI was done to RCA with one drug-eluting stent DES, and TIMI III flow was achieved. Case 3: (e) an attempt with balloon angioplasty was done to the thrombotic stenosis in mid-RCA but failed to achieve TIMI III flow. Case 4: (f) caudal projection showing 100% thrombotic stenosis in distal left coronary circumflex LCx; (g) successful PCI to distal LCx with one drug-eluting stent (DES) with TIMI III flow. Case 5: (h) total mid-RCA occlusion; (i) successful PCI to mid-RCA with one DES insertion.

11. Discussion

Atrioventricular blocks are relatively common as a complication of acute myocardial ischemia; despite the marked improvements in the management of acute coronary syndromes, complete (AV) block can still be seen in the context of acute myocardial infarction (MI), especially inferior STEMIs.

The incidence rates of third-degree AV block in patients with inferior/posterior wall AMI were twice compared with patients with anterior wall AMI. Third-degree AV block in context of acute inferior wall STEMI is usually transient, supra-Hisian in origin, narrow QRS escape junctional rhythm, and usually the risk of mortality is low. Anterior wall infarctions, on the other hand, are usually infra-Hisian, have a wide QRS escape rhythm, and carry a much higher

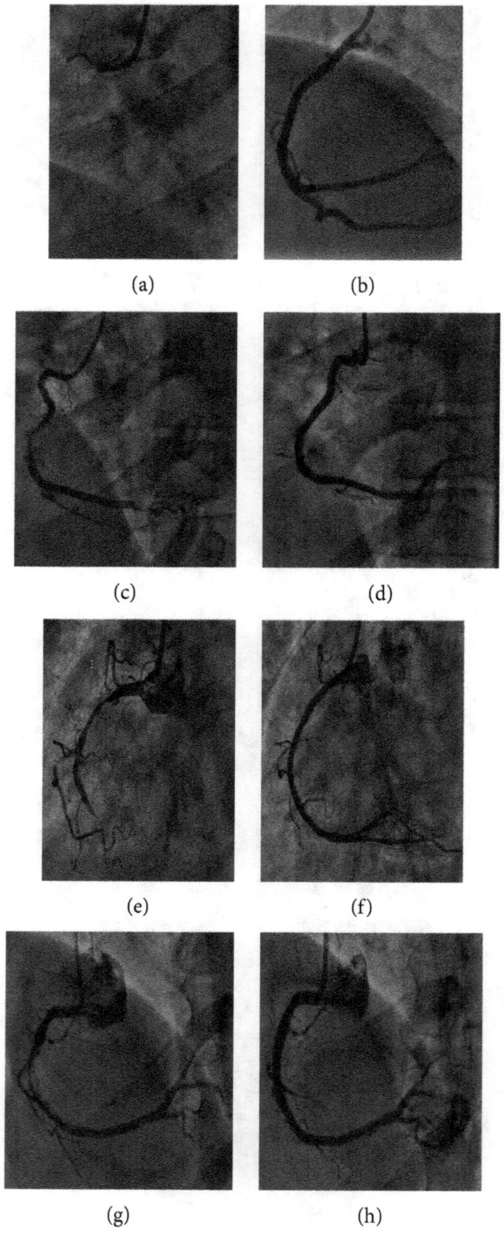

FIGURE 3: Coronary angiography to the culprit lesion. Case 6: (a) complete thrombotic occlusion in the very proximal segment of right coronary artery (RCA) with TIMI 0 flow; (b) successful PCI to proximal to mid-RCA with one drug-eluting stent DES, and TIMI III flow was achieved. Case 7: (c) severe thrombotic stenosis in mid-RCA with complete occlusion in the distal part due to distal embolization from the proximal thrombotic lesion; (d) successful thrombus aspiration and PCI to mid-RCA with one DES, and TIMI III flow was achieved distally. Case 8: (e) left anterior oblique (LAO) projection for right coronary artery (RCA) showed severe stenosis in the proximal segment followed by thrombotic occlusion from mid to distal RCA segment; (f) successful PCI to the proximal and distal RCA with 2 drug-eluting stent DES, and TIMI III flow was achieved. Case 9: (g) severe thrombotic stenosis in mid-RCA segment with TIMI III flow, a large thrombus burden in mid-RCA; (h) successful thrombus aspiration and PCI to RCA with 2 overlapping drug-eluting stent DES, and TIMI III flow was achieved.

mortality rate because of the wide extension of myocardial damage [11].

In the prethrombolytic era, both Goldberg RJ et al. and Rathore SS et al. reported that the overall incidence of second- or third-degree AV block was recorded in 5% to 7% of patients presenting with acute MI [12, 13] and reached 28% in those with acute inferior STEMI [14]. In the thrombolytic era, no significant change in the rate of incidences of second- or third-degree AV block. It was recorded in 6.9% of patients presenting with acute inferior STEMI [15].

In the current modern era of primary percutaneous coronary intervention, the incidence and in-hospital mortality rate of complete atrioventricular block in patients with STEMI who underwent primary PCI was reduced compared to the data from the thrombolytic era, and the incidence of complete atrioventricular block (CAVB) dropped to 3.2 and 4.6% [16] and 3.2% [17] in 2 separate studies. The risk factors of CAVB are age, worse Killip class at presentation, female sex, smoking, hypertension, and diabetes [16.17].

COVID-19 outbreak has introduced new clinical and logistical challenges in the treatment of STEMI and related complications. We still have no clue about conduction abnormalities as one of the complications of STEMI in patients who tested positive for the COVID-19 infection regardless of COVID-19 infection symptoms.

All patients who presented with inferior MI without evidence of viral infection did not develop any type of atrioventricular block, while all documented cases with complications related to conduction abnormalities in the settings of inferior MI have tested positive for the COVID-19 infection.

The factors that can stand behind the high incidence of AV block (61%) are theoretically due to:

(1) Some STEMI patients were presented to the hospital later than usual; this could be due to the new policies that took place over the country to minimize the risk of COVID infection transmission and spread like the lockdown areas

(2) Patient fears of getting the COVID-19 infection if they seek medical help, assuming that the risk of infection is higher in places that provide health care like hospitals. It is known that stress and anxiety can trigger cardiovascular problems like heart attacks. It is no doubt that the COVID-19 outbreak carries lots of social and financial negative impacts that could lead to an increase in the risk of cardiovascular events and related complications in general

(3) The COVID-19 infection itself might be associated with larger MI extension, high burden clots, and more active inflammatory process, which can be measured by elevated CRP, ferritin, and IL6

(4) High burden clots also could be a potential factor. Four patients (22%) underwent thrombus aspiration despite the current international guidelines do not support the routine thrombus aspiration in the context of acute STEMI. It is worldwide accepted that thromboembolic events and pulmonary embolism are common in very critical COVID-19 patients. Most of the current regimens encourage the use of anticoagulation as part of management protocols with antiviral agents, especially in the high-risk patients [18]

We also noted that patient's age was lower than what was watched previously in Meine et al. study [15] even all of them were male with lower Killip class at presentation. In most cases, AV block recovered with conservative or invasive treatments, and only one patient required a transvenous temporary pacemaker.

Only one patient (less than 1% of the total) died because of multiorgan failure caused by COVID-19 infection complications in the context of acute inferior STEMI.

12. Conclusion

Based on our findings, the incidence of atrioventricular blocks is higher than the incidence of AV block even in the prethrombolytic era. In almost 24 months of COVID-19 outbreaks worldwide, we are still lacking understanding of the aspects of COVID-19 behavior. While more recent studies provide more details of how the infection invades body organs in general, the cardiac manifestations of COVID-19 infections are still unclear, especially those related to the conduction system. The higher rate of patients with inferior STEMI who tested positive for COVID-19 infection developed conduction system abnormalities, even double the incidence of such a complication in the prethrombolytic era. Further studies with larger numbers are recommended to clarify why the incidence of AV blocks is higher in COVID-19 infection patients.

References

[1] "COVID-19 dashboard by the Center for Systems Science Engineering (CSSE) at Johns Hopkins University (JHU)," 2020, https://www.arcgis.com/apps/opsdashboard/index.html#/bda7594740fd40299423467b48e9ecf6.

[2] L. Pan, M. Mu, P. Yang et al., "Clinical characteristics of COVID-19 patients with digestive symptoms in Hubei, China: a descriptive, cross-sectional, multicenter study," *The American Journal Of Gastroenterology*, vol. 115, no. 5, pp. 766–773, 2020.

[3] A. Filatov, P. Sharma, F. Hindi, and P. S. Espinosa, "Neurological complications of coronavirus disease (COVID-19): encephalopathy," *Cureus*, vol. 12, no. 3, article e7352, 2020.

[4] E. Terpos, I. Ntanasis-Stathopoulos, I. Elalamy et al., "Hematological findings and complications of COVID-19," *American Journal of Hematology*, vol. 95, no. 7, pp. 834–847, 2020.

[5] C. Zhang, L. Shi, and F. S. Wang, "Liver injury in COVID-19: management and challenges," *The Lancet Gastroenterology & Hepatology*, vol. 5, no. 5, pp. 428–430, 2020.

[6] Y. Cheng, R. Luo, K. Wang et al., "Kidney disease is associated with in-hospital death of patients with COVID-19," *Kidney International*, vol. 97, no. 5, pp. 829–838, 2020.

[7] S. Shi, M. Qin, B. Shen et al., "Association of cardiac injury with mortality in hospitalized patients with covid-19 in wuhan, china," *JAMA Cardiology*, vol. 5, no. 7, p. 802, 2020.

[8] D. Wang, B. Hu, C. Hu et al., "Clinical characteristics of 138 hospitalized patients with 2019 novel coronavirus–infected pneumonia in Wuhan, China," *JAMA*, vol. 323, no. 11, p. 1061, 2020.

[9] F. G. P. Welt, P. B. Shah, H. D. Aronow et al., "Catheterization laboratory considerations during the coronavirus (COVID-19) pandemic: from the ACC's Interventional Council and SCAI," *Journal of the American College of Cardiology*, vol. 75, no. 18, pp. 2372–2375, 2020.

[10] R. M. Inciardi, L. Lupi, G. Zaccone et al., "Cardiac involvement in a patient with coronavirus disease 2019 (COVID-19)," *JAMA Cardiology*, vol. 5, no. 7, pp. 819–824, 2020.

[11] B. Ibanez, S. James, S. Agewall et al., "2017 ESC guidelines for the management of acute myocardial infarction in patients presenting with ST-segment elevation: the task force for the management of acute myocardial infarction in patients pre-

senting with ST-segment elevation of the European Society of Cardiology (ESC)," *European Heart Journal*, vol. 39, no. 2, pp. 119–177, 2018.

[12] R. J. Goldberg, J. C. Zevallos, J. Yarzebski et al., "Prognosis of acute myocardial infarction complicated by complete heart block (the Worcester heart attack study)," *The American Journal of Cardiology*, vol. 69, no. 14, pp. 1135–1141, 1992.

[13] S. S. Rathore, B. J. Gersh, P. B. Berger et al., "Acute myocardial infarction complicated by heart block in the elderly: prevalence and outcomes," *American Heart Journal*, vol. 141, no. 1, pp. 47–54, 2001.

[14] P. B. Berger and T. J. Ryan, "Inferior myocardial infarction. High-risk subgroups," *Circulation*, vol. 81, no. 2, pp. 401–411, 1990.

[15] T. J. Meine, S. M. Al-Khatib, J. H. Alexander et al., "Incidence, predictors, and outcomes of high-degree atrioventricular block complicating acute myocardial infarction treated with thrombolytic therapy," *American Heart Journal*, vol. 149, no. 4, pp. 670–674, 2005.

[16] H. H. Chera, C. A. Mitre, J. Nealis, A. Mironov, and A. S. Budzikowski, "Frequency of complete atrioventricular block complicating ST-elevation myocardial infarction in patients undergoing primary percutaneous coronary intervention," *Cardiology*, vol. 140, pp. 146–151, 2018.

[17] U. J. O. Gang, A. Hvelplund, S. Pedersen et al., "High-degree atrioventricular block complicating ST-segment elevation myocardial infarction in the era of primary percutaneous coronary intervention," *Europace*, vol. 14, no. 11, pp. 1639–1645, 2012.

[18] C. T. Rentsch, J. A. Beckman, L. Tomlinson et al., "Early initiation of prophylactic anticoagulation for prevention of coronavirus disease 2019 mortality in patients admitted to hospital in the United States: cohort study," *BMJ*, vol. 372, 2021.

41

Acute Device-Related Thrombus after Watchman Device Implant

Muhammad Ajmal[1,2] **and Vijendra Swarup**[1,3]

[1]*St. Joseph's Hospital and Medical Center, Phoenix, Arizona, USA*
[2]*Cardiology Fellow, Creighton University School of Medicine, Phoenix, Arizona, USA*
[3]*Arizona Heart Rhythm Center, Phoenix, Arizona, USA*

Correspondence should be addressed to Muhammad Ajmal; drajmal207@gmail.com

Academic Editor: Konstantinos P. Letsas

Atrial fibrillation is characterized by irregularly irregular heart rhythm with an increased morbidity and mortality. It is associated with an increased risk of thromboembolism due to formation of blood clot in the left atrium. Most of these blood clots are formed in the left atrial appendage. The risk of blood clot formation is reduced with the use of anticoagulants. The patients who cannot take anticoagulants due to an increased bleeding risk can undergo percutaneous left atrial appendage (LAA) closure. A Watchman device is used for this purpose. LAA closure with the Watchman device is associated with some adverse effects, and one of them is device-related thrombus. Currently, there are no specific guidelines for the management of device-related thrombus. We present a case of Watchman device-related thrombus which developed 16 hours after the device placement. We will also discuss various options for the management of acute thrombosis.

1. Introduction

Atrial fibrillation (AF) is the most common arrhythmia which is strongly associated with thromboembolism. The risk for thromboembolism is determined by the CHA2DS2-VASc score, and this risk is reduced with the use of anticoagulation. But anticoagulants increase the risk of bleeding. Patients with a high CHA2DS2-VASc score and a high risk of bleeding had limited options in the past. But after the successful trial of left atrial appendage (LAA) closure with the Watchman device for nonvalvular AF, now these patients can be managed with occlusion of left atrial appendage [1]. The Watchman device like other prosthetic material used for various cardiac indications is associated with an increased risk of device-related thrombus (DRT) [2]. The incidence of DRT is reported variably in different studies, but acute thrombosis within 24 hours after the device placement has never been reported before.

2. Case Report

A 79-year-old male with a past medical history significant for the long-term persistent atrial fibrillation with a CHA2DS2-VASc score of 4, essential hypertension, hemorrhagic stroke, and dyslipidemia was referred to our electrophysiology clinic for the evaluation of left atrial appendage (LAA) closure. The patient had been taking Warfarin for 10 years, and it was discontinued 3 months ago at the time of cerebral hemorrhage. He was deemed a high risk for the recurrent bleeding. The lab work showed normal complete metabolic panel but had anemia with a hemoglobin level of 9.5 g/dl (N 13.5-17.5 g/dl) on a complete blood count. Because of the high risk for recurrent ischemic stroke and also for bleeding, he was considered a good candidate for the LAA closure with the Watchman device. Transesophageal echocardiogram (TEE) done before the procedure showed mildly dilated left atrium without left atrial thrombus and normal left ventricular and valvular

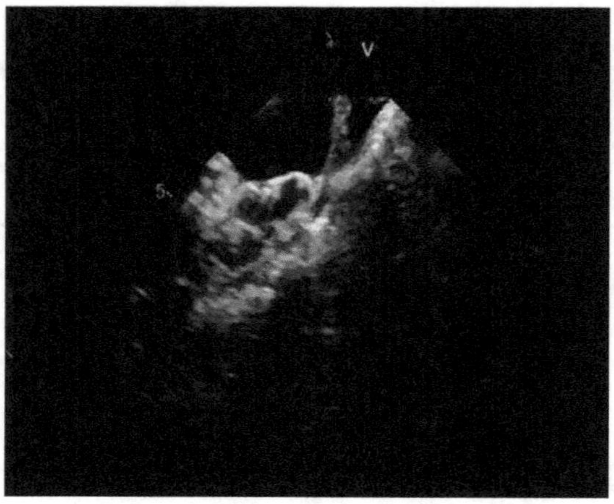

FIGURE 1: Intraoperative TEE showing a well-positioned Watchman device without thrombus.

function. The left atrial appendage dimensions were 23 mm osteal diameter and 27 mm depth. He underwent successful placement of the 27 mm Watchman, Boston Scientific device, compressed to a final diameter of 24 mm with a compression factor of 11%. There was no evidence of left atrial thrombus during and after the procedure as shown in Figure 1, and his activated clotting time was measured throughout the procedure which remained therapeutic. There was also no peridevice leak noted on TEE.

After the procedure, Warfarin was started along with aspirin for the prevention of DRT. Next day, he started complaining of chest discomfort and echocardiogram was done to rule out postprocedure complications. Transthoracic echocardiogram showed moderate pericardial effusion which was likely related to device implant. To better visualize the device, transesophageal echocardiogram was done about 16 hours after the procedure and it showed laminar thrombus on the device as shown in Figure 2.

He underwent drainage of about 150 cc of hemorrhagic pericardial effusion. Anticoagulation regimen was not interrupted, and we bridged low molecular weight heparin with Warfarin after the diagnosis of DRT. Heparin bridging was continued until the therapeutic level of international normalized ratio (INR) 2.2 was achieved on day 5. The patient had a close follow-up at clinic in a week after the discharge and did not demonstrate thromboembolic or bleeding complications. We continued the Warfarin with aspirin for 45 days following the procedure. Repeat TEE after 45 days showed a well-positioned device with resolution of thrombus and no peridevice leak as shown in Figure 3. The INR level was therapeutic at 2.3. At this stage, we switched Warfarin to clopidogrel 75 mg daily and continued it with aspirin 81 mg daily until 6 months after procedure. At 6-month follow-up, TEE showed no thrombus and normal functioning device without leak. Clopidogrel was discontinued, and he is kept on lifelong aspirin 81 mg daily.

3. Discussion

Atrial fibrillation is associated with an increased risk of stroke and systemic thromboembolism. This risk is reduced with the use of anticoagulation. Traditionally, Warfarin has been used as an anticoagulant in atrial fibrillation to prevent thromboembolism. Although effective, Warfarin has a narrow therapeutic profile, need lifelong monitoring, and has food and drug-drug interactions. It has been reported that approximately 40% eligible patients do not receive anticoagulation, leaving them at a substantial risk for stroke. Echocardiographic and autopsy studies have suggested that left atrial appendage (LAA) is the main source of thromboembolism in patients with AF. The PROTECT AF trial showed noninferiority of left atrial appendage closure with Watchman to Warfarin in the prevention of thromboembolism [3]. US Food and Drug Administration (FDA) approved the Watchman device in March 2015 to reduce the risk of thromboembolism in patients with nonvalvular AF. These patients are at an increased risk for thromboembolism based on the CHADS2 or CHA2DS2-VASC score with an appropriate rationale for seeking nonpharmacological alternative to Warfarin, taking into account the safety and efficacy of the device compared to Warfarin. But these prosthetic devices have some risks too, and one of them is device-related thrombosis (DRT). Ideally, anticoagulation should be continued until complete occluder endothelialization occurs. Anticoagulation regimen after placement of the Watchman device is Warfarin with aspirin for 45 days. After 45 days, Warfarin is switched to clopidogrel after ruling out device-related thrombosis and significant peridevice leak (>5 mm) on TEE. After 6 months, clopidogrel is stopped and patients are kept on lifelong aspirin. Despite using this regimen, thrombus formation on the Watchman device is not uncommon. Predisposing factors for the development of thrombus are multifactorial including patient- and device-related factors [4]. These factors include but are not limited to prior thromboembolism, high CHA2DS2-VASC score, and deeply implanted device or large device [5, 6]. The device-related thrombosis is reported early (at 1.5 months), late (at 3-6 months), and very late (at 12 months). Acute thrombosis within 24 hours has not been reported in literature. The exact etiology for the acute thrombosis is not known but is likely patient related and device related as described above. The management strategy for the device-related thrombosis is challenging as there are no set of guidelines about the choice and duration of anticoagulant. Although classically Warfarin was studied in the trials but as we know, direct oral anticoagulants (DOACs) have been effective in nonvalvular AF and there are small studies which showed promising results after Watchman device placement. Although it needs further research to explore the duration and choice of anticoagulants for DRT, we have few options to prevent the acute thrombosis. The literature search has showed that patients with a high CHA2DS2-VASC score have a high risk for DRT so the anticoagulation regimen should be individualized accordingly. Patients who are at a high risk for thrombosis and lower risk for bleeding should be bridged with parenteral anticoagulants when using Warfarin, as Warfarin can take a few days to be therapeutic. The bridging can be done by using intravenous heparin if the patient is admitted in the hospital or with low molecular weight heparin if the patient is discharged. Second option is the use of DOACs which will

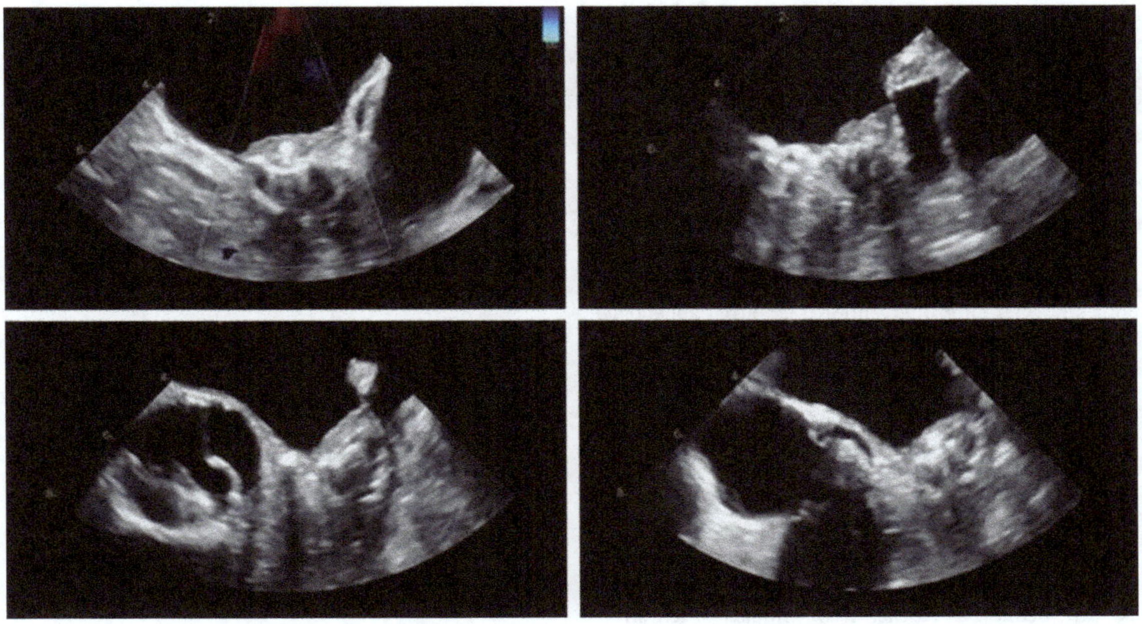

Figure 2: 16 hours postoperative TEE showing thrombus on a Watchman device.

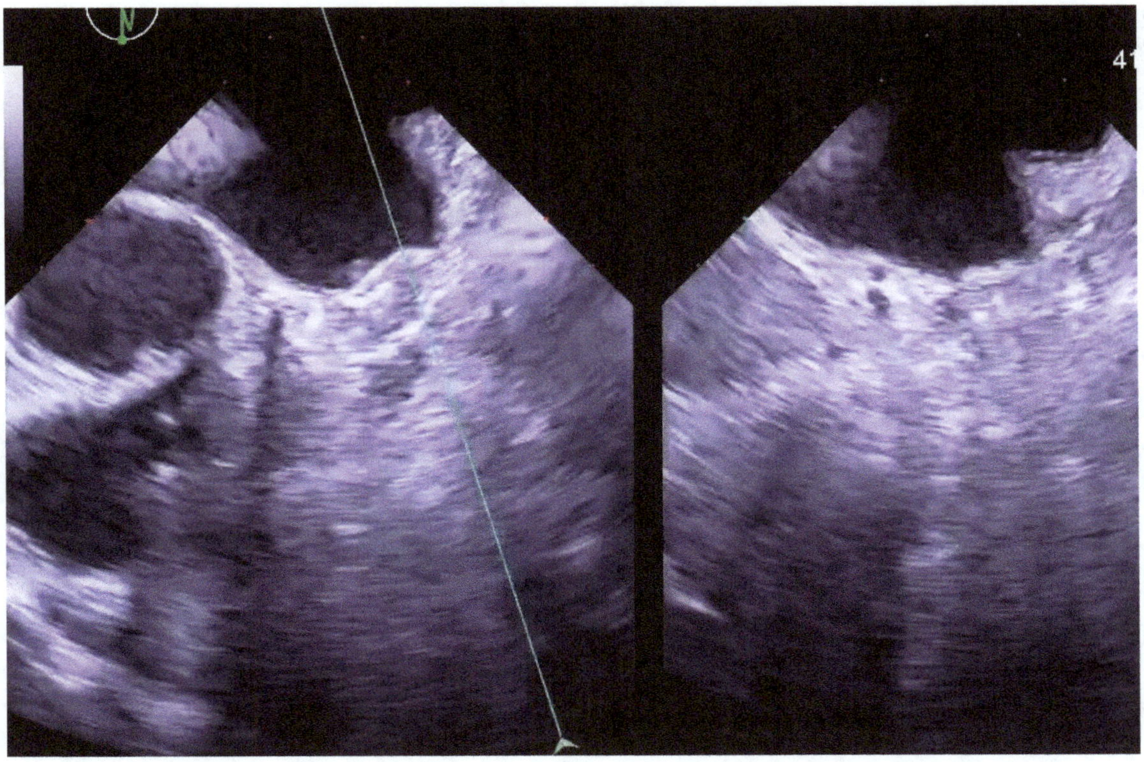

Figure 3: 45 days postoperative TEE showing a well-positioned Watchman device without thrombus.

be effective in preventing acute DRT because of their rapid onset of action [7]. In our patient, we bridged it with low molecular weight heparin till the INR was therapeutic.

4. Conclusion

Percutaneous closure of left atrial appendage for AF has a risk of device-related thrombosis. This complication can occur at any time after the procedure, and the shortest duration as reported in our case can be a few hours. Although it was an incidental finding in our case, it demonstrates the importance of follow-up imaging in days rather than weeks (45 days) especially for the patients who are at a high risk for thrombosis. The real challenge is the choice and duration of anticoagulation for acute DRT. We propose that acute thrombosis should be treated either with Warfarin bridged with heparin until the INR is therapeutic or with DOACs which have rapid onset of action. The duration of anticoagulation should be based on the resolution of thrombus on follow-up imaging. Future studies will be helpful in the management of DRT.

References

[1] S. Chen, F. K. Weise, K. R. J. Chun, and B. Schmidt, "Antithrombotic strategies after interventional left atrial appendage closure: an update," *Expert Review of Cardiovascular Therapy*, vol. 16, no. 9, pp. 675–678, 2018.

[2] L. Fauchier, A. Cinaud, F. Brigadeau et al., "Device-related thrombosis after percutaneous left atrial appendage occlusion for atrial fibrillation," *Journal of the American College of Cardiology*, vol. 71, no. 14, pp. 1528–1536, 2018.

[3] V. Y. Reddy, H. Sievert, J. Halperin et al., "Percutaneous left atrial appendage closure vs warfarin for atrial fibrillation," *JAMA*, vol. 312, no. 19, pp. 1988–1998, 2014.

[4] W. Dieker, M. Behnes, C. Fastner et al., "Impact of left atrial appendage morphology on thrombus formation after successful left atrial appendage occlusion: assessment with cardiac-computed-tomography," *Scientific Reports*, vol. 8, no. 1, 2018.

[5] H. Kaneko, M. Neuss, J. Weissenborn, and C. Butter, "Predictors of thrombus formation after percutaneous left atrial appendage closure using the WATCHMAN device," *Heart and Vessels*, vol. 32, no. 9, pp. 1137–1143, 2017.

[6] R. Pracon, S. Bangalore, Z. Dzielinska et al., "Device thrombosis after percutaneous left atrial appendage occlusion is related to patient and procedural characteristics but not to duration of postimplantation dual antiplatelet therapy," *Circulation: Cardiovascular Interventions*, vol. 11, no. 3, article e005997, 2018.

[7] C. K. Wong, P. H. Chan, C. C. Lam, O. H. Kwok, Y. Y. Lam, and C. W. Siu, "WATCHMAN device-related thrombus successfully treated with apixaban: a case report," *Medicine*, vol. 96, no. 47, article e8693, 2017.

Submitral Aneurysm in a Patient with a Normal Electrocardiogram

Carlos A. Solis-Olivares ,[1] **Irene Meester** ,[2] **and Juan M. Solis-Soto** [3]

[1] *Instituto Mexicano del Seguro Social, Hospital General de Zona 67, Apodaca, Nuevo León 66600, Mexico*
[2] *Universidad de Monterrey, Escuela de Medicina, San Pedro Garza Garcia 66238, Mexico*
[3] *Universidad Autonoma de Nuevo Leon, Facultad de Odontologia, Monterrey 64460, Mexico*

Correspondence should be addressed to Carlos A. Solis-Olivares; caso105@hotmail.com

Academic Editor: Man-Hong Jim

A ventricular aneurysm entails well-known risks for the patient such as heart failure, potentially lethal arrhythmias, and systemic embolic phenomena. The submitral or posterolateral ventricular aneurysm is a very rare variety, usually of congenital etiology, which may also have other causes, including ischemic heart disease. The present case is about a 76-year-old male with the antecedent of an acute myocardial infarction 3 years ago. He presented with intermittent, brief, and self-limiting episodes of severe dyspnea, intense desperation, and accelerated palpitations, with a nonspecific electrocardiogram. An echocardiography revealed a large submitral aneurysm, with a good clinical response to the specific treatment of heart failure, antiarrhythmics, and oral anticoagulation therapy. We analyze the implications of an aneurysm in the context of an ischemic etiology, with special attention to the limitations of the electrocardiogram in the diagnosis of occlusions of the circumflex artery that irrigates the posterolateral region of the heart. We suspect that a greater number of patients with a culprit circumflex artery could receive appropriate coronary interventionism or thrombolysis if decision-making in the emergency room would not depend mainly on the electrocardiogram. Better stratification tools are needed to prevent late complications of infarction, such as those observed in this patient.

1. Introduction

Prior to current modern treatment of acute coronary syndromes, it was estimated that a ventricular aneurysm (VA) developed in 30-35% of patients with acute myocardial infarction (AMI) with an elevated ST-T segment. With the advent of fibrinolysis and coronary angioplasty, the incidence of VA has decreased to 8-15% [1]. The most common etiology of these aneurysms is ischemic heart disease, although there may be other causes.

According to the Mexican Health Secretary, 70-85% of VAs occur in the apical and anterior region of the left ventricle, whereas the lateral wall is the least common location [1]. Also worldwide, VAs most often involve the apex (31.7%), the posterior wall (23.8%), and the anterior wall (9.5%), but only 1% of cardiac aneurysms affect the lateral region of the left ventricle and these aneurysms tend to be small-sized [2].

The clinical importance of VA ranges from asymptomatic to potentially lethal ventricular arrhythmias; sometimes, there are signs and symptoms of heart failure or episodes of arterial embolism.

We present the case of a septuagenarian male patient who was evaluated at a private cardiology clinic because of frequent and severe paroxysmal symptoms of heart failure and palpitations, which were strikingly brief and self-limiting, with nonspecific findings in the electrocardiogram (ECG). Finally, a VA with an unusual submitral or posterolateral location was detected by echocardiography.

2. Case

A 76-year-old Mexican man, from the state of San Luis Potosí, Mexico, was examined at a private cardiology clinic in the Mexican state of Nuevo Leon in April 2018 because

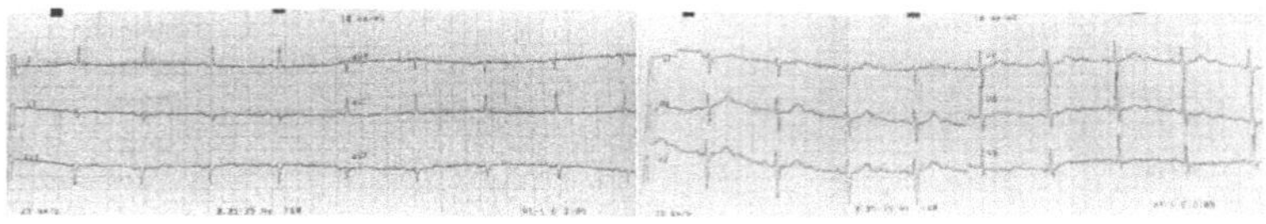

Figure 1: Admission ECG without abnormalities.

of episodes of excessive dry cough, severe dyspnea, and accelerated palpitations as of the previous day. These episodes were frequent and of sudden onset and short duration, without angina, lipothymia, or syncope. He was asymptomatic between episodes.

There were no nonpathological antecedents of importance; he had worked as a farmer until his retirement; he did not smoke nor consume alcohol or drugs; and he was neither diabetic nor hypertensive. The only personal pathological antecedent of interest was a hospitalization due to an AMI 3 years ago, which had been attended in the patient's native state. Access to his medical file was not an option at the moment of the consult.

Upon arrival at the clinic, he was calm and symptom-free. However, at the start of the clinical interview, he suddenly presented a new episode of severe dyspnea accompanied by intense desperation, which lasted less than 1 minute, after which he remained calm and asymptomatic. The physical examination did not yield relevant data, except for arrhythmic heart sounds due to premature beats. The pulmonary fields were considered clean and well-ventilated, abdominal visceromegalies were not found, and no edema was detected in the lower limbs. The blood pressure was 120/80 mmHg, the heart rate 76 bpm, and the respiratory rate 20 respirations per minute.

The initial ECG revealed a sinus rhythm with a heart rate of 55 bpm, PR 0.18, QRS 0.08, AQRS at -30 degrees, and tracing without significant abnormalities (Figure 1). A ventricular arrhythmia was suspected, but a 24 h Holter monitoring was discarded because of the apparent urgency of the situation. Instead, a color Doppler echocardiography was performed immediately. The echocardiogram revealed a left ventricular ejection fraction (LVEF) of 34% and a large submitral aneurysm in the posterolateral basal-medial region of the left ventricle, as well as severe anterior and inferior basal-medial hypokinesia, mild mitral valve insufficiency, and no pulmonary artery hypertension (Figures 2 and 3).

As the patient presented symptoms of intermittent heart failure probably due to paroxysmal tachycardia, which, in the context of a cardiac posterolateral submitral VA (SVA), could be potentially lethal, medical treatment was initiated with spironolactone (50 mg/day), furosemide (20 mg/day), amiodarone (200 mg every 12 hours for 2 weeks and then a single 200-mg dose daily), nitroglycerin patches (5 mg/day), and apixaban (5 mg every 12 hours, orally).

On a control visit three weeks later, the patient had no cardiovascular symptoms (New York Heart Association (NYHA) functional class I) and had not experienced recurrence of palpitations nor episodes of sudden dyspnea. The laboratory blood values were as follows: hemoglobin, 16.4 gr/dL; leukocytes, 7,400/mm^3; platelets, 261,000/mm^3; glucose, 108 mg/dL; creatinine, 1.16 mg/dL; uric acid, 5.5 mg/dL; total cholesterol, 207 mg/dL; triglycerides, 147 mg /dL; low-density lipoprotein cholesterol (LDL-c), 144. 3 mg/dL; and high-density lipoprotein cholesterol (HDL-c), 51 mg/dL. Hepatic function tests and serum electrolytes were normal, except for an elevated thyroid-stimulating hormone (TSH) level (45 mIU/mL). Urinalysis was without significant abnormalities: pH, 7.5 and density, 1.010. The posteroanterior chest radiograph (Figure 4) revealed grade II cardiomegaly with a rounded growth on a left profile, compatible with VA, without further abnormalities.

Levothyroxine (first week, 50 μg/day; from second week onwards, 75 μg/day) and simvastatin (20 mg/day) were added to the treatment. With this therapeutic scheme, the patient remained asymptomatic until August 2018, month of the last follow-up visit at this private clinic. At the beginning of this month, the last monitored TSH level was 7.48 mUI/mL. The good clinical response to treatment and the tendency to a sinus bradycardia did not seem to justify the inclusion of beta-blockers.

The patient, with low economic resources, will continue his follow-up and treatment at a third-level public hospital in Monterrey, Mexico. Cardiac gammagraphy, cardiac catheterization, and electrophysiological monitoring were recommended.

3. Discussion

SVA is a peculiar pathology, which is rarely detected worldwide. The majority of cases occur in the African population and in a lesser proportion in the Indian population [3, 4]. SVA can be defined as a dilation of the ventricle and a thinning of the ventricular wall below the mitral valve apparatus, due to a weak union of the cardiac muscle to the fibrous tissue adjacent to the posterolateral mitral valve. Most often, there is a congenital etiology, but any of the following may be an alternative cause: infection, for example, tuberculosis and endocarditis; inflammation as in rheumatic fever or Takayasu disease; neoplasia; post-AMI; and idiopathic causes [5, 6]. Patients with this problem may be asymptomatic or have symptoms of heart failure, palpitations, lipothymia, syncope, or sudden death, in addition to systemic embolic phenomena. The ECG often shows nonspecific findings, unlike VA cases due to ischemia of the apical or anterior wall, which are detected by a persistent ST-T segment elevation and the presence of Q waves in electrocardiographic derivations corresponding to the affected area. In fact, localization of aneurysms in the posterolateral region of the left ventricle, as in the present case, is very rare.

The initial objective when detecting a SVA is to corroborate an ischemic etiology and rule out other potential

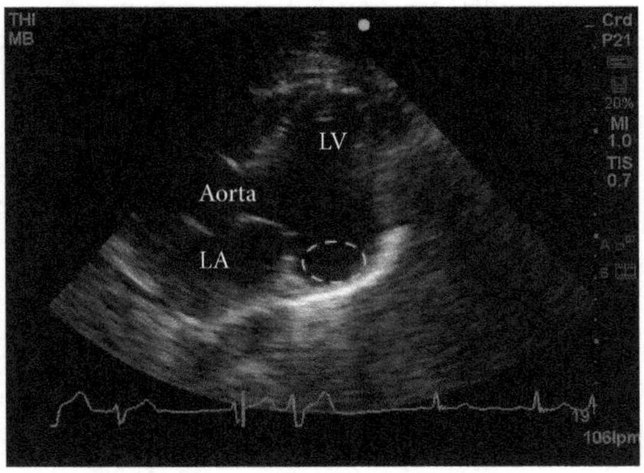

FIGURE 2: Transthoracic echocardiogram, parasternal long axis view. Notice the large submitral aneurysm (diameter, 3 cm) in the posterolateral basal-medial region of the left ventricle (encircled area). LA: left atrium; LV: left ventricle.

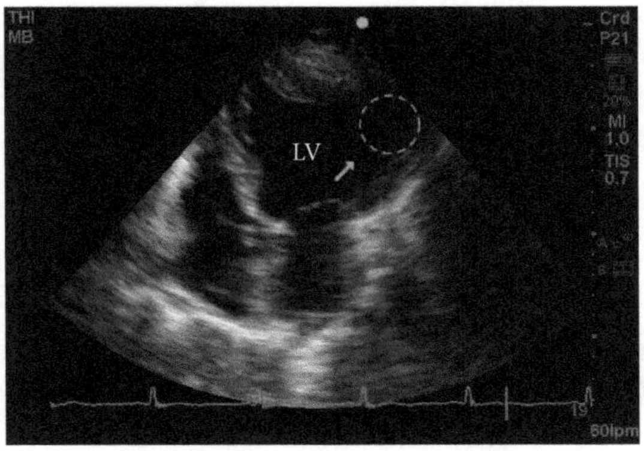

FIGURE 3: The echocardiogram reveals a large aneurysm (diameter, 3 cm; encircled area) in the lateral basal-medial region of the ventricle without apparent thrombus (arrow). LV: left ventricle.

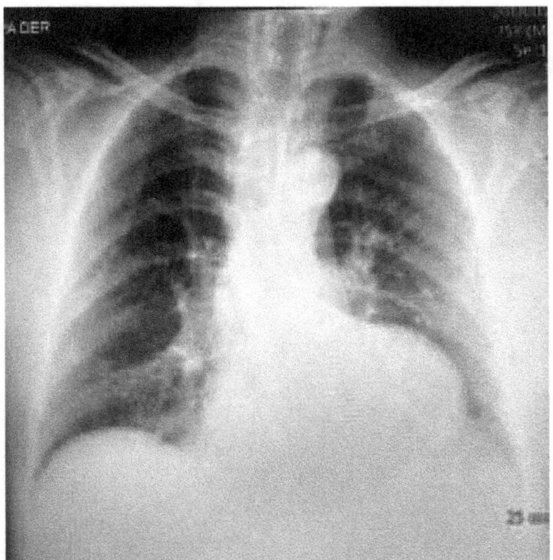

FIGURE 4: Posteroanterior thoracic radiography denotes cardiomegaly imparted mostly by the low left cardiac bulging.

causes.The therapy goal is to offer interventional or surgical treatment of coronary vessels with critical lesions and/or myocardial ischemia and viability, resection of the SVA, or, if surgery seems too risky, a cardioverter defibrillator implant.

Considering that this case concerns a senile patient with a clinical history of hospitalization due to an AMI 3 years ago, combined with the echocardiographic findings of segmental alterations of left ventricle mobility in regions other than the VA area, it seems most probable that ischemia had caused this SVA, although a congenital or other origin cannot be ruled out completely. It is known that 40% to 50% of the occlusions of the circumflex left coronary artery (LCA) in the context of myocardial infarction do not alter the ST-T segment in the ECG [7]. The ECG, therefore, is insufficient to detect a narrowing or occlusion of the LCA and can lead to a wrong classification of risk and a delay in the performance of coronary angiography and interventional procedures [8]. This situation probably applies to this case. Patients with an AMI due to an occluded LCA tend to have a worse evolution than patients with an occluded right coronary artery. Among other reasons, this could be because of a delay in the establishment of fibrinolytic or interventional reperfusion therapy in cases with an ECG with nonspecific findings, which is more common when the culprit occlusion occurs in the LCA [9]. Finally, supposing that the posterolateral SVA of this case is due to ischemia, the issue that deserves attention is the inadequate procedure of risk stratification of emergency room patients with chest pain and a suspect of cardiac ischemia. Up to 10% of patients with thoracic pain and the suspicion of cardiac ischemia are dismissed because of a normal ECG but return within 24 to 48 hours with an established AMI and are no longer within the therapeutic window for fibrinolytic or interventional reperfusion therapy [10].

In clinical practice, the LCA is the least frequent culprit vessel among patients treated invasively for AMI. Patients with LCA occlusion may present an acute non-ST segment elevation myocardial infarction and require emergency coronary intervention [11]. The consequences of this inadequate risk stratification, based mainly on a normal ECG but without considering an adequate semiology of chest pain, which should include studies such as troponin levels, echocardiography, and nuclear medicine studies, can lead to a substantial delay in reperfusion therapy and the appearance of late complications such as VA.

4. Conclusion

SVA, usually congenital in origin and peculiar for its rare occurrence and particular anatomical location in the heart, may also be of ischemic origin. Occlusions of the circumflex artery as a culprit lesion of myocardial infarction, often invisible in an ECG, could lead to the development of VA in elderly patients whom were not treated timely with coronary reperfusion therapy. This case demonstrates the need to improve clinical risk categorization strategies in patients evaluated for chest pain in an emergency service.

References

[1] Instituto Secretaría de Salud, *Diagnóstico y Tratamiento del Aneurisma Ventricular Mexico*, Instituto Secretaría de Salud, 2011.

[2] M. Ruhela, D. Kumar, S. Choudhary, R. Bagarhatta, and A. Jain, "Post myocardial infarction submitral aneurysm causing stroke in an elderly patient- a rare case report," *American Journal of Medical Case Reports*, vol. 3, no. 1, pp. 23–26, 2015.

[3] D. K. Baruah, P. V. N. Kumar, G. S. P. Reddy, and V. R. Babu, "Submitral aneurysm of the left ventricle," *Indian Heart Journal*, vol. 64, no. 1, pp. 77–79, 2012.

[4] A. A. Abdusamed, H. A. Mulatu, and R. N. Martinez, "Submitral left ventricular aneurysm associated with thrombus," *Ethiopian Journal of Health Sciences*, vol. 28, no. 1, pp. 93–96, 2018.

[5] P. J. d. F. Ribeiro, R. G. G. Mendes, W. V. d. A. Vicente, A. C. Menardi, and P. R. B. Evora, "Submitral left ventricular aneurysm. Case report and review of published Brazilian cases," *Arquivos Brasileiros de Cardiologia*, vol. 76, no. 5, pp. 399–402, 2001.

[6] J. S. Pahwa, D. Patil, J. Kohli, M. S. Phadke, C. P. Lajewar, and P. G. Kerkar, "Giant ischemic left ventricular submitral aneurysm," *Indian Heart Journal*, vol. 68, pp. S168–S169, 2016.

[7] W. K. Stribling, A. Abbate, M. Kontos, G. W. Vetrovec, and K. Lotun, "Myocardial infarctions involving acute left circumflex occlusion: are all occlusions created equally?," *Interventional Cardiology*, vol. 2, no. 5, pp. 695–704, 2010.

[8] M. Kozuch, P. Kralisz, M. Rog-Makal, H. Bachorzewska-Gajewska, and S. Dobrzycki, "Significant narrowing of the circumflex artery leads to worse outcomes than right coronary artery narrowing in patients with anterior myocardial infarction treated invasively," *Netherlands Heart Journal*, vol. 23, no. 5, pp. 258–262, 2015.

[9] W. K. Stribling, M. C. Kontos, A. Abbate et al., "Left circumflex occlusion in acute myocardial infarction (from the National Cardiovascular Data Registry)," *The American Journal of Cardiology*, vol. 108, no. 7, pp. 959–963, 2011.

[10] D. Bialostozky, "Chest pain syndrome with normal or non-diagnostic ECG in the emergency service. Assessment with myocardial perfusion (SPECT) and ventricular function (gated-SPECT)," *Archivos de Cardiología de México*, vol. 74, no. 1, pp. S18–S31, 2004.

[11] A. M. From, P. J. M. Best, R. J. Lennon, C. S. Rihal, and A. Prasad, "Acute myocardial infarction due to left circumflex artery occlusion and significance of ST-segment elevation," *The American Journal of Cardiology*, vol. 106, no. 8, pp. 1081–1085, 2010.

43

Solely MRI-Guided Cardiac Catheterization for Assessment of Pulmonary Hypertension in a Pregnant Lady with Undiagnosed Congenital Heart Disease

Aphrodite Tzifa,[1,2] **Ioannis Polymerou**,[2] **and Dimitra Loggitsi**[3]

[1]*Department of Congenital Heart Disease, Mitera Children's Hospital, Athens, Greece*
[2]*Biomedical Engineering & Clinical Sciences, King's College London, UK*
[3]*Department of Radiology, Mitera Children's Hospital, Athens, Greece*

Correspondence should be addressed to Aphrodite Tzifa; a.tzifa@btinternet.com

Academic Editor: Aiden Abidov

Pregnancy in women with complex congenital heart disease (CHD) can be poorly tolerated. Amongst pregnant women with CHD and pulmonary hypertension (PH), the mortality rate can be as high as 30%. Cardiac catheterization procedures for assessment of haemodynamics and pulmonary vascular resistance (PVR) are often required in this patient population for risk stratification. However, during the first few weeks of pregnancy, this should better be avoided due to the known adverse effects of the ionizing radiation to the immature fetus. In this setting, a solely MRI-guided catheterization may present as a better alternative.

1. Introduction

Persistent exposure of the pulmonary vasculature to increased blood pressure or blood flow from a systemic to pulmonary shunt can lead to pulmonary arterial hypertension (PAH) which is classified in Group 1 of the PH clinical classification. Some of these shunts can go unrecognized for years. In a retrospective cohort study on the prevalence of PAH in adults with a cardiac septal defect, PH was present in 28% of all patients or in 34% of patients with an open ASD and in 28% of patients with an open VSD and in 12% and 13% of patients with a closed defect, respectively [1].

Pregnant women with pulmonary hypertension have a high mortality and morbidity rate. Careful assessment of haemodynamics is crucial for their consultation with regard to pregnancy planning. However, on occasion, the diagnosis of pulmonary hypertension in the setting of congenital heart disease may be made for the first time during pregnancy. Risk stratification in such cases may require a cardiac catheterization procedure that normally exposes the woman and her fetus to ionizing radiation. We report on the case of a pregnant woman with newly diagnosed complex congenital heart disease and pulmonary hypertension who underwent solely magnetic resonance imaging- (MRI-) guided catheterization using real-time interactive imaging in order to ascertain anatomy, as well as haemodynamics and pulmonary vascular resistance, due to her wish to maintain pregnancy. To our knowledge, this is the first reported case of solely MRI-guided cardiac catheterization in pregnancy, expanding further the potentials of magnetic resonance imaging in cardiovascular disease.

2. Case Report

A 33-year-old woman presented with newly diagnosed pulmonary hypertension (PH) and significantly dilated right heart structures. She had been investigated in childhood for situs inversus abdominalis, but no definitive cardiac diagnosis was made. At presentation, she was 10 weeks pregnant and completely asymptomatic. Electrocardiogram showed negative p waves in lead II. Transthoracic echocardiography showed a large atrial septal defect with exclusive left to right shunt and severely dilated right ventricle with tricuspid valve velocity of 5 m/sec. The hepatic veins were imaged to drain directly into the right-sided atrium with no inferior

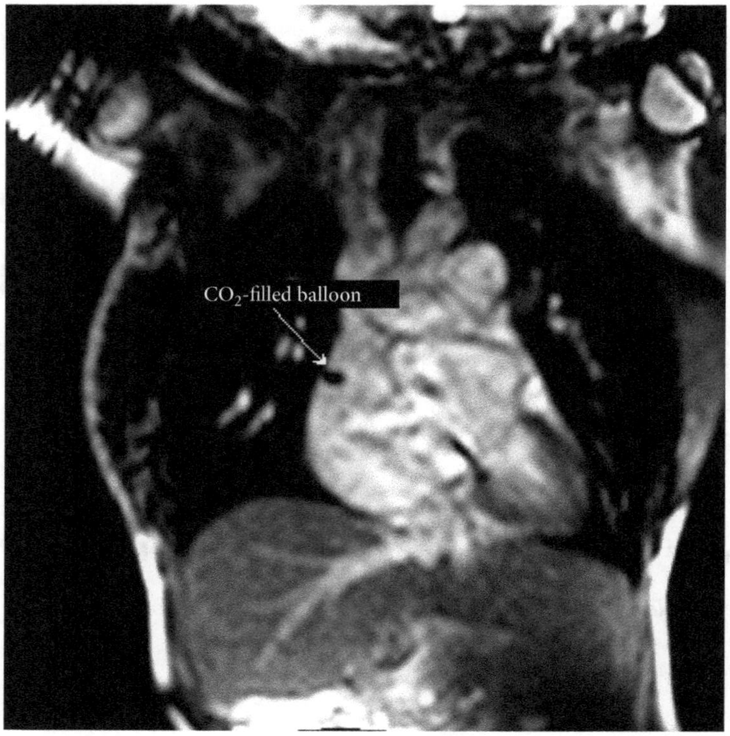

FIGURE 1: The balloon of the wedge catheter appears as a black circle in the white blood pool in the right-sided atrium. The hepatic veins appear to drain directly to the atrium.

vena cava flow seen; hence, the suspicion of left atrial isomerism was raised.

Due to evidence of pulmonary hypertension and her wish to maintain pregnancy, a cardiac catheterization procedure was advised, to assess the pulmonary arterial (PA) pressures and PVR. To avoid fluoroscopy at this early stage of pregnancy, we planned to perform a solely MRI-guided right heart catheterization, with which accurate PVR as well as the rest of the anatomy could be ascertained. The procedure was performed on the 15th week of pregnancy in a High-Field Open MR Scanner (1.0T, Panorama, Philips). The following sequences were used: interactive planning for real-time imaging (TR-TE shortest, Act. TR/TE (ms) = 3.1/1.56, flip angle 45°), phase contrast flow sequences for Q flow measurements (TR-TE shortest, Act. TR/TE (ms) = 5.7/3.5, flip angle 15°), BTFE sequences for cine imaging (TR-TE shortest, Act. TR/TE (ms) = 5.1/2.1, flip angle 75°), and T1-weighted black blood sequences for anatomical imaging (TR = 667 ms,TE = 37 ms, flip angle 90°).

The catheterization took place through the internal jugular vein, due to IVC interruption. An 8 French sheath was inserted into the right internal jugular vein under local anesthetic. The patient was transferred to the magnetic resonance suite where baseline real-time interactive imaging was initially performed. This confirmed IVC interruption with azygos continuation to the superior vena cava. The patient's hepatic veins drained directly to the right-sided atrium (Figure 1) whilst the liver extended from right to left throughout the upper abdomen. Polysplenia was also noted, and therefore, the diagnosis of heterotaxy/left atrial isomerism with an atrial septal defect was confirmed.

Under magnetic resonance guidance, a CO_2-filled balloon wedge catheter was inserted through the internal jugular vein without a guidewire, and the positioning of the balloon was confirmed on MRI as a black spot in the white blood pool (Figures 1 and 2). The imaging planes that were used to monitor the balloon position were the 4 chamber views, the right vertical long axis, right ventricular outflow tract, main pulmonary artery (MPA) bifurcation, and right pulmonary artery coronal views. Simultaneous recordings of the pressure waveforms in the right heart were performed. After obtaining the haemodynamic data in the MPA, the branches, and the wedge position (Figure 3), the wedge catheter was left in the MPA (Figure 4) and the pulmonary flow (Qp) was estimated using the phase contrast flow sequence. MPA pressure measured 93/29/52 mmHg against systemic pressure of 96/65 mmHg, whilst wedge pressure measured 20 mmHg. Right heart cardiac output, as estimated from the volumetric analysis of the right ventricle, was 15.5 l/min, which coincided with Qp of 15 l/min as measured by the pulmonary artery through plane flows (PA-TP) during phase contrast sequences. In comparison, LV stroke volume on the volumetric analysis was measured at 6 l/min, which coincided with Qs of 6 l/min as measured by the aortic artery through plane flows (Ao-TP) during phase contrast sequences. The estimated Qp : Qs was 2.6 : 1 with PVR of 3.3 WU·m^2. The patient was therefore diagnosed with high pulmonary flow but sufficiently low pulmonary vascular resistance to allow her to carry on with pregnancy and plan for transcatheter closure of her atrial septal defect at a later stage.

Indeed, she carried on with pregnancy and delivered a healthy child by planned caesarean section at term. Her

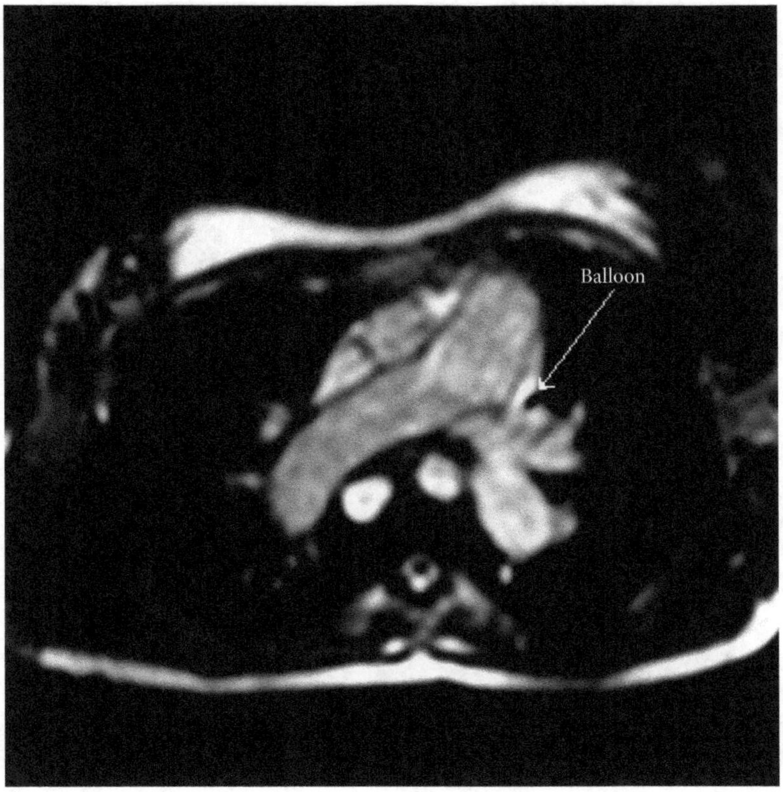

FIGURE 2: The CO_2-filled balloon appears black in the SSFP images. The image shows the CO_2-filled balloon of the wedge catheter in the left pulmonary artery.

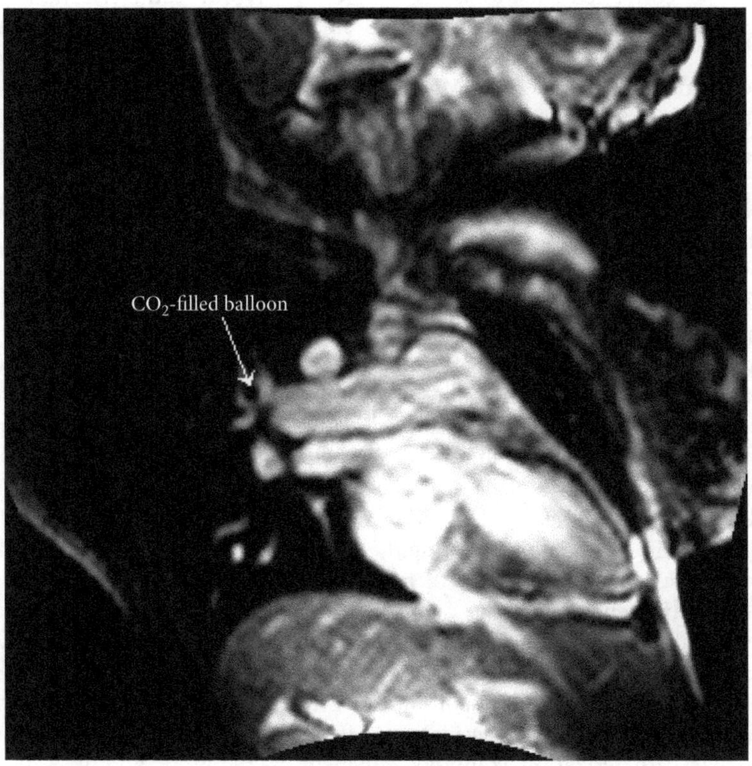

FIGURE 3: The balloon of the wedge catheter appears in the wedge position of the right pulmonary artery.

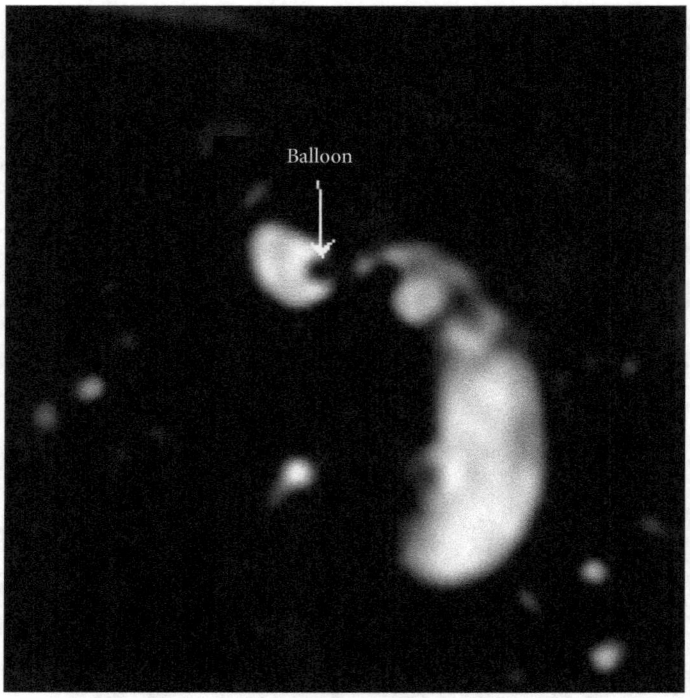

FIGURE 4: At the end of the right heart catheterization, the CO_2-filled balloon was left inflated and the wedge catheter was left in the main pulmonary artery for simultaneous pressure measurement whilst the pulmonary flow was obtained with the phase contrast flow sequence.

pulmonary arterial pressures as estimated by the TR Dopplers and oxygen saturation remained unchanged throughout pregnancy and postpartum. She received low-weight heparin during the last trimester and was converted back to aspirin after delivery. She did not suffer from any postpartum haemorrhage.

The patient was started on Sildenafil 10 mg ×2 and Macitentan 10 mg ×1 after delivery, but Sildenafil was discontinued due to nausea and hot flushes. She therefore continued with Macitentan monotherapy. She underwent repeat cardiac catheterization 2.5 years later in order to assess her PVR and suitability for transcatheter closure of the atrial septal defect. Main pulmonary artery pressures measured 72/16/40 mmHg with wedge pressure of 16 mmHg. Test balloon occlusion of the atrial septal defect was performed, which showed stable systemic pressures without increase of the venous pressures. Repeat PA pressure with the balloon occluding the defect reduced to 55/20/28 mmHg, suggesting significant flow-related element for the increased pulmonary artery pressures, as demonstrated previously during MRI-guided catheterization. PVRi was measured as 6 WU·m^2 at baseline and dropped to 4 WU·m^2 after reversibility testing. We therefore proceeded with closure of the defect with a 27 mm Occlutech device with a 6 mm fenestration.

At the age of 37 years, 4 years after the initial MRI-guided catheterization and 1.5 years after the fenestrated device closure, she presented for a repeat cardiac assessment in order to quantify the risk for another pregnancy. Once again, she underwent a hybrid cardiac catheterization combined with MRI assessment. Main pulmonary artery pressure at baseline measured 48/11/31 mmHg with wedge pressure of 15 mmHg, Qp : Qs of 1.22 : 1, and PVRi of 4.1 WU·m^2, all based on MRI flows and crosschecked with catheterization data. With FiO_2 of 100% and 20 ppm NO, repeat MPA pressures measured 43/10/28 mmHg and Qp : Qs remained at 1.2 : 1, accounting for a drop in PVRi to 3.4 WU·m^2. The repeat hybrid catheterization procedure demonstrated a small decrease of the MPA pressure and unchanged PVR after the fenestrated device closure.

3. Discussion

Adults with congenital heart disease are an ever-growing population. It is estimated that in the United States, there are more adults with congenital heart disease than infants and children with the disease. Approximately half of the grown-up CHD population are women, most of whom are of childbearing age [2]. Cardiac catheterization procedures are often required, particularly when there is suspicion of pulmonary hypertension. However, this may not be feasible in pregnant women within the first few weeks of pregnancy, due to the deleterious effects of ionizing radiation on the fetus during organogenesis. We report on the technique of performing a right heart catheterization under sole MRI guidance in a pregnant woman with severe pulmonary hypertension and CHD. Solely MRI-guided diagnostic catheterizations were first introduced in children with congenital heart disease in 2003 [3], whilst MR-guided interventions were made possible by the authors' group in 2010 [4]. Performing a cardiac catheterization under MRI is quite different from fluoroscopy. MRI-compatible monitoring equipment is required, and it is essential for the monitoring equipment to have 2 ports, where invasive blood pressure measurements can be transduced from the arterial and the venous system. Although pressure monitoring can be done smoothly with the use of a balloon catheter, this type of procedure would not provide accurate flow measurements and PVR, as well as the anatomical and structural details that were required for our congenital heart disease patient.

To this end, we decided to apply a solely MRI-guided catheterization procedure. She tolerated pregnancy extremely well due to the large ASD and the ability to offload the right heart.

We watched her carefully throughout pregnancy, due to the known fact that pregnancy in women with haemodynamically significant congenital heart disease can be poorly tolerated due to the increase in blood volume and cardiac output. In this patient group, who also has pulmonary hypertension, the maternal mortality is 30-50% in older series and 9-33% in more recent papers, placing them in a high-risk category [5–7]. As pulmonary vascular disease is considered to be the worst risk factor for pregnancy and the postpartum period [8] with a 40% risk for maternal death or heart failure, despite the recent advances in pre- and postpartum care for these patients [7], assessment of pulmonary artery pressures and vascular resistance via cardiac catheterization is essential for risk stratification and appropriate consultation and therapy (class of recommendation I, level of evidence C) [9]. Traditionally, fluoroscopy has been used to guide catheters around the cardiac structures and vessels. In the recent years with the development of MRI hardware and software, it is possible to obtain real-time imaging of the heart in order to guide a cardiac catheterization procedure using MRI-compatible catheters, whilst also obtaining advanced imaging datasets (3D, flow quantification, and tissue characterization).

MRI-guided catheterization in our patient facilitated accurate measurement of haemodynamics and PVR, in a situation where fluoroscopy was a relative contraindication. Although the pulmonary arterial pressures were found to be at the systemic level, accurate measurement of cardiac output by volumetry and pulmonary flows established that the PVR was sufficiently low for pregnancy to be continued. This case depicts the various and important applications of MRI-guided catheterization that can offer unique anatomic as well as physiologic information in cases where ionizing radiation is best to be avoided.

4. Conclusion

The adoption of MRI-guided catheterizations for patients with CHD, who undergo multiple tests involving ionizing radiation throughout their lifetime, is a promising and safe alternative in terms of limiting radiation exposure. As the effects of ionizing radiation are increasingly deleterious with younger age, fetuses are the most vulnerable population. To this end, MRI-guided catheterization could provide a good alternative for pregnant women with cardiovascular disease who have to undergo invasive haemodynamic evaluation.

Abbreviations

PH: Pulmonary hypertension
MRI: Magnetic resonance imaging
CHD: Congenital heart disease
PAH: Pulmonary arterial hypertension
PVR: Pulmonary vascular resistance
PVRi: Indexed pulmonary vascular resistance
MPA: Main pulmonary artery
IVC: Inferior vena cava
TR: Tricuspid regurgitation
NO: Nitric oxide.

Consent

Informed consent was obtained from the patient for the publication of this case report and any accompanying images. A copy of the written consent is available for review with the Editor-in-Chief of this journal.

Authors' Contributions

All authors had access to all the data and a role in writing this manuscript.

References

[1] P. M. Engelfriet, M. G. Duffels, T. Möller et al., "Pulmonary arterial hypertension in adults born with a heart septal defect: the Euro Heart Survey on adult congenital heart disease," *Heart*, vol. 93, no. 6, pp. 682–687, 2007.

[2] R. A. Curry, C. Fletcher, E. Gelson et al., "Pulmonary hypertension and pregnancy – a review of 12 pregnancies in nine women," *BJOG*, vol. 119, no. 6, pp. 752–761, 2012.

[3] R. Razavi, D. L. Hill, S. F. Keevil et al., "Cardiac catheterisation guided by MRI in children and adults with congenital heart disease," *The Lancet*, vol. 362, no. 9399, pp. 1877–1882, 2003.

[4] A. Tzifa, G. A. Krombach, N. Krämer et al., "Magnetic resonance–guided cardiac interventions using magnetic resonance–compatible devices," *Circulation: Cardiovascular Interventions*, vol. 3, no. 6, pp. 585–592, 2010.

[5] B. M. Weiss, L. Zemp, B. Seifert, and O. M. Hess, "Outcome of pulmonary vascular disease in pregnancy: a systematic overview from 1978 through 1996," *Journal of the American College of Cardiology*, vol. 31, no. 7, pp. 1650–1657, 1998.

[6] E. Bédard, K. Dimopoulos, and M. A. Gatzoulis, "Has there been any progress made on pregnancy outcomes among women with pulmonary arterial hypertension?," *European Heart Journal*, vol. 30, no. 3, pp. 256–265, 2009.

[7] J. R.-H. L. B. M. Johnson, J. De Backer, C. Otto et al., "Pregnancy outcomes in women with cardiovascular disease: evolving trends over 10 years in the ESC Registry Of Pregnancy And Cardiac disease (ROPAC)," *European Heart Journal*, vol. 40, no. 47, pp. 3848–3855, 2019.

[8] A. Chamaidi and M. A. Gatzoulis, "Heart disease and pregnancy," *Hellenic Journal of Cardiology*, vol. 47, no. 5, pp. 275–291, 2006.

[9] V. Regitz-Zagrosek, J. W. Roos-Hesselink, J. Bauersachs et al., "ESC guidelines for the management of cardiovascular diseases during pregnancy," *European Heart Journal*, vol. 39, no. 34, pp. 3165–3241, 2018.

The Unmasking Effect: Propofol-Induced Brugada Pattern in a Critically Ill Patient

Esiemoghie Akhigbe,[1] Ebubechukwu Ezeh,[1] Benjamin Dao,[2] Kelechukwu Okoro,[2] and Paul Okhumale[2]

[1]*Department of Internal Medicine, Marshall University Joan C. Edwards School of Medicine, Huntington, WV, USA*
[2]*Department of Cardiovascular Services, Marshall University Joan C. Edwards School of Medicine, Huntington, WV, USA*

Correspondence should be addressed to Esiemoghie Akhigbe; akhigbe@marshall.edu

Academic Editor: Christopher S. Snyder

Brugada syndrome is a known cause of dysrhythmias and sudden cardiac death. It is linked to mutations in myocardial sodium channel leading to hyperexcitable cardiac myocytes. The use of this sedative has been linked to the development of inducible Brugada via blockade of sodium currents in cardiac myocytes. Although propofol is usually avoided in patients with known Brugada syndrome, some patients might have undiagnosed Brugada syndrome and thus are at risk for complications. We present a case of propofol induced Brugada in a critically ill patient.

1. Introduction

Brugada syndrome (BrS) is an autosomal dominant genetic disorder that is associated with malignant arrhythmias and sudden cardiac death [1, 2]. The enhanced myocardial excitability is largely attributed to mutations in the myocardial sodium channel. Due to antagonization of sodium channels, propofol's use as an induction and sedation agent in patients with BrS has traditionally been avoided. In fact, the Brugada-Drugs.org Advisory Board recommends avoiding administration of propofol in patients with Brugada syndrome [3]. However, recent case reports and case studies have described the safe use of propofol without arrhythmic sequelae [4]. We describe a case of unmasked type I Brugada pattern electrocardiogram (EKG) due to prolonged propofol infusion in a critically ill patient.

2. Case Presentation

Patient is a 35-year-old man with no known past medical history presented from an outside facility on account of with epigastric abdominal pain, nausea, and vomiting of 3 days duration. He was subsequently diagnosed with gallstone pancreatitis for which he was taken to the operating room for a laparoscopic cholecystectomy. Patient was induced with propofol and intubated perioperatively but aspirated during intubation. During the laparoscopy, the patient was noted to have dilated small bowel loops, and the cholecystectomy was terminated. The patient was extubated postoperatively. A follow-up computed tomography (CT) scan demonstrated necrotizing pancreatitis, and the patient was transferred to our facility.

After arrival at our facility, the patient was again induced with propofol for cholecystectomy. The patient was noted to have dense intra-abdominal adhesions necessitating the need for an open cholecystectomy. The patient tolerated the procedure well and was extubated. On postoperative day (POD) 3, the patient developed acute respiratory failure secondary to hypovolemic shock. He was reintubated and again induced with propofol. Patient was later found to have a pancreatic hematoma with no active bleeding and was treated medically. Patient postoperative period was also complicated by an extensive pulmonary embolus for which he underwent pulmonary artery thrombectomy and inferior vena cava filter placement after which he remained intubated and sedated. On POD 11, patient developed abdominal

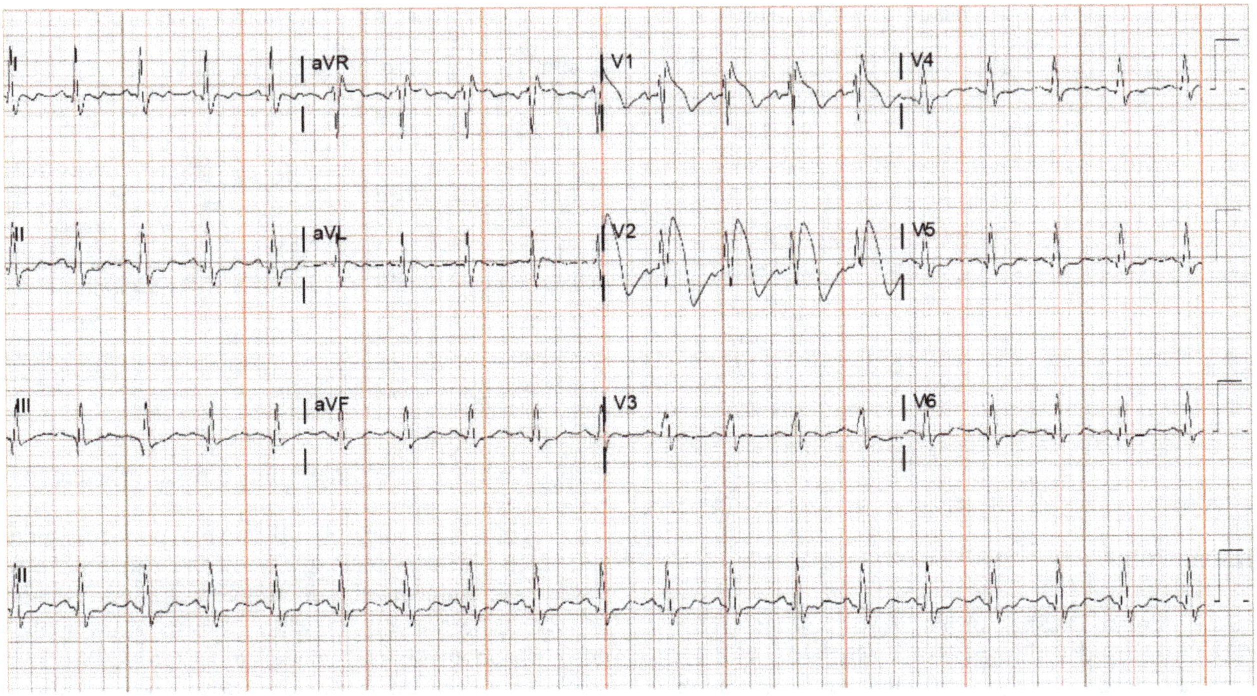

FIGURE 1: Electrocardiogram on day 12 of admission showing characteristic type 1 coved shaped ST segment elevation in leads V1 and V2.

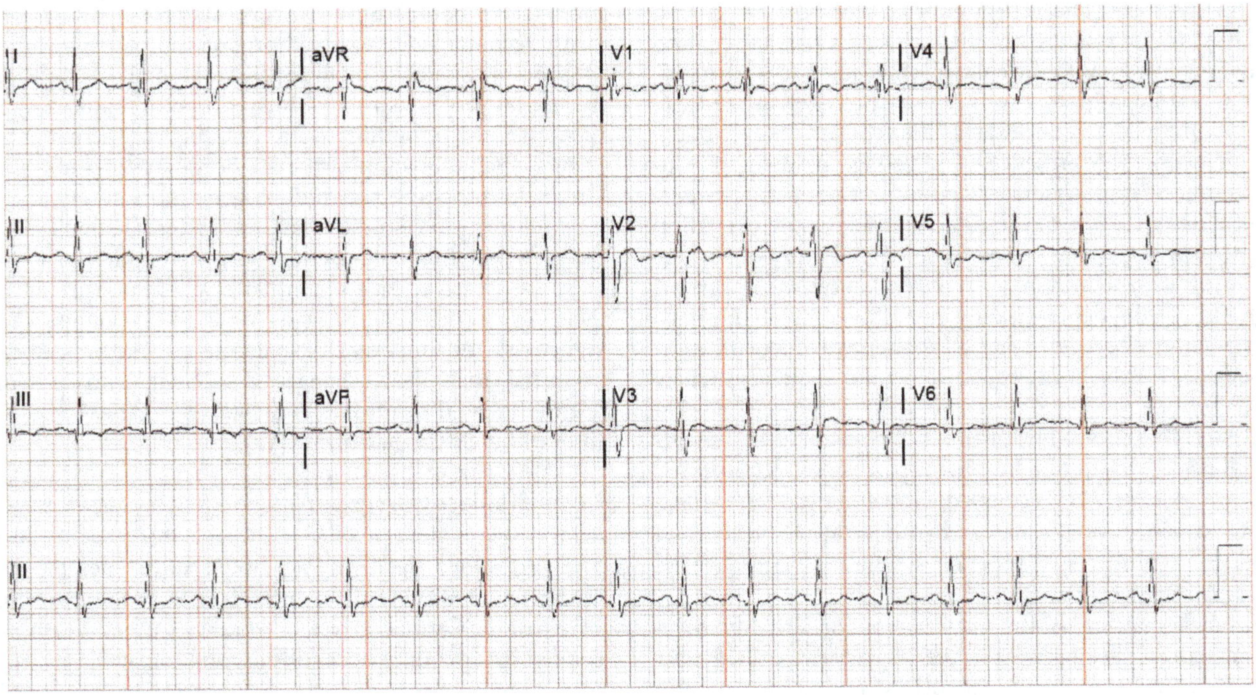

FIGURE 2: EKG 10 hours following cessation of propofol administration showing reversal of Brugada pattern.

distension with anuria and was taken back to the OR where a decompressive exploratory laparotomy with evacuation of an intra-abdominal hematoma was performed. On POD 12, an EKG was obtained and demonstrated type I Brugada pattern (Figure 1). After identification of type I Brugada pattern, propofol was discontinued, and EKG changes resolved within 10 hours (Figure 2). The patient received a total of 12880 mg of propofol (Table 1). The patient had a prolonged hospital course that lasted a total of 83 days and underwent other multiple interventions. The remainder of hospitalization was not complicated by any cardiac arrest or malignant arrhythmia.

Table 1: Table showing total amount of propofol received by patient during hospital course.

POD	Propofol dose (mg)
1	180
2	20
3	1070
4	1430
5	1680
6	1440
7	1680
8	1680
9	1680
10	1480
11	540

Table 2: Patterns of ST abnormalities in leads V1-V3.

Feature	Type 1	Type 2	Type 3
J wave amplitude	≥2 mm	≥2 mm	≥2 mm
T wave	Negative	Positive or biphasic	Negative, positive, or biphasic
ST-T configuration	Coved	Saddle-back	Coved or saddle-back
Terminal portion of ST segment	Gradually descending	Elevated ≥1 mm	Gradually descending or elevated ≥1 mm

3. Discussion

Brugada syndrome (BrS) is an autosomal dominant channelopathy associated with malignant arrhythmias and sudden cardiac death [2]. It is known to have variable penetrance with a strong male predominance [5]. BrS has been linked to a myriad of etiologies, but it is widely associated with mutations in the genes encoding the cardiac sodium channels. The genes implicated are the SCN5 and SCN10A. Mutations in this channel lead to an unopposed potassium current into the epicardium leading to its instability. Various hypotheses have been used to explain the ECG changes in BrS. These include (a) the repolarization hypothesis, involving the presence of a voltage gradient due to transmural or transregional dispersion of the action potential of different layers of the right ventricle at the beginning of repolarization, as a consequence of a loss of Na current combined with a dominant transient outward K current (Ito) and (b) the depolarization hypothesis, involving right ventricular conduction delay at the end of depolarization combined probably with subtle structural right ventricular anomalies [5].

BrS is characterized by distinct ST segment changes with appearance of a right bundle branch pattern and ST segment elevation in leads V1-V3 coupled with either sudden cardiac arrest, sustained ventricular arrhythmia, atrial fibrillation, nocturnal agonal respiration, or symptoms suggestive of ventricular arrhythmias. [6]

Brugada pattern is the presentation of EKG findings without clinical features. Like BrS, It is subclassified into three types depending on phenotypic appearance on the EKG (Table 2). Type I Brugada pattern is characterized by coved ST-segments in V1 and V2, and type II Brugada pattern is characterized by saddle-back ST segments where the ST segment descends before rising again to an upright or biphasic T wave, while type III is a combination of both types 1 and 2 without satisfying the criteria for either type 1 or 2 [5–7]. Multiple factors have been identified to precipitate BrS including fever, sodium channel blockers, anesthetics, tricyclic antidepressants, and cocaine [8]. Drug-induced Brugada syndrome from noncardiac drugs occurs predominantly in adult males and is frequently due to drug toxicity [9].

Propofol is a widely used sedative-hypnotic in surgeries and in the management of critically ill patients. Since its widespread implementation, propofol infusion syndrome (PRIS) has been identified, which consists of metabolic acidosis, rhabdomyolysis, hyperkalemia, and sudden cardiac death. These sudden cardiac deaths have been attributed to malignant arrhythmias. Propofol has been demonstrated to have sodium channel blocking properties. Multiple case reports have identified Brugada patterns in patients with prolonged propofol infusion and/or induction [10]. It is currently recommended to avoid propofol in patients with BrS to prevent inducing malignant arrhythmia [3]. Although the exact mechanism in which propofol induces BrS is unknown, the resolution of EKG findings in the patient following discontinuation of the medication points to a possible role of propofol in arrhythmogenesis.

Multiple case studies have, however, demonstrated a Brugada type EKG change heralding ventricular arrhythmia or sudden cardiac arrest. Junttila et al. demonstrated with their case series that Brugada type EKG changes are at higher risk for sudden cardiac arrest [11]. It has been demonstrated that EKG changes associated with propofol-related infusion syndrome is a sign of electrical instability and can herald cardiac arrest [12].

There have been multiple other cases describing propofol-induced Brugada pattern EKG changes, but these were in the context of PRIS. Although this patient did not have any other signs of PRIS, our patient demonstrated Brugada-type EKG changes secondary to prolonged propofol infusion. Cardiac arrest or sudden cardiac death were avoided by discontinuation of propofol infusion.

3.1. Follow-Up. Patient was scheduled for outpatient follow-up upon discharge for genetic testing and repeat EKG. However, patient was lost to follow-up.

4. Conclusions

Propofol has traditionally been avoided in patients with BrS. Although recently, there have been multiple reports of patients with Brugada syndrome that have safely tolerated propofol infusion or induction without any arrhythmia. This case demonstrates that sudden cardiac death, cardiac death, or malignant arrhythmia can be avoided in propofol-induced type I Brugada pattern with discontinuation and avoidance of propofol.

Abbreviations

BrS: Brugada syndrome
EKG: Electrocardiogram
CT: Computerized tomography
POD: Postoperative day.

Disclosure

The abstract of this case was accepted and has been presented as a poster at ACC National Conference 2022.

References

[1] E. J. Akhigbe, E. Ezeh, B. Dao, K. U. Okoro, and P. I. Okhumale, "The unmasking effect: propofol induced Brugada pattern in a critically ill patient," *Journal of the American College of Cardiology*, vol. 79, no. 9, p. 2452, 2022.

[2] Y. Minoura, Y. Kobayashi, and C. Antzelevitch, "Drug-induced Brugada syndrome," *Journal of Arrhythmia*, vol. 29, no. 2, pp. 88–95, 2013.

[3] P. G. Postema, C. Wolpert, A. S. Amin et al., "Drugs and Brugada syndrome patients: review of the literature, recommendations, and an up-to-date website," *Heart Rhythm*, vol. 6, no. 9, pp. 1335–1341, 2009.

[4] P. Flamee, C. De Asmundis, J. T. Bhutia et al., "Safe single-dose administration of propofol in patients with established Brugada syndrome: a retrospective database analysis," *Pacing and Clinical Electrophysiology*, vol. 36, no. 12, pp. 1516–1521, 2013.

[5] A. B. de Luna, J. Brugada, A. Baranchuk et al., "Current electrocardiographic criteria for diagnosis of Brugada pattern: a consensus report," *Journal of Electrocardiology*, vol. 45, no. 5, pp. 433–442, 2012.

[6] A. A. M. Wilde, C. Antzelevitch, M. Borggrefe et al., "Proposed diagnostic criteria for the Brugada syndrome," *Auropean Heart Journal*, vol. 23, no. 21, pp. 1648–1654, 2002.

[7] A. De Gasperi, G. Spagnolin, M. Ornaghi, L. Petrò, and G. Biancofiore, "Preoperative cardiac assessment in liver transplant candidates," *Best Practice & Research Clinical Anaesthesiology*, vol. 34, no. 1, pp. 51–68, 2020.

[8] Y. G. Yap, E. R. Behr, and J. A. Camm, "Drug-induced Brugada syndrome," *Europace*, vol. 11, no. 8, pp. 989–994, 2009.

[9] M. Konigstein, R. Rosso, G. Topaz et al., "Drug-induced Brugada syndrome: clinical characteristics and risk factors," *Heart Rhythm*, vol. 13, no. 5, pp. 1083–1087, 2016.

[10] A. R. P. Riera, A. H. Uchida, E. Schapachnik, S. Dubner, C. Ferreira Filho, and C. Ferreira, "Propofol infusion syndrome and Brugada syndrome electrocardiographic phenocopy," *Cardiology Journal*, vol. 17, no. 2, pp. 130–135, 2010.

[11] M. J. Junttila, M. Gonzalez, E. Lizotte et al., "Induced Brugada-type electrocardiogram, a sign for imminent malignant arrhythmias," *Circulation*, vol. 117, no. 14, pp. 1890–1893, 2008.

[12] K. Vernooy, T. Delhaas, O. L. Cremer et al., "Electrocardiographic changes predicting sudden death in propofol-related infusion syndrome," *Heart Rhythm*, vol. 3, no. 2, pp. 131–137, 2006.

Anomalous Origin of the Right Coronary Artery Causing Myocardial Ischemia: A Case for a Multimodality Imaging Approach

Fatimah A. Alkhunaizi,[1] **Karan Kapoor**,[2] **Vincent Pallazola**,[1] **Edward P. Shapiro**,[2] **Peter V. Johnston**,[2] **Joban Vaishnav**,[2] **Nisha A. Gilotra**,[2] **Ahmet Kilic**,[3] **and Rosanne Rouf**[2]

[1]*Department of Medicine, Johns Hopkins Hospital, Baltimore, MD, USA*
[2]*Division of Cardiology, Department of Medicine, Johns Hopkins Hospital, Baltimore, MD, USA*
[3]*Division of Cardiothoracic Surgery, Department of Surgery, Johns Hopkins Hospital, Baltimore, MD, USA*

Correspondence should be addressed to Fatimah A. Alkhunaizi; falkhun1@jhmi.edu
Academic Editor: Christopher S. Snyder

A 46-year-old man was admitted with non-ST elevation myocardial infarction and newly diagnosed acutely decompensated heart failure. Echocardiogram demonstrated left ventricular ejection fraction of 30% with basal inferior and inferolateral akinesis. Coronary angiography showed mild diffuse coronary artery disease and an anomalous right coronary artery arising from the left coronary cusp. Further imaging was consistent with ischemia in the right coronary distribution. Etiology of ischemia was thought to be the anomalous right coronary artery, and surgical unroofing of the right coronary ostium was performed. Here, we report a multimodality imaging approach, including cardiac magnetic resonance, cardiac computed tomographic angiography, and single-photon emission computed tomography, to support the diagnosis and management of a patient with anomalous right coronary artery arising from the left coronary cusp.

1. History of Presentation

A 46-year-old man from Honduras with no prior medical history presented with two weeks of crescendo angina, exertional dyspnea, two-pillow orthopnea, and paroxysmal nocturnal dyspnea. He took no medications and had no history of alcohol or illicit substance use. He had no family history of cardiovascular disease. He reported an active childhood and adolescence and was employed in a labor-intensive profession installing fiber optic cables for a telecommunication company. Physical examination was notable for a blood pressure of 178/81 mmHg, heart rate of 100 beats/min, a third heart sound, and mild jugular venous distention. The lung fields were clear, and there was no peripheral edema. Resting electrocardiogram showed sinus tachycardia and flattened T-waves in leads II, III, aVF, V5, and V6. Troponin-I was initially 0.35 ng/mL, peaking at 7.16 ng/mL upon serial assessment. Pro-BNP was elevated at 3961 pg/mL.

2. Investigations

Transthoracic echocardiogram (TTE) showed severe left ventricular dilatation (end-diastolic diameter of 6.6 cm) with normal wall thickness and ejection fraction (LVEF) of 30% with basal inferior and inferolateral akinesis. Coronary angiography showed mild nonobstructive coronary artery disease and an anomalous right coronary artery (ARCA) arising from the left coronary cusp (Figure 1 and Video 1). Iron and thyroid indices, hepatitis serologies, and antibodies against HIV and *Trypanosoma cruzi* were unremarkable. Cardiac magnetic resonance imaging (CMR) was obtained given suspicion for myocarditis as a cause of dilated cardiomyopathy which corroborated severe left ventricular dysfunction with ejection fraction of 16% (Video 2), but no myocardial edema on T2-weighted images or late gadolinium enhancement (LGE) (Figures 2(a) and 2(b)). Axial scout images again demonstrated an ARCA arising from the left

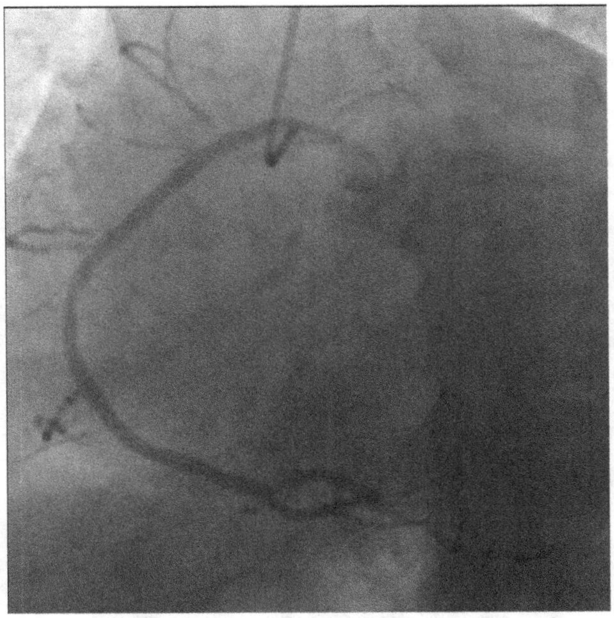

FIGURE 1: Still frame image of the RCA in the right anterior oblique (RAO) projection. The RCA is seen arising from the left coronary cusp prior to taking a usual course through the atrioventricular groove.

coronary cusp, but now clearly appearing to take an intra-arterial course between the aorta and the main pulmonary artery (Figure 3). Cardiac computed tomographic angiography (CCTA) was obtained to better delineate its course, confirming a slit-like proximal orifice arising at an acute angle and an intramural and intra-arterial course between the great vessels (Figures 4(a)–4(d)). Exercise single-photon emission computed tomography (SPECT) demonstrated a mild-to-moderate-sized reversible defect in the inferolateral wall referable to the territory supplied by the ARCA (Figures 5(a) and 5(b)).

3. Management

The patient's presenting symptoms eventually improved with a medical regimen including a diuretic, beta-blocker, ACE-inhibitor, and aldosterone antagonist. His chest pain, biomarker elevation, and inducible ischemia on SPECT were hypothesized as consequential to his ARCA, albeit disproportionate to the degree of left ventricular dysfunction, which was ascribed to a more global, nonischemic cardiomyopathic process. Given the presence of inducible ischemia in the RCA territory, there was a consensus to proceed with surgical unroofing of the right coronary ostium. He tolerated the operation well and was discharged on postoperative day 7 on a guideline-directed regimen for heart failure.

4. Follow-Up

He was seen in a follow-up three weeks after discharge with complete resolution of his exertional chest pain and shortness of breath. He returned back to work and remained asymptomatic.

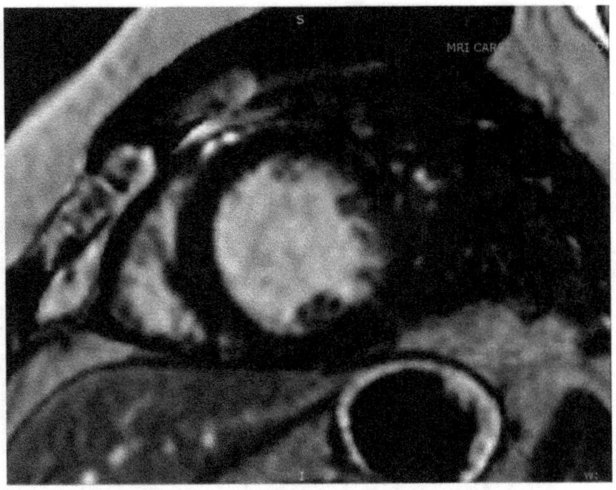

(a)

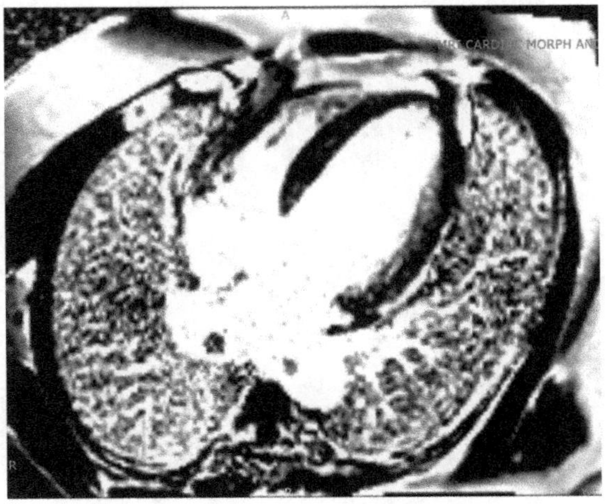

(b)

FIGURE 2: (a, b) Short-axis and four-chamber myocardial delayed enhancement imaging performed 10 minutes following injection of gadolinium contrast demonstrated no evidence of late gadolinium enhancement.

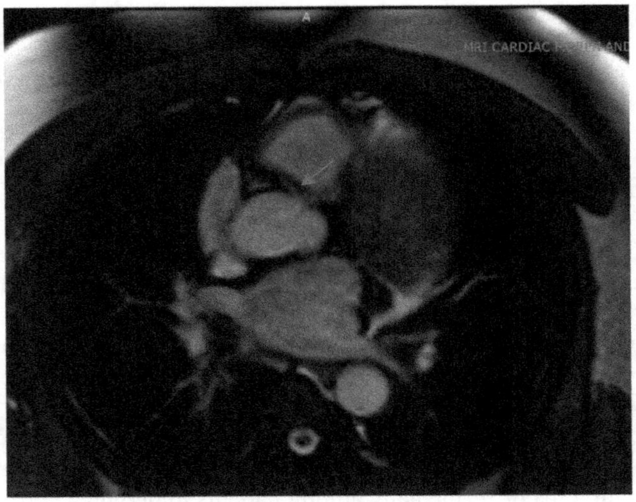

FIGURE 3: Axial CMR images corroborating the anomalous RCA (arrow) arising from the left coronary cusp and appearing to take an intra-arterial course.

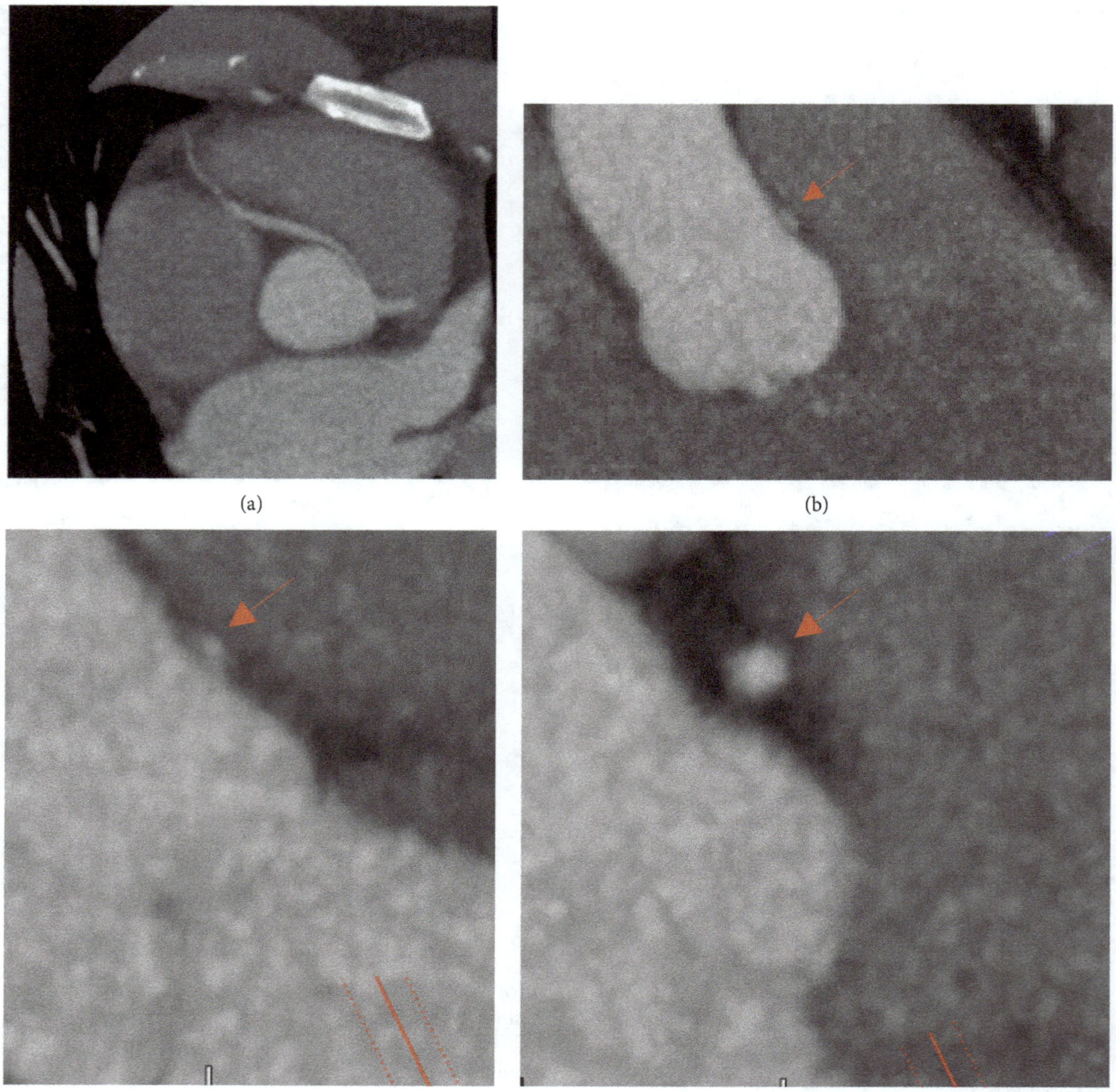

(a) (b) (c) (d)

Figure 4: (a–d) Axial CCTA images demonstrating the anomalous RCA arising from the left coronary cusp and taking an intra-arterial course. The extent of the proximal and mid-vessel is better delineated than in CMR (a). The slit-like configuration of the ostial RCA, as well as the acute angulation of its takeoff, is seen in this en-face coronal view (b). Cross sections of the RCA are shown, demonstrating the intramural portion (c) and just distally (d).

5. Discussion

Congenital coronary anomalies (CA) refer to a family of aberrations including anomalies of the origin, course and number of epicardial coronary arteries [1]. They have an estimated prevalence of 0.2-1.0%, with a slight male predilection reported in observational series [2]. ARCA arising from the left sinus of Valsalva is more common than anomalous left coronary artery (ALCA) from the right sinus of Valsalva [3]. CA are usually diagnosed on the basis of their presenting symptoms or incidentally among patients undergoing coronary angiography, CCTA, or at autopsy [4]. Whereas most CA are asymptomatic, presentation with arrhythmia, syncope, myocardial infarction, or sudden death has been described. For patients who present with sudden death, mean age of presentation is reported in various studies to range from teenage years to the fourth decade [5]. Patients who present with ischemia generally do so before the fifth decade, and the degree of troponin elevation is highly variable [6]. Systolic dysfunction and heart failure are rare consequences of CA, with most reported cases associated with anomalous left coronary artery arising from the pulmonary artery (ALCAPA) [7]. To the best of our knowledge, this case is the first report of systolic dysfunction and dilated cardiomyopathy associated with ARCA.

Our patient presented with angina, signs and symptoms of heart failure, and profound systolic dysfunction with inferior ischemia on SPECT imaging. Following an initial ischemic evaluation with coronary angiography (which first disclosed the ARCA), his degree of the ventricular

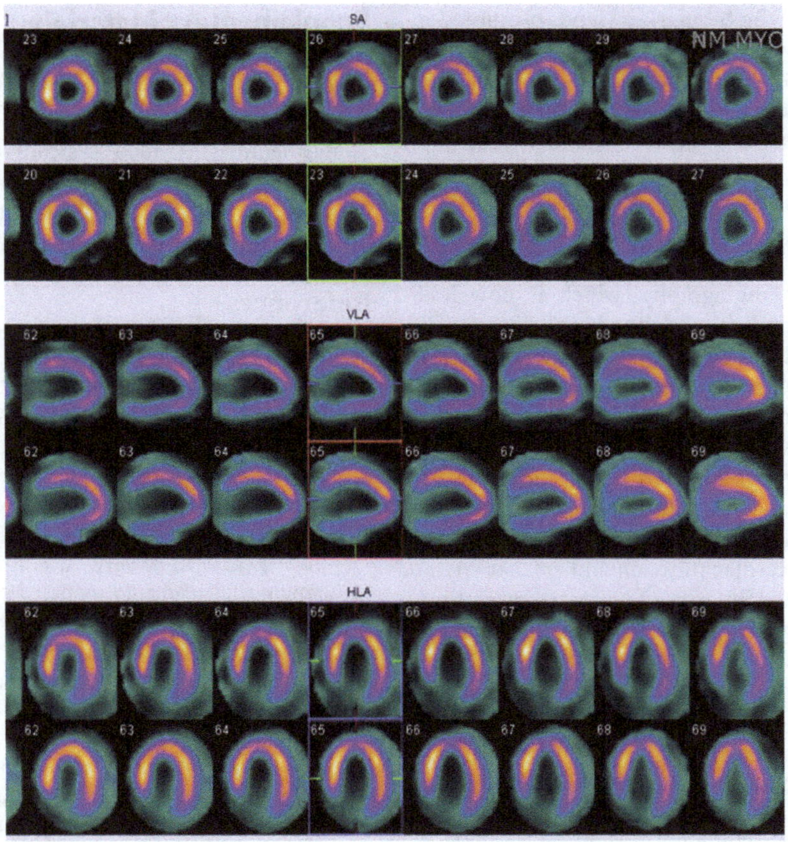

(a)

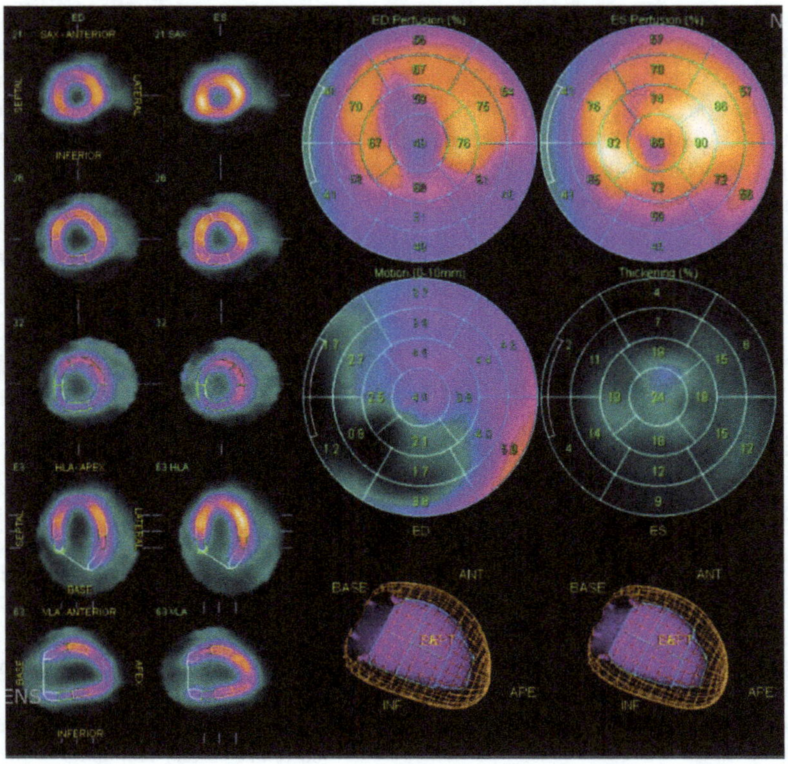

(b)

Figure 5: (a, b) The patient achieved 11 METS on a modified Bruce protocol but developed symptomatic chest discomfort and inferior lead ST-segment depressions at peak exercise persisting 1 minute into recovery. SPECT images demonstrated a reversible inferior wall perfusion deficit.

dysfunction, coupled with the biomarker trend, prompted a diagnostic workup for myocarditis with CMR. CCTA was subsequently needed to delineate the distal course of the ARCA and to identify possible high-risk features. Finally, SPECT perfusion imaging was needed to identify inducible ischemia.

A multimodal imaging approach as exemplified in this case is often required to comprehensively risk stratify patients with CA. In our patient, ARCA was first detected incidentally via coronary angiography, which is now less commonly utilized as a first-line modality due to its invasive nature and limited ability to assess the full course of the vessel and surrounding noncoronary anatomy [8]. CCTA has thus emerged as the first-line imaging modality to assess the origin and course of CA [9]. This is owing to its high spatial resolution and ability to identify high-risk features including a slit-like orifice, acute angle takeoff, or intramural course [10]. CMR is another noninvasive method that has the added benefit of being able to assess cardiac function and areas of myocardial fibrosis, but is limited in terms of its spatial resolution and ability to track the arterial course beyond the proximal aspect [11].

The functional relevance of any detected CA, especially when incidental, often requires further clarification with myocardial perfusion imaging. This can be done using SPECT, positron emission tomography (PET), or CMR. Notable anatomic factors associated with high risk for ischemia on perfusion imaging include an intramural and intra-arterial course between the great vessels, acute angulation at the ostium, and a slit-like orifice, all features which were present in our patient [12].

Management strategies for CA include observation, medical therapy with beta-blockers, stenting, and surgical unroofing [13]. In cases of ARCA with evidence of ischemia, surgical revascularization is a class I recommendation per the joint guidelines of the American College of Cardiology and American Heart Association [14].

6. Conclusions

ARCA is a well known cause of myocardial ischemia. A multimodal imaging approach is often required in order to rule out concomitant diagnoses and to definitively delineate the anomalous course. Surgical correction should be pursued in symptomatic patients or in those with evidence of myocardial ischemia attributed to the anomalous coronary artery.

Abbreviations

TTE: Transthoracic echocardiography
CMR: Cardiac magnetic resonance
CCTA: Coronary computed tomographic angiography
SPECT: Single-photon emission computed tomography
CA: Coronary anomalies
ARCA: Anomalous right coronary artery
ALCA: Anomalous left coronary artery
LGE: Late gadolinium enhancement
LVEF: Left ventricular ejection fraction
MPI: Myocardial perfusion imaging.

Supplementary Materials

Supplementary 1. Video 1: cine-angiographic images demonstrating the anomalous RCA in the RAO projection.

Supplementary 2. Video 2: steady-state free precession cine images in the four-chamber view demonstrating severely reduced biventricular systolic function.

References

[1] P. Angelini, "Coronary artery anomalies," *Circulation*, vol. 115, no. 10, pp. 1296–1305, 2007.

[2] C. Graidis, D. Dimitriadis, V. Karasavvidis et al., "Prevalence and characteristics of coronary artery anomalies in an adult population undergoing multidetector-row computed tomography for the evaluation of coronary artery disease," *BMC Cardiovascular Disorders*, vol. 15, no. 1, 2015.

[3] R. E. Eckart, E. A. Shry, A. P. Burke et al., "Sudden death in young adults: an autopsy-based series of a population undergoing active surveillance," *Journal of the American College of Cardiology*, vol. 58, no. 12, pp. 1254–1261, 2011.

[4] A. Yildiz, B. Okcun, T. Peker, C. Arslan, A. Olcay, and V. M. Bulent, "Prevalence of coronary artery anomalies in 12, 457 adult patients who underwent coronary angiography," *Clinical Cardiology*, vol. 33, no. 12, pp. E60–E64, 2010.

[5] G. Finocchiaro, E. R. Behr, G. Tanzarella et al., "Anomalous coronary artery origin and sudden cardiac death: clinical and pathological insights from a national pathology registry," *JACC: Clinical Electrophysiology*, vol. 5, no. 4, pp. 516–522, 2019.

[6] C. Basso, B. J. Maron, D. Corrado, and G. Thiene, "Clinical profile of congenital coronary artery anomalies with origin from the wrong aortic sinus leading to sudden death in young competitive athletes," *Journal of the American College of Cardiology*, vol. 35, no. 6, pp. 1493–1501, 2000.

[7] L. L. B. Trevizan, A. Nussbacher, M. C. B. Da Silva et al., "Anomalous origin of the left coronary artery from the pulmonary artery as a rare cause of left ventricular dysfunction," *Circulation. Cardiovascular Imaging*, vol. 12, no. 12, article e009724, 2019.

[8] C. Gräni, R. R. Buechel, P. A. Kaufmann, and R. Y. Kwong, "Multimodality imaging in individuals with anomalous coronary arteries," *JACC: Cardiovascular Imaging*, vol. 10, no. 4, pp. 471–481, 2017.

[9] J. R. Ghadri, E. Kazakauskaite, S. Braunschweig et al., "Congenital coronary anomalies detected by coronary computed tomography compared to invasive coronary angiography," *BMC Cardiovascular Disorders*, vol. 14, no. 1, 2014.

[10] M. A. Harris, K. K. Whitehead, D. C. Shin, M. S. Keller, P. M. Weinberg, and M. A. Fogel, "Identifying abnormal ostial morphology in anomalous aortic origin of a coronary artery," *The Annals of Thoracic Surgery*, vol. 100, no. 1, pp. 174–179, 2015.

[11] D. A. Bluemke, S. Achenbach, M. Budoff et al., "Noninvasive coronary artery imaging," *Circulation*, vol. 118, no. 5, pp. 586–606, 2008.

[12] A. Jegatheeswaran, P. J. Devlin, B. W. McCrindle et al., "Features associated with myocardial ischemia in anomalous aortic origin of a coronary artery: a Congenital Heart Sur-

geons' Society study," *The Journal of Thoracic and Cardiovascular Surgery*, vol. 158, no. 3, pp. 822–834.e3, 2019.

[13] C. Gräni, P. A. Kaufmann, S. Windecker, and R. R. Buechel, "Diagnosis and management of anomalous coronary arteries with a malignant course," *Interventional Cardiology Review*, vol. 14, no. 2, pp. 83–88, 2019.

[14] K. K. Stout, C. J. Daniels, J. A. Aboulhosn et al., "2018 AHA/ACC guideline for the management of adults with congenital heart disease: a report of the American College of Cardiology/American Heart Association task force on clinical practice guidelines," *Circulation*, vol. 139, no. 14, pp. e698–e800, 2019.

Permissions

All chapters in this book were first published by Hindawi Publishing Corporation; hereby published with permission under the Creative Commons Attribution License or equivalent. Every chapter published in this book has been scrutinized by our experts. Their significance has been extensively debated. The topics covered herein carry significant findings which will fuel the growth of the discipline. They may even be implemented as practical applications or may be referred to as a beginning point for another development.

The contributors of this book come from diverse backgrounds, making this book a truly international effort. This book will bring forth new frontiers with its revolutionizing research information and detailed analysis of the nascent developments around the world.

We would like to thank all the contributing authors for lending their expertise to make the book truly unique. They have played a crucial role in the development of this book. Without their invaluable contributions this book wouldn't have been possible. They have made vital efforts to compile up to date information on the varied aspects of this subject to make this book a valuable addition to the collection of many professionals and students.

This book was conceptualized with the vision of imparting up-to-date information and advanced data in this field. To ensure the same, a matchless editorial board was set up. Every individual on the board went through rigorous rounds of assessment to prove their worth. After which they invested a large part of their time researching and compiling the most relevant data for our readers.

The editorial board has been involved in producing this book since its inception. They have spent rigorous hours researching and exploring the diverse topics which have resulted in the successful publishing of this book. They have passed on their knowledge of decades through this book. To expedite this challenging task, the publisher supported the team at every step. A small team of assistant editors was also appointed to further simplify the editing procedure and attain best results for the readers.

Apart from the editorial board, the designing team has also invested a significant amount of their time in understanding the subject and creating the most relevant covers. They scrutinized every image to scout for the most suitable representation of the subject and create an appropriate cover for the book.

The publishing team has been an ardent support to the editorial, designing and production team. Their endless efforts to recruit the best for this project, has resulted in the accomplishment of this book. They are a veteran in the field of academics and their pool of knowledge is as vast as their experience in printing. Their expertise and guidance has proved useful at every step. Their uncompromising quality standards have made this book an exceptional effort. Their encouragement from time to time has been an inspiration for everyone.

The publisher and the editorial board hope that this book will prove to be a valuable piece of knowledge for researchers, students, practitioners and scholars across the globe.

List of Contributors

Varun Kumar
Department of Cardiology, Orchid Medical Centre, Ranchi, India

Shalini Gupta and Krishna Prasad
Department of Anaesthesia, Orchid Medical Centre, Ranchi, India

Franz Haertel, P. Christian Schulze, Anett Große and Ralf Surber
University Hospital Jena, Department of Internal Medicine I, Cardiology, Am Klinikum 1, 07743 Jena, Germany

Dirk Prochnau
Department of Internal Medicine, Cardiology, Sophien- und Hufeland-Klinikum, Henry-van-de-Velde-Straße 2, 99425 Weimar, Germany

J. Mannion, L. Chapman, K. Deasy and N. S. Colwell
Cardiology Department, Tipperary University Hospital, Clonmel, Tipperary, Ireland

Monique Oye
Department of Internal Medicine, UF Health Jacksonville, Jacksonville, FL, USA

Aaron Richardson, Edin Sadic and Gladys Velarde
Division of Cardiology, UF Health Jacksonville, Jacksonville, FL, USA

Ahmad Alkhasawneh
Department of Pathology, University of Florida Health Jacksonville, Jacksonville, FL, USA

Daniel Barnebee
University of South Florida College of Medicine, Tampa, FL, USA

Brian Morse and Daniel Jeong
Department of Diagnostic Imaging and Interventional Radiology, H. Lee Moffitt Cancer Center and Research Institute, Tampa FL, USA

Jonathan R. Strosberg
Department of Gastrointestinal Oncology, H. Lee Moffitt Cancer Center and Research Institute, Tampa FL, USA

Marijan Pejic
Department of Radiology, University of South Florida College of Medicine, Tampa, FL, USA

H. Sharma
Institute of Cardiovascular Sciences, University of Birmingham, Birmingham, UK

S. N. Doshi and M. A. Nadir
Cardiology Department, Queen Elizabeth Hospital, Birmingham, UK

Vy A. Pham and Evan S. Manning
Department of Medicine, University of Colorado, 12631 E. 17th Ave, Room 8601, Aurora, CO 80045, USA

Christopher P. Kovach, Karl Gordon Patti and James E. Carter Jr.
Division of Cardiology, Department of Medicine, University of Colorado, 12631 E. 17th Ave, B130, Aurora, CO 80045, USA

Stephen J. Slade and Elena Weinstein
Division of Rheumatology, Department of Medicine, University of Colorado, 1775 Aurora Court, B115, Aurora, CO 80045, USA

Rebecca Pollard and Jennifer Simpson
Division of Neurology, Department of Medicine, University of Colorado, 12700 E. 19th Ave, Room 5018, Aurora, CO 80045, USA

Seong Hyeon Bu
Division of Cardiology, Department of Internal Medicine, Uijeongbu St. Mary's Hospital, College of Medicine, The Catholic University of Korea, Uijeongbu-si, Gyeonggi-do, Republic of Korea

Sung-Hwan Kim
Division of Cardiology, Department of Internal Medicine, Seoul St. Mary's Hospital, College of Medicine, The Catholic University of Korea, 222 Banpo-daero, Seocho-gu, Seoul, 06591 Seoul, Republic of Korea

Imran Zainal Abidin
Division of Cardiology, Department of Medicine, University Malaya Medical Centre, 59100 Kuala Lumpur, Malaysia

Mohd Ridzuan Mohd Said
Department of Internal Medicine, Kulliyyah of Medicine, International Islamic University Malaysia, 25200 Kuantan, Pahang, Malaysia

Nor Saadah Idris
Department of Radiology, University Malaya Medical Centre, 59100 Kuala Lumpur, Malaysia

Mohd Al-Baqlish Mohd Firdaus
Division of Cardiology, Department of Medicine, University Malaya Medical Centre, 59100 Kuala Lumpur, Malaysia
Department of Internal Medicine, Kulliyyah of Medicine, International Islamic University Malaysia, 25200 Kuantan, Pahang, Malaysia

Nur Syahirah Abdul Rahim and Nurtasneem Rusdi
Department of Internal Medicine, Kulliyyah of Medicine, International Islamic University Malaysia, 25200 Kuantan, Pahang, Malaysia

Hussein Daoud, Ashraf Abugroun and Shruti Erramilli
Department of Internal Medicine, Advocate Illinois Masonic Medical Center, 836 W Wellington Ave., Chicago, IL 60657, USA

Surender Kumar
Department of Cardiology, Advocate Illinois Masonic Medical Center, 836 W Wellington Ave., Chicago, IL 60657, USA

Ju Young Bae and Khalil Ian Hussein
Department of Medicine, Greenwich Hospital, Yale-New Haven Health System, 5 Perryridge Road, Greenwich, CT 06830, USA

Christopher John Howes and John Francis Setaro
Department of Medicine, Greenwich Hospital, Yale-New Haven Health System, 5 Perryridge Road, Greenwich, CT 06830, USA
Section of Cardiovascular Medicine, Department of Internal Medicine, Yale University School of Medicine, 333 Cedar St, New Haven, CT 06510, USA

Alia Arif Hussain and Erik Kovacs
Emergency Department, North Denmark Regional Hospital, Denmark

Jeppe Nygaard and Celi Anne Schoenike
Department of Abdominal Surgery, North Denmark Regional Hospital, Denmark

Kasper Kofod Pedersen
Department of Radiology, North Denmark Regional Hospital, Denmark

Steen Hylgaard Jørgensen
Department of Cardiology, North Denmark Regional Hospital, Denmark

Matthew R. Petersen
Department of Internal Medicine, University of Florida, USA

Christopher Perry
Department of Cardiology, University of Florida, USA

Rachel Nickels
United States Department of Veterans Affairs, North Florida South Georgia VA Hospital, USA

Bisher Sawaf, Wael Kanjo, Yasir Alabbas and Ahmad Hatim
Internal Medicine, Department of Medical Education, Hamad Medical Corporation, Doha, Qatar

Unus K. Bedardeen and Wafer A. Dabdoob
Department of Cardiology, Heart Hospital, Hamad Medical Corporation, Doha, Qatar

Vrijraj Sinhji Rathod, Tanmay Kanitkar and Grigoris Karamasis
Essex Cardiothoracic Centre, Basildon University Hospital, Nethermayne, Basildon, UK SS16 5NL

Hendrik Lapp, Marcel Keßler, Thomas Rock, Dong-In Shin, Heinrich G. Klues and Christian Blockhaus
Department of Cardiology, Heart Centre Niederrhein, Helios Clinics Krefeld, Germany

Franz X. Schmid
Department of Cardiothoracic Surgery, Heart Centre Niederrhein, Helios Clinics Krefeld, Germany

Alexander Bufe
Department of Cardiology, Heart Centre Niederrhein, Helios Clinics Krefeld, Germany University Witten/ Herdecke, Germany

Anh Tuan Vo, Thu Trang Nguyen, Thanh Thuy Tran and Dinh Hoang Nguyen
Department of Cardiovascular Surgery, University Medical Center, University of Medicine and Pharmacy at Ho Chi Minh City, Ho Chi Minh City, Vietnam

Chirik-Wah Lau
Cardiovascular Research Center, Department of Cardiology, OLV Ziekenhuis Aalst-Asse-Ninove, Aalst, Belgium

Ward Heggermont
Cardiovascular Research Center, Department of Cardiology, OLV Ziekenhuis Aalst-Asse-Ninove, Aalst, Belgium
Cardiovascular Research Institute Maastricht, Maastricht, Netherlands

Pham Anh Hong Nguyen
Department of Respiratory Medicine, OLV Ziekenhuis Aalst-Asse-Ninove, Aalst, Belgium

Kurt Tournoy
Department of Respiratory Medicine, OLV Ziekenhuis Aalst-Asse-Ninove, Aalst, Belgium
Faculty of Medicine and Life Sciences, Ghent University, Ghent, Belgium

Jemimah Nallarajah and M. I. Mujahieth
Department of Medicine, Colombo South Teaching Hospital, Sri Lanka

S. Ashwin Reddy
Papworth Hospital, Papworth Everard, Cambridge, UK

David J. Sanders, Joanne S. Sutter, Tisha M. Suboc and Anupama K. Rao
Department of Internal Medicine, Section of Cardiology, Rush University Medical Center, Chicago, IL, USA

Antone Tatooles
Department of Cardiovascular and Thoracic Surgery, Rush University Medical Center, Chicago, IL, USA

Zahra Khajali, Homa Ghaderian, Ata Firoozi and Zahra Hosseini
Rajaie Cardiovascular Medical and Research Center, Iran University of Medical Sciences, Tehran, Iran

Maryam Aliramezany
Cardiovascular Research Center, Institute of Basic and Clinical Physiology Sciences, Kerman University of Medical Sciences Kerman, Iran

Harish Sharma
Institute of Cardiovascular Sciences, University of Birmingham, Birmingham, UK
University Hospitals Birmingham NHS Foundation Trust, Mindelsohn Way, Birmingham B15 2TH, UK

Sudhakar George
University Hospitals Birmingham NHS Foundation Trust, Mindelsohn Way, Birmingham B15 2TH, UK

Sally Harrison
Dunedin Public Hospital, Dunedin, New Zealand

John Eliveh, Shravani Vindhyal and Mohinder Vindhyal
Department of Internal Medicine, University of Kansas, 1001 N Minneapolis St., Wichita, KS 67214, USA

Mahmood Abu Akel, Yaron M. Hellman, Amnon Eitan and Moshe Y. Flugelman
Department of Cardiovascular Medicine, Lady Davis Carmel Medical Center and Rappaport Faculty of Medicine, Technion Israel Institute of Technology, Haifa, Israel

Shtiwi Sawaed and Erez Sharoni
Department of Cardiothoracic Surgery, Lady Davis Carmel Medical Center and Rappaport Faculty of Medicine, Technion Israel Institute of Technology, Haifa, Israel

Amer Aljundi, Alaa Rahhal
Pharmacy Department, Heart Hospital, Hamad Medical Corporation, Doha, Qatar

Wafer Dabdoob
Cardiology and Cardiovascular Surgery Department, Heart Hospital, Hamad Medical Corporation, Doha, Qatar

Deborah Adepoju, Jamie A. L. Smith and Stephen J. Leslie
Cardiac Unit, Raigmore Hospital, Inverness IV2 3UJ, UK

Ammar Ahmed
Department of Internal Medicine, Ascension Providence Hospital, Southfield, MI, USA

Andrew Assaf and Marcel Zughaib
Department of Cardiovascular Disease, Ascension Providence Hospital, Southfield, MI, USA

Aditi Shankar
Department of Internal Medicine, Texas Health Presbyterian Dallas, Dallas, TX, USA

Mary Lark, Phillip Rideout and David Gregg
College of Medicine, Medical University of South Carolina, Charleston, SC 29425, USA

Amanda Cai and Valerian L. Fernandes
Department of Cardiology, Medical University of South Carolina, Charleston, SC 29425, USA

Pal Suranyi
Department of Cardiology, Medical University of South Carolina, Charleston, SC 29425, USA
Department of Radiology, Medical University of South Carolina, Charleston, SC 29425, USA

Fred A. Crawford
Department of Surgery, Medical University of South Carolina, Charleston, SC 29425, USA

Luigi Rivetti, Roberto Mantovan, Nadir Sitta, Ricarda Marinigh, Giuseppe Allocca, Moemen Mohammed, Fausto Pizzino and Giuseppe Nucifora
Department of Cardiology, "S. Maria dei Battuti" Hospital, AULSS 2 Veneto, Via Brigata Bisagno, Conegliano (TV), Italy

Mohamed E. Taha
Department of Internal Medicine, University of Nevada, Reno, NV, USA

Ammar Eljack
Department of Internal Medicine, Beaumont Health, Detroit, MI, USA

Hisham Ibrahim
Department of Internal Medicine, University of Iowa, IA, USA

Chanwit Roongsritong
Department of Heart and Vascular Health, Renown Regional Medical Center, Reno, NV, USA

Mariano Rillo, Zefferino Palamà, Giulia My, Raffaele Punzi and Luigi My
Cardiology Unit "Villa Verde", Taranto, Italy

Francesco Zonno
Abbott Medical Italia, Sesto San Giovanni, Italy

Luigi Sciarra
Cardiology Unit "Policlinico Casilino", Rome, Italy

Ayman R. Fath, Hemalatha Narayanasamy, Farouk Mookadam, Nithin R. Venepally, Sudheer Konduru, Reza Arsanjani and Luis R. Scott
Department of Cardiovascular Diseases, Mayo Clinic Arizona, USA

Amro Aglan
Beth Israel Deaconess Medical Center, Harvard Medical School, Boston, MA, USA

Clinton E. Jokerst
Department of Radiology, Mayo Clinic Arizona, USA

Nawfal Mihyawi
Department of Internal Medicine, Creighton University Arizona Health Alliance, USA

Padma Shenoy, Taher Tayeb, Pedro Covas, Nardos Temesgen and Cynthia Tracy
The George Washington University Hospital, Washington, DC, USA

Mahmood Mubasher, Ashfaq Patel, Mohamed Magdi and Tahir Hamid
Hamad Medical Corporation, Qatar

Rafał Januszek and Magdalena Jędrychowska
2nd Department of Cardiology and Cardiovascular Interventions, University Hospital, Krakow, Poland

Piotr Jankowski
1st Department of Cardiology, Jagiellonian University Medical College, Krakow, Poland

Dariusz Dudek and Stanisław Bartuś
2nd Department of Cardiology and Cardiovascular Interventions, University Hospital, Krakow, Poland
Department of Interventional Cardiology, Jagiellonian University Medical College, Krakow, Poland

Pratik K. Dalal, Amy Mertens and Dinesh Shah
Department of Cardiovascular Medicine, Beaumont Health System, Royal Oak, MI, USA

Ivan Hanson
Department of Cardiovascular Medicine, Beaumont Health System, Royal Oak, MI, USA
Oakland University William Beaumont School of Medicine, Royal Oak, MI, USA

Shaohui Wu, Xu Liu, Weifeng Jiang, Mu Qin and Daoliang Zhang
Shanghai Chest Hospital, Shanghai Jiao Tong University, Shanghai, China

Guangchen Zou
Danbury Hospital, Danbury, Connecticut, USA

Yaser Alahmad, Hassan Al-Tamimi, Fadi Khazaal, Mawahib Elhassan, Abdulrahman Arabi, Jassim Al Suwaidi, Awad AlQahtani and Nidal Asaad
Hamad Medical Corporation, Heart Hospital, Doha, Qatar

Muhammad Ajmal
St. Joseph's Hospital and Medical Center, Phoenix, Arizona, USA
Cardiology Fellow, Creighton University School of Medicine, Phoenix, Arizona, USA

Vijendra Swarup
Arizona Heart Rhythm Center, Phoenix, Arizona, USA

Carlos A. Solis-Olivares
Instituto Mexicano del Seguro Social, Hospital General de Zona 67, Apodaca, Nuevo León 66600, Mexico

Irene Meester
Universidad de Monterrey, Escuela de Medicina, San Pedro Garza Garcia 66238, Mexico

Juan M. Solis-Soto
Universidad Autonoma de Nuevo Leon, Facultad de Odontologia, Monterrey 64460, Mexico

Aphrodite Tzifa
Department of Congenital Heart Disease, Mitera Children's Hospital, Athens, Greece
Biomedical Engineering & Clinical Sciences, King's College London, UK

Ioannis Polymerou
Biomedical Engineering & Clinical Sciences, King's College London, UK

Dimitra Loggitsi
Department of Radiology, Mitera Children's Hospital, Athens, Greece

Esiemoghie Akhigbe and Ebubechukwu Ezeh
Department of Internal Medicine, Marshall University Joan C. Edwards School of Medicine, Huntington, WV, USA

Benjamin Dao, Kelechukwu Okoro and Paul Okhumale
Department of Cardiovascular Services, Marshall University Joan C. Edwards School of Medicine, Huntington, WV, USA

Fatimah A. Alkhunaizi and Vincent Pallazola
Department of Medicine, Johns Hopkins Hospital, Baltimore, MD, USA

Karan Kapoor, Edward P. Shapiro, Peter V. Johnston, Joban Vaishnav, Nisha A. Gilotra and Rosanne Rouf
Division of Cardiology, Department of Medicine, Johns Hopkins Hospital, Baltimore, MD, USA

Ahmet Kilic
Division of Cardiothoracic Surgery, Department of Surgery, Johns Hopkins Hospital, Baltimore, MD, USA

Index

www.ingramcontent.com/pod-product-compliance
Lightning Source LLC
LaVergne TN
LVHW082225200926
848484LV00008B/2309